THE PSYCHOBIOLOGY OF DOWN SYNDROME

Issues in the Biology of Language and Cognition
John C. Marshall, editor

THE PSYCHOBIOLOGY OF DOWN SYNDROME

edited by Lynn Nadel

A Bradford Book
The MIT Press
Cambridge, Massachusetts
London, England

This book was printed and bound by Halliday Lithograph,
in the United States of America.

Library of Congress Cataloging-in-Publication Data

The Psychobiology of Down syndrome / edited by Lynn Nadel
     p.   cm. -- (Issues in the biology of language and
cognition)
    "A Bradford book."
     Based on papers presented at the National Down
Syndrome Society Conference on the Psychobiology of Down
Syndrome, held in New York in Dec. 1987.
    Bibliography: p.
    Includes index.
    ISBN 0-262-14043-8
    1. Down's syndrome--Congresses. 2. Down's syndrome-
-Patients-Language--Congresses. 3. Psychobiology-
-Congresses. 4. Down's syndrome--Patients--Longitudinal
studies--Congresses. I. Nadel, Lynn. II. National Down
Syndrome Society Conference on the Psychobiology of Down
Syndrome (1987 : New York, N.Y.) III. Series.
     [DNLM: 1. Down's Syndrome--psychology--congresses.
2. Language Development--congresses.   WS 107 P974 1987]
RJ506.D68P78 1988
616.85'8842--dc19
DNLM/DLC
for Library of Congress   88-12999
                                                    CIP

CONTENTS

Series Foreword

The MIT Press series on Issues in the Biology of
Language and Cognition brings new approaches, concepts,
techniques, and results to bear on our understanding of
the biological foundations of human cognitive
capacities. The series will include theoretical,
experimental, and clinical work that ranges from the
basic neurosciences, clinical neuropscyhology, and
neurolinguistics to formal modeling of biological
systems. Studies in which the architecture of the mind
is illuminated by both the fractionation of cognition
after brain damage and formal theories of normal
performance are specifically encouraged.

John C. Marshall

ACKNOWLEDGMENTS

The Conference on the Psychobiology of Down Syndrome was sponsored by the National Down Syndrome Society, under the leadership of Elizabeth Goodwin, President. The organization of the conference was flawlessly executed by Donna M. Rosenthal, Executive Director of the Society. Without her careful attention neither the conference nor this book would have been possible. Special thanks are due to Peter Mangan and Mary Newman for their compilation of the bibliography, and to Jane Clark for her perseverance and dedication at the computer.

Both the conference and this volume were made a reality by the generous support of the Ambrose Monell Foundation, Republic New York Corporation and the Down Syndrome Northeast Regional Coalition.

Additional information about the work of the National Down Syndrome Society can be obtained from the Society at 141 Fifth Avenue, New York, NY 10010. [The telephone numbers of the Society are (212)460-9330 and (800)221-4602 (outside New York State).]

THE PSYCHOBIOLOGY OF DOWN SYNDROME

INTRODUCTION

Until recently, individuals with Down Syndrome were
routinely institutionalized, their lives usually fulfil-
ling the direst of expectations. Deinstitutionization has
changed this picture in a number of dramatic ways. First,
many individuals with Down Syndrome are living longer,
healthier lives. This is generally good news, though it
has a recently discovered down side -- it has become
clear that most if not all Down Syndrome individuals have
extensive Alzheimer-like brain pathology by the age of
35. Second, there has been a shattering of the barriers
assumed to drastically limit the potential of Down Syndrome individuals. We are no longer so sure just how subnormal they must be. In this atmosphere of new possibilities and potential, research studies aimed at more accurately characterizing the precise developmental abnormalities associated with Down Syndrome serve a critical role.
They suggest specific intervention techniques to help
every individual achieve his/her maximum potential. Quite
often, basic research and intervention strategies go
hand-in-hand. Unfortunately, we are quite ignorant of
many of the most basic facts about Down Syndrome. We do
not know what the cognitive and functional limits are,
how these limits change during the lifespan, and what
kinds of interventions can help reach or perhaps even expand these limits.

The past decade has seen a surge of interest in Down
Syndrome, and a great deal of research, much of it done
with children reared in relatively normal, or even en-
riched, circumstances. These studies are beginning the
much-needed job of working out the actual developmental
problems faced by Down Syndrome children when they are
reared under the best, rather than the worst, of conditions. These recent historical trends helped to shape the
workshop at which the papers in this volume were presented. The National Down Syndrome Society Conference on
The Psychobiology of Down Syndrome was held in New York
in December, 1987. There were three major themes to the

conference.

First: What do we currently know of the extent, and qualitative nature of the deficits seen in Down Syndrome? Is there a general "developmental delay" which manifests across all forms of psychological function, or are there more specific problems related only to certain kinds of abilities?

Second: How does the development of language in Down Syndrome differ from that seen normally? Does the language defect cut across the board or is it related to certain areas of verbal function? Could more 'peripheral' problems with hearing/vision be important? Are there interventions that can work to improve verbal ability?

Third: What is the progress of Down Syndrome through the life-span? Can learning continue through adolescence and into adulthood? What are the consequences of approaching age 35, at which time all Down Syndrome individuals apparently have "Alzheimer-like" brain profiles?

While we certainly did not generate final answers to any of these questions, the conference participants expressed the feeling that there have been significant gains in our insight into many of the critical issues. The book is divided into two sections, followed by an extensive bibliography prepared especially for this volume. The first section is concerned with cognitive development in general, and language development and function in particular. Chapters in this part of the book focus on the development of the object concepts, number concepts, basic categories, and word use. They provide, in their totality, a picture of selective rather than general, deficits, and a highly variable pattern across the life-span. They offer cause for great hope, in that progress seems possible even in adolescents, but they caution against false hopes -- arriving at the best intervention strategies will be difficult, and there are no certain guarantees that parents will correctly apply these strategies. Optimism is warranted, on balance, and these chapters provide a rich source of ideas about cognitive development in Down Syndrome and normally developing infants, ideas which one imagines will contribute to progress in the creation of effective intervention techniques. The second section contains chapters concerned with the neurobiological underpinnings of Down Syndrome, and the relation between Down Syndrome and Alzheimer's disease. They confirm the sense provided in the first section of selective deficit: only certain portions of the central nervous system are affected. And though the strong linkage between Down Syndrome and Alzheimer's disease stands confirmed, interesting and perhaps critical differences are beginning to emerge in the precise nature and sequence of neurological defects observed in the two cases. Some such difference would provide a basis for understanding another recently established fact: though 100% of Down Syndrome individuals older than 35 years are assumed to have Alzheimer-like pathology, only 30% or so show signs of clinically-defined dementia. This uncoupling of the brain pathology and dementia in Down Syndrome is most intriguing, and will certainly be a focus of intense research interest in the future.

There has been a revolution in the past 20 years in our understanding of the nervous system and its normal and abnormal function. From genetic and molecular to systems and behavioral neuroscience, recent technical and conceptual advances have created new opportunities for unexpected insights in the clinic. The chapters in this volume evaluate what is currently known about the psychobiological status of Down Syndrome individuals throughout life, identify areas where more information is needed, and provide directions that should facilitate the direct application of research results to the lives of affected individuals. Participants at the conference left with renewed enthusiasm, and it is hoped that this enthusiasm is communicated in the chapters that follow. Though we have a long way to go before our understanding is complete, tremendous strides have been made.

Lynn Nadel
Professor of Psychology and
Research Cognitive Scientist,
University of Arizona

PART 1

COGNITIVE AND BEHAVIORAL PERSPECTIVES

1

Early Learning in Infants and Young Children with Down Syndrome

Dr. Jennifer G. Wishart
Department of Psychology
University of Edinburgh
7 George Square
Edinburgh EH8 9JZ, Scotland

Introduction

This paper falls into three sections. The first gives a basic introduction to Down Syndrome (DS) and evaluates the likelihood of biomedical research leading either to effective preventive measures or to discovery of a "cure" for children born with this condition. The second section looks at the role of environmental factors in determining developmental outcome in DS and at the contrast between difference and delay accounts of psychological development in children with mental handicap. The final section presents an overview of a longitudinal study of early learning in infants and young children with DS which revealed higher than expected levels of cognitive ability but a style of learning which failed to make efficient use of that ability.

Down Syndrome

Down Syndrome is the best known - and probably the most misunderstood - of all of the mental handicapped conditions. It is the most common cause of mental handicap in developed countries, accounting for around one third of all children with severe handicap. Incidence is approximately 1/600 live births: in the UK, around 1000 babies are born with DS each year and in the US, about 7000. The mental handicap associated with DS is frequently aggra-

vated by the presence of additional health problems: a-
round 1/3 of children with DS also have congenital heart
disease, defects in hearing and vision are common, and
mortality rates from respiratory diseases and leukemia
are significantly elevated. In the 1950s, only 50% of
babies born with DS survived infancy but recent advances
in medicine, particularly in cardiology and immunology,
have increased life expectancy dramatically. Many people
with DS now survive into their fifties and even sixties
and as a result, prevalence has increased fourfold over
the last decade.

DS arises from a chromosomal abnormality, the presence
in triplicate, rather than duplicate, of all or part of
chromosome 21. DS is therefore a condition in which an
extra complement of normal genetic material is present:
the child with DS does not have defective genes - he or
she simply has too many. The cumulative effect of the re-
sultant increase in concentration of a large number of
gene products, compounded by secondary reactions triggered by the imbalance of the genome, results in a highly
complex phenotype (Patterson, 1987). Chromosome 21 is the
smallest of the 23 human chromosomes, representing only
1.5% of the total genetic material. Gene mapping studies
indicate, moreover, that only 10-20% of chromosome 21 -
the 21q22 band on the long arm - is actually implicated
in DS. Nonetheless, the presence of an extra copy of this
tiny chromosome appears to have a swamping effect on abnormal mental development and mental handicap (Breg,
1977).

*Current Prospects for Preventing Down Syndrome or
Discovering a "Cure"*

Although our understanding of the underlying genetics and
neurochemistry of DS has vastly increased in recent years
(for review, see Smith, 1985), prospects for either cure
or prevention are, it would seem, still remote. DS is only very rarely an inherited condition. Most cases arise
de novo, usually caused by non-disjunction during gamete
formation, by a failure of division at meiosis I or II.
Screening for DS is now possible early in pregnancy, using either amniocentesis or chorion villus sampling meth-

ods. Both techniques are costly and both carry a small but significant risk of miscarriage; together these factors dictate, for the moment, that screening be restricted to pregnancies known to be at risk for DS. Women over 35 or women who have already given birth to a child with DS - the only known high risk categories - account for only 1/3 of DS births. Even within this high risk group, it would appear that a significant proportion of women are either not offered screening or do not take up that offer (Walker & Howard, 1986). The majority of children with DS - two thirds - are born to mothers for whom there are no known predisposing genetic or environmental factors (Miller & Farmer, 1982).

Until some less invasive and less expensive form of pre-natal diagnosis can be found, DS will continue to remain undetected in the majority of affected pregnancies. For the meantime, hopes lie in finding some form of inexpensive pre-screening test for identifying younger mothers at risk, mothers for whom at present the risks of amniocentesis would normally outweigh the risk of having a DS baby. Findings of reliably low levels of maternal serum alphafetaprotein (MSAFP) in affected pregnancies led to the suggestion that the use of a combination at-risk index might be the answer in such cases, an index derived from a number of simple, non-invasive measures easily obtainable during pregnancy without risk to the foetus - for example, a weighted combination of MSAFP level, gestational age and maternal age and weight. Trials have shown, however, that such indices are insufficiently discriminating to justify referral for amniocentesis, falsely identifying an unacceptably high number of pregnancies as being at-risk where no risk in fact existed.

All of the presently-available preventive measures are applied during pregnancy. If DS is detected or suspected, abortion of the fetus is the only preventive route. For many parents, especially when the pregnancy is already well under way, this is not a satisfactory option. Even if termination is decided upon, anxiety and distress is an almost inevitable consequence. Ideally then, some form of screening should be available prior to pregnancy, at the stage of planning a family. Unfortunately, we still do not have any insight into what predisposes certain

couples to having a child with DS. Cytogenetic and biochemical data drawn retrospectively from the parents of
children born with DS have been compared with data drawn
from parents whose children were born without DS. Although significant differences between the two parent
groups have been found in protein levels and in gene cut
patterns, these possible "markers" were also found to occur at a sufficiently high level of frequency in control
parents to make them unsuitable for either genetic coun-
selling purposes or for recommending pre-natal diagnostic
screening. In the search for the cause (or causes) of DS,
numerous environmental factors have also been examined -
length of use of the contraceptive pill, exposure to ra-
diation, even the season at time of conception. Once a-
gain, none has shown a sufficiently high correlation to
be of use in identifying at-risk groups (Hook, 1982).

For present, the best predictor of DS is still maternal
age although we still do not know why the older mothers
should be more at risk of giving birth to a baby with DS.
Although awareness of this age-link has led to a fall in
DS births to women in older age groups there is little
evidence of overall incidence rates falling. A number of
studies suggest that this may be due to an increase in
the occurrence of DS in babies born to younger mothers
although the evidence is still inconclusive (Abroms &
Bennett, 1983; Stratford & Steele, 1985). Even if maternal age trends in DS births remain constant, there would
still be cause to predict an overall increase in DS in
the 1980s and 1990s. Two major reasons, both age-related,
stand out. One is that the very large number of women
born in the "baby boom" post-war period are now reaching
35 (Heuther, 1983). The other is the trend towards delaying the child-bearing years. Average maternal age, having
dipped dramatically in the 70s (Shepperdson, 1985), is a-
gain rising slowly but steadily. An increase in the number of DS births unfortunately seems inevitable.

There has recently been a great deal of media attention
to the possibility of finding a "cure" for DS, some form
of genetic engineering or biochemically-based therapy
that could correct the adverse developmental effects of
DS. It is indeed possible in principle that research in
the neurosciences could identify methods of intervention
to counteract or at least modify the effects of the chro-

mosomal   imbalance in the children born with DS. While not
wishing   to   quash   the   optimism   of those of us who work
with   children   with DS, it would nonetheless be unrealis-
tic   not to acknowledge the enormous practical problems in
implementing   any   therapy. In most cases of DS, the genetic   abnormality   acts on developmental processes from the
very   earliest   point,   we are unaware that a new affected
life   is   about   to begin and cannot therefore know of the
need   to   intervene.   By the time pregnancy is recognized,
development   is   already well under way; the original trisomic   cell   has   divided and multiplied itself many thou-
sands   of   times,   each new copy carrying the extra chromosomal material.

Understanding   the genetic mechanisms and the underlying
biochemistry   of DS and being able to apply that knowledge
to   prevent   it   taking its usual developmental course are
two   quite   different   matters.   Whether future biomedical
research   will   lead eventually either to prevention of DS
births   or   to some form of corrective therapy must remain
an   open question. DS is obviously going to be with us for
some   time   yet. As long as prevalence and incidence rates
are   high and likely to remain so, it is essential to continue   our efforts to understand DS more adequately and to
try   to   find ways to enhance development in children born
with   this condition. It seems particularly important that
we   attempt to find some way to counteract the progressive
decline   in the rate of mental development generally found
with increasing age (Gibson, 1978).

Enhancing Development in Children with Down Syndrome

Even   if   we have to acknowledge that DS may be a condition   that   is likely to remain with us in future decades,
increasingly   understood   but   effectively   beyond medical
prevention   or   cure, there is still reason to be optimistic   about   the prospects for improving developmental outcome   in DS. All development comes from an interaction between   genes   and   environment, an interaction between the
child's   genetic makeup and the physical and psychological
environment   in which the child grows up. All the children
with   DS   have   extra   genetic   material on 21 and yet the
range   of   achievement   seen   is very wide (Melyn & White,

12 Jennifer G. Wishart

1973; Morgan, 1979); this is not the case with most other forms of mental handicap of known aetiology, where developmental range is typically very restricted.

Recent years have seen a major impact on development as a result of children with DS being brought up in the parental home rather than in an institutional setting (Carr, 1975, 1985; Centerwall & Centerwall, 1960). Some children have progressed to an extent that has called into question our previous estimations of the developmental limits imposed by the genetic component in DS (Rynders et al., 1978). In normal children, variations in ability, particularly in IQ, are often associated with factors such as parental IQ and social class. This relationship does not generally hold true in DS (Carr, 1975; Gibson, 1978) although, interestingly, exceptions to this trend have recently been reported (Cunningham, 1986; Sharev et al., 1985). Given the wide variation in learning ability found in the children with DS and the absence of any clear, straightforward relationship with environmental factors usually closely associated with developmental outcome, it would seem that other, less obvious factors must be influencing development in DS. If these could be identified, appropriate fine-tailoring of the environment to the particular needs and skills of the child with DS might well improve on presently achieved levels of development. Support for this more optimistic viewpoint comes from recent results from a number of training studies and intervention studies carried out with young DS subjects (Duffy & Wishart, 1987; Haydn & Haring, 1977; McConkey, 1980; Morss, 1984; Wishart, 1986). Processes of early development in children with DS do seem to be responsive to intervention - although how long early gains are maintained has recently been called into question (Halpern, 1984; Simeonsson et al., 1982; Sloper, Glenn & Cunningham, 1986).

DS is primarily a mental handicap and its associated anomalies are expressed behaviorally. Psychology can, therefore, contribute much to attempts at facilitative intervention. If intervention programs are to have any chance of effecting long-term amelioration in development, however, they must be firmly based on an understanding of early psychological development in DS, an understanding of the exact nature of processes operating in handicap. It is important to be realistic about what may be achieved: the genetic component in DS must inevitably impose some upper limit on the extent to which environmentally-based intervention methods can improve on developmental outcome. Nonetheless, there seems to be reason to believe that with appropriately sensitive teaching methods, more children with DS could be encouraged to develop to their full potential.

The Psychological Environment of the Child with DS

Recent years have seen an upsurge in both media and scientific interest in mental handicap. DS, being the most common and most easily recognized form of mental handicap, has probably received a disproportionate share of this attention. It is now in the unfortunate position of being a condition with which everyone claims familiarity while in reality, still only a small minority of the general public have had any direct personal experience of either children or adults with DS. There are many misconceptions still held about DS, about the condition itself and about the level of ability generally associated with it. The move towards community care will inevitably rectify some of these misconceptions. The general public, however, is not alone in holding ill-informed views. Professional ignorance of DS is also surprisingly high. Despite its high incidence and increasing prevalence, many doctors, scientists and psychologists have little more than a textbook acquaintance with the condition; often the textbook from which that knowledge is drawn is at best out of date, at worst, seriously inaccurate. Many professionals consequently hold unnecessarily pessimistic views on the developmental potential of children with DS. These views are passed on to parents, often insensitively and with little consideration of the negative effects such information may have on the way parents will then respond to and interact with their child. Lowered expectations often adversely influence the psychological environment in which the child's learning must take place. Opportunities for learning may be adversely affected, leading to self-fulfilling prophecy of slow and unsatisfactory development.

It might be expected that the parents of a child with DS would be less likely than others to hold stereotyped views on DS and would be more willing to reserve judgement about their own particular child's learning abilities until it became clear how he or she was progressing. An interesting study by Krasner (1985) suggests that this may not be the case, with parents of children with DS just as susceptible as others to the effects of labelling a child as having DS. Krasner showed mothers films of two babies, one baby supposedly "normal", the other said to have DS. The films she used were actually of two non-retarded six-month-olds, the so-called DS baby being the more developmentally advanced of the two. She demonstrated that simply labelling a child as DS led to underestimates of both ability and stage of development, the non-DS baby consistently being rated as more advanced than the "DS" baby. Surprisingly perhaps, the mothers of toddlers with DS were as susceptible to this effect as the mothers of ordinary children.

There were similar results produced in a second study in which mothers were asked to play separately with each of two non-identical 4-year-old twins, one of whom - again the more able - was identified as having DS. In this study, it was again clear that the behavior of the mothers varied according to which child was the "DS" child. Mothers used more commands and far fewer complex wh-type questions ("where?", "what?", "why?", "who?", "when?") when interacting with the "DS" child. They also responded much more to her sister's attempts to start up a conversation, ignoring many of the "DS" sister's attempts to do the same. In Krasner's work, neither "DS" child actually either had DS or looked as if they might have DS. Real DS children are easily recognizable. This probably acts against their best interests, lowering people's expectations of their ability level before they have had a chance to demonstrate what they can or cannot do. The importance of this point will hopefully become more evident later, when the approach to learning which seems to characterize early cognitive development in DS is described. Young children with DS seem to learn quickly that others' expectations of them are low, that help will be forthcoming even when unneeded - "help" which can only in the long run be counterproductive, reducing both

the   reliance on and development of efficient, self-initiated learning strategies.

Learning in Children with Down Syndrome

Many different theories of cognitive functioning in
mental handicap exist. Few are based in developmental research although many of the issues central to competing
theories could in principle be resolved by such research.
Assessment of those theories which _are_ developmentally-
based - mainly learned helplessness or motivation-based
theories - is hampered by the limited amount of experimental and normative data available on mentally-handi-
capped subjects in the lower age ranges. Problems in arriving at a sound, well-established database have been
compounded by the instability which seem to characterize
development in mental handicap (Carr, 1985; Shapiro,
1983). This limits the confidence that can be placed in
cross-sectional data, both within and across age-groups.
Longitudinal studies seem essential to identifying the
developmental processes underlying poor progress but are
time-consuming, costly and therefore rare. Developmental
research into learning in children with DS starts off
with several advantages, however. In the majority of cases of mental handicap, aetiology is unknown; in many cases, the handicap may go undetected for many months or
even years, diagnosed only when it becomes clear that the
child is consistently failing to reach the developmental
milestones on schedule. DS, by contrast, can be confi-
dently identified at birth, is of known genetic origin
and occurs in sufficiently large numbers and with sufficient variation in developmental outcome to enable proper
scientific investigation. It should be emphasized, however, that there is no strong evidence as yet to suggest
that early cognitive development in children with DS differs in any radical way from development in children with
other forms of mental handicap.

Is Development Different or Simply Slow?

Much research on learning disabilities in children with

DS assumes there to be some basic and irremediable central deficit in processing environmental input (see e.g. Benda, 1954; Illingworth, 1972). This deficit is expressed in the increasingly delayed appearance of recognized developmental milestones. Achievement of milestones can only ever be part of any account of development, however; insight into the processes underlying each new cognitive step is much more crucial to our understanding of development in mental handicap. Despite the relative absence of firm developmental data, deficit accounts simply as- sume that these processes are identical in non-handicapped and handicapped children: development in mental handicap is seen as a slowed-down version of normal cognitive development - equivalent in structure and organization, only progressing more slowly to a lower ceiling (Illingworth, 1980; Mans et al., 1978). Any study which uses psychometrically-based mental age (MA) scores to measure developmental progress, to evaluate intervention programs or to match handicapped and non-handicapped subjects by definition subscribes to this viewpoint (Duffy & Wishart, 1987; Wishart, 1987). The near-universal use of the word "retarded" to describe those with mental handicap also reflects how widely this assumption is made, by professionals and the general public alike.

Deficit theories, by their very nature, leave little room for optimism over the chances of ameliorating development in children with DS. Until recently, very little direct evidence existed either to support or to refute the "slow development" theory. Most studies of mental handicap had concentrated on the end product rather than the dynamics of learning, providing developmental information on milestone achievement consistent with a slow development theory but telling us little about early cognitive processing in the child with a mental handicap (Weisz & Zigler, 1979). If, however, we entertain the possibility that DS development is not only slower but may also be quite _different_ from processes of normal development, there is less cause for pessimism. Research in several areas of psychological development has already shown that the same developmental milestones can be successfully reached by a number of different developmental routes (Bower, 1982). There is now a growing body of evidence suggesting that learning in children with mental

handicap may well differ in very fundamental ways from
that seen in normal development, with important qualitative as well as quantitative differences in learning processes existing in the two populations (Cherkes-Julkowski
et al., 1986; Duffy & Wishart, 1987; Macpherson, 1984;
Morss, 1983, 1985; Moss & Hogg, 1987; Rogers, 1977;
Rondal, 1984; Wishart, 1986, 1987; Zigler & Balla, 1982).
If processes of cognitive development are different in DS
infants, it may be possible to improve further on their
developmental prospects by more careful structuring of
the learning environment to their particular needs and
skills.

In evaluating recent evidence relevant to the differ-
ence-delay debate, two factors should be borne in mind.
Firstly, delay in appearance of a particular stage or
skill in any area of development can in itself lead to
significant differences in the unfolding of subsequent
developmental processes: the late appearance of that particular ability may throw out of synchrony the normally
well-geared meshing of progress within and between developmental areas. Secondly, and possibly more importantly,
it may well turn out that the contrast between differences and delay theories of development hinges ultimately
on the level of analysis used: studies in which the evidence appears to support a slow development theory may,
on more detailed analysis, reveal the existence of important differences (Kiernan, 1984). The presence of two apparently conflicting accounts of the nature and course of
development in children with mental handicap can be highly productive; different questions yield different answers, all of which can contribute to our aim of understanding developmental processes in DS to better effect.
Trying to decide between them, however, may well turn out
to be a fruitless pursuit, not unlike trying to portion
out the exact and relative contributions of genes and environment to development.

One of the most recent theoretical attempts at modelling cognitive deficit in mental handicap incorporates
structures and mechanisms which would allow both qualitative differences in performance profiles to emerge,
thereby amalgamating the stronger aspects of both difference and delay theories (Anderson, 1986). Evaluation of
this and other competing theories is presently limited,

however, by the poor database against which they can be tested. The study outlined below hoped to go some way towards remedying that deficit.

Cognitive Development in Infants with Down Syndrome

The milestones of motor development in infancy - reaching, sitting unsupported, crawling and so forth - have long been charted. Research into mental development in infancy, however, is a relatively new area of investigation. Until recently, the mental life of babies seemed an impenetrable mystery to psychologists; some would have disputed that infants were actually capable of thought. Even if the capacity to think were conceded, the problems of investigating mental ability in infancy seemed insurmountable. Infants, by definition, cannot talk - how then could we ever know what they were thinking? In adult or child psychology, it was accepted that thinking could be inferred from the subject's behavior in a given experimental situation. The limited response repertoire of the infant, it seemed, apparently severely restricted even this possible avenue of access to early thought.

The development of new, simple - and inexpensive - recording techniques has transformed infancy research. The advent of first the 16mm and then the 8mm film, followed quickly by video, has made possible the reliable recording of even the smallest change in a baby's behavior; that behavior can then be subsequently analysed and re-analysed in the minutest of detail. Use of these new facilities, coupled with some ingenious experimental design, has uncovered previously unsuspected levels of cognitive ability in the young infant; some surprising gaps in early understanding have also been revealed (see e.g. Bower, 1982). In a comparatively short period of time, a large body of normative data on many important aspects of early development has been established and we now have considerable insight into cognitive processing in young infants.

Unfortunately, present-day tests of mental ability in infants reflect few of these advances in our understanding of development in infancy. The most widely used test of infant ability - the Bayley Scales of Infant Development (Bayley, 1969) - was first devised in the thirties; norms have been updated several times but test items and materials have remained essentially unchanged. As with most other scales of infant ability, test items from the mental scale, particularly in the lower age ranges, often turn out to be little more than measures of the physical abilities and coordinations; few have even face validity as measures of cognitive functioning. Not surprisingly, the predictive validity of such tests is low: average correlation with later intelligence, even just two years later, is only .14 (Fagan, 1984, 1985).

Test items in scales like the Bayley are normatively derived, selected for their ability to characterize average developmental level at any given age while distinguishing between ability levels at different ages. Physical and mental development are assumed to go hand-in-hand in such scales: the average 18 month old child would be expected to reach the 18 month level on both the mental and motor scales of the Bayley. Although in normal development this will usually be the case, poor motor development does not always necessarily imply correspondingly poor mental development (or, indeed, vice versa). Because of the need to infer a baby's mental ability from his or her behavior, however, any baby whose motor development is impaired will necessarily be at a disadvantage in any Bayley-type test of "mental" ability (Zelazo, 1979).

DS babies do perform poorly on both the mental and motor scales of these early "IQ" tests in comparison to non-handicapped babies (for an excellent review, see Carr, 1985). This is hardly surprising given the poor muscle tone generally present and the motor skills required for success on many of the mental scale test items. Several studies, however, have shown a relative superiority of "mental" development over motor development in the first years of DS. In one study of children between 12 and 36 months of age, motor scores lagged behind mental scores by as much as ten months (LaVeck & LaVeck, 1977). As the authors point out, this mismatch may lead to serious underestimation of mental competence and of the readiness to acquire cognitive skills.

In all but the severest of cases, DS children do reach all of the important milestones in early motor development, albeit later than the average child. The delayed appearance of these abilities must, however, mean that making use of whatever mental ability is present is an uphill struggle for the child with DS, particularly in the earliest months; the baby's own ability to explore and to initiate learning situations is obviously severely restricted. Given this and the lowered parental expectations of learning ability described above, it is perhaps not surprising that we see a rapid and marked decline in rate of development, both mental and motor, as children with DS grow older (Carr, 1985; Harris, 1981; Piper et al., 1986). Development would appear to be further compromised by a learning style which apparently fails to take maximum use of learning situations (to be described below).

If a major aim of early intervention is to prevent or stem this decline in rate of development, we shall need to build up a detailed data base on early learning processes in DS. It is now well-established that the first two years of life are normally the most active - and vulnerable - periods in brain development. Within this short period, the brain reaches 80% of adult size, tripling in bulk as it constructs the complex networks of neuronal interconnections required for advanced behaviors. These early years are obviously also crucial to psychological growth - possibly particularly so in the case of children with mental handicaps. Research has shown that advances made during this period underlie much of later learning and that early losses cannot easily be made up for later. More critically, perhaps, there is considerable evidence that experience in these early years may determine subsequent learning style: a form of learned helplessness may set in, with increasing awareness of low personal efficacy being generalized to areas of comparative - or untested - strength (Kearsley, 1979; Seligman, 1975). We obviously need a clearer description of the nature, course and parameters of learning during this period in children with DS. This will require not only investigating the level of mental ability present at different ages but also discovering how the child with DS approaches learning at different stages in his or her development. The Edinburgh longitudinal study hoped to make some contribution to this end.

fficult manual search tasks. In these tasks, a toy is
idden in some way either inside, under or behind some
orm of occluder (usually a cup, cloth or screen); the
nfant then has to remove the occluder in order to re-
rieve the toy. In all but the simplest task, the infant
ust choose between one of two identical occluders; un-
ess he or she fully comprehends the relevant hiding se-
uence, performance can only be at chance level.
We used 4 different hiding tasks in our longitudinal
tudy (in ascending order of difficulty):

Task 1: a one cup, Stage III-VI task
Task 2: a two cup, Stage IV-V AAB task
Task 3: a two cup, Stage V-VI inference task
Task 4: a two cup, Stage V-VI switching task

Order of difficulty of these particular tasks had been
scertained in a normative study of object concept devel-
pment in which 228 babies aged between 4 and 22 months
ere tested on each of the four tasks (Wishart & Bower,
984). Tasks 3 and 4 are alternative versions of Piaget's
nvisible displacement task: Task 3 proved to be the
asier of these two tasks. All four tasks are described
n full in Wishart & Bower and so will be only briefly
lescribed here.

Task 1: involves a simple hiding of a toy under one cup.
All babies, handicapped or non-handicapped, pass through
a stage in their development when they will make no attempt to retrieve the hidden object; although well able
to reach and pick up the toy from the table, they act as
if that same toy had disappeared when put under the cup.
This behavior has frequently been described as "out-of-
sight, out-of-mind" behavior.

Task 1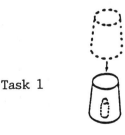

*The Edinburgh Longitudinal Study of Earl]
Infants and Young Children with Down Syndrome*

Development of the Object Concept - For the
practical reasons, the Edinburgh longitudin
concentrated on object concept development, a
step in early cognitive development, normal:
by around two years of age. Reasons for cl
particular area of conceptual development are
but the term "object concept development" pe
needs some explanation.

To understand even the simplest event, an i
to acquire an understanding of physical rea
the laws which determine that reality. Basic
derstanding is learning the defining propertie
ject.Infants must learn, for example, that ob_
independently of our actions, that they contin:
even when we cannot see them or act upon them
also learn that every object has a unique ide:
two objects which are identical in every respe
in any way the same object. They must come to
that objects are subject to the laws of space
causality - that the same object cannot be in
simultaneously, that one object must have con
other for it to have caused its movement, t
ject placed inside another object will share
ments made by that object, and so on. Learning
jects and their properties is an essential fir:
early understanding; without a fully developed (
an object, the acquisition of many more advance(
would be impossible.

Development of the Object Concept: Object Concep
Development of the object concept is indexed by
ance on a number of object search tasks in which
ing sequence increases in complexity accordi:
stage of object concept development being tested
1937). The earliest stages, Stage I-II (0-4 1/2
are defined by visual search behaviors (e.g. :
the path of an object which falls out of si{
study, however, concentrated on Stages III-VI o1
ject concept (4 1/2 - 24 months). These later st
indexed by success or failure on a number of incr

Task 2: known as the AAB task, involves two cups. The toy is hidden twice under one of these cups (A); if the baby successfully retrieves the toy from A on both occasion, the toy is then hidden under the second, identical cup (B). Again, all infants at some point in their development make the error of looking for the toy on the third trial under A, the first cup; despite having seen it disappear under B only a moment earlier, they search in the place where they have always previously found the toy, under the first rather than second cup.

Task 2

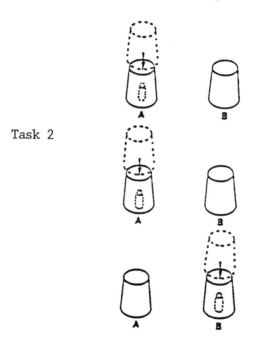

Task 3: requires the infant to make a deduction. The experimenter shows the infant the toy in the palm of her hand. She then closes her hand slowly over the toy and places her closed hand in one of two identical upturned cups, one to either side of her hand. There, she silently releases the toy, recloses her empty hand and returns it to the center position. The first reaction of the infant should be to look in the experimenter's hand for the toy, the place where he last saw it. When, however, he discovers that it is no longer there, he will have to deduce or infer that it can only be in the cup into which the ex-

perimenter's hand disappeared during the hiding sequence.

Task 3

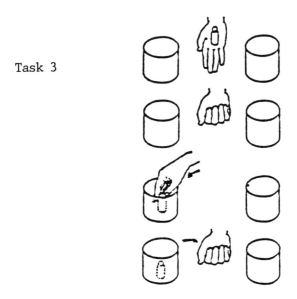

Task 4:   the "switching' task, is by far the most difficult of the tasks. The toy is put under one of two cups
and then the positions of these transposed. To succeed on
this task, the baby must ignore the fact that an identical cup is now in the place where he saw the toy disappear and work out that, even although he did not see it
move, the toy has switched position and is still to be
found in the original cup.

Task 4

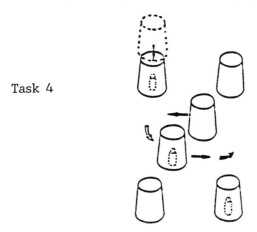

These search tasks, simple to the adult mind, pose enormous difficulties for all babies during their development, no matter how intelligent they may be. Task 1 can be passed by the majority of babies by around 5 months of age, Task 2 by 10 months and Task 3 by 15 months; Task 4 however, presents infants with considerable problems even at two years of age (Wishart & Bower, 1984, op. cit.). Video tapes of the babies' behavior in response to these tasks make it clear that these tasks do tap early thought processes. Babies also clearly enjoy taking part in these "tasks". Even babies who are going through a stage of extreme wariness of strangers will quickly engage in object concept tasks; although at first unwilling even to touch an attractive toy proffered encouragingly - and unconditionally - by a friendly experimenter, they cannot resist searching for that self-same toy when it is hidden by the very same person; for trial after trial, natural curiosity wins out over reluctance to interact with a stranger.

Development of the Object: Success/Failure Criteria for the Tasks - All tasks are presented four times, with side of hiding randomized over trials. To score a pass on any of the tasks, the infant must succeed on all four trials. Although there is a 50/50 probability of chance success on any one of the two-cup problems, there is only a very small chance - 1 in 16 - that a score of 4/4 could result from guessing rather than from a true understanding of the problem presented by the task. In the longitudinal studies, all-correct performance in two successive testing sessions is required (a more detailed discussion of these criteria can be found in Wishart & Bower (1984, op. cit.).

Why Select These Particular Tasks in an Investigation of Early Learning in Children with Down Syndrome?

Development of the object concept is already known to be a major hurdle to children with mental handicap; it would seem that many children, even those with fairly well developed motor and social skills, never reach its highest stages (Silverstein et al., 1975; Wohlheuter & Sindberg, 1975). Why, though, favor these particular

tasks in a study of mental development in children with
DS? Clearly, object concept tasks require minimal motor
skills and so are particularly suited for use with young
DS children. There are, however, three further and more
important reasons to believe these tasks to be ideal for
any attempt at investigating cognitive processes in a
young handicapped population.

The first is that development of the object concept is
considered by many to be prototypical of all later processes of cognitive development. Object concept development has become one of the most widely researched and
well described areas of cognitive development in infancy
(see recent reviews by Harris, 1986; Schuberth, 1982). As
a result, we have highly detailed, up-to-date information
not only on typical ages of achievement of the stages indexed by each of the tasks but also of the processes of
learning normally leading up to achievement of each of
the stages of object concept development (Piaget, 1937;
Uzgiris & Hunt, 1975; Wishart & Bower, 1984). Such high-
ly-detailed information on other areas of early learning
simply does not yet exist. While wishing to reserve our
options on the possibility that important qualitative
differences in performance might distinguish DS and non-
handicapped infants, it is nevertheless useful, indeed
essential, to carry out research into early cognitive
processes in DS against a background of understanding of
cognitive processes in normal development.

A second reason for focussing on object concept devel-
ment is that numerous studies have shown it to be a universal cognitive process: under standard testing situations, all infants in all cultures at some point in their
development make the same object concept errors in exactly the same sequence. Babies who do well on these tasks,
however, also tend to do well when given more traditional
intelligence tests at a later age (Birns & Golden, 1972;
Wachs, 1975; Wishart, 1979). This makes object concept
behavior one of the very few cognitively-directed behaviors of infancy which have any predictive validity for
later intellectual development.

Rate of development of the object concept has been
shown to be highly susceptible to environmental influences. In normal infants, for instance, naturally-occur-
ring variations in upbringing have been shown to lead to

differences of up to nearly two years in the age of a-
chievement of the highest stage in object concept development; in a study by Hunt et al. (1975), middle class
American babies passed the Stage V-VI tasks at 73 weeks
of age on average while babies brought up in an under-
staffed Greek orphanage did not succeed on these same
tasks until 182 weeks of age. Experimental work has also
shown that repeated exposure to a conceptually-rich, visual tracking task can almost double the normal rate of
object concept development (Wishart & Bower, 1985). This
susceptibility of rate of development to environmental
input, when taken in conjunction with the apparent importance of object concept development to subsequent cognitive development, gives us a third reason for selecting
it for detailed longitudinal study - we can improve performance on these tasks by altering the conditions under
which babies learn them.

  This last reason for selecting object concept development is particularly important in view of our longer-term
interest in amelioration of development in DS. The object
concept development meets all of the criteria recently
advanced by Fagan & Singer (1981) for any individual differences, it is known to have alterable components and it
is amenable to theoretical interpretation (see Wishart &
Bower, 1984, op. cit.). The study to be reported here, it
should be emphasized, was purely an observational study;
no attempt at intervention was made. Some small-scale
training studies have been carried out using the tasks
described above, some with encouraging results (see e.g.
Morss, 1984; Wishart, 1986), but the primary purpose of
this particular study was to provide a detailed description of the natural course of early learning in children
with DS. It hoped to identify the processes which impede
learning in DS, an essential prerequisite to any attempt
to generate training procedures which might improve that
learning.

The Edinburgh Study

A total of 50 infants and young children with DS participated in the Edinburgh longitudinal study of object concept development. Subjects ranged between 4 months and 5 years of age on entry to the study. All children had been volunteered by their parents in response to an approach from either the local maternity hospital or from the Scottish Down Syndrome Association, a parent-professional self-help group. With the exception of only one child, an adopted child whose early medical records were not available, the presence of DS was in all cases confirmed by karyotyping. Most children, as would be expected, had standard Trisomy 21; DS in one child was due to a translocation while two other children had a mosaic form of DS. (One of these latter two other children had to be dropped from the study when it became clear that his development was unaffected by this partial presence of DS). In addition to DS, fifteen children in the study also had congenital heart disease (in three cases, inoperable); eleven had some degree of either hearing or vision loss diagnosed during infancy. Two children unfortunately died during the course of the study, one of leukemia, one from respiratory complications following an attack of pneumonia.

All testing sessions took place in the Psychology Department infant lab. Sessions were scheduled for a time of day at which the parent thought the child would be the most likely to be cooperative, neither too hungry nor too tired to be interested in the tasks. Data were collected on performance on all four levels of task at fortnightly intervals. Both qualitative and quantitative aspects of performance were monitored over periods ranging from 3 months to 3 years, length of participation in the study being determined by age and development stage at entry. In all but the oldest and most capable subjects, both pre- and post-acquisition performance on the developmental sequence tapped by object concept tasks was thus monitored over several stages in development.

There were two control groups of non-handicapped infants and young children, one matched with the DS group for age at entry to the study, the other matched for developmental stage. Chronological age-matching was considered the less important of the two matching procedures, likely only to tell us what we already know - that children with DS perform poorly on these tasks in comparison

to non-handicapped   children of similar age. Matching for
developmental   stage was achieved retrospectively. Records
were   matched   by   transition points in development of the
object   concept: the session in which the target stage was
first   achieved   was identified and data from the two subject   groups then compared over equivalent numbers of sessions before   and   after   this   point. This method allows
precise   matching   on specific tasks at specific points in
development while   leaving   open the option that behavior
in   the   DS   group   prior and subsequent to acquisition of
any   stage   in development might differ significantly from
that seen in the non-handicapped subjects.

Results

Final   detailed   results   form   the study are not yet a-
vailable   as   data collection from some late-entering subjects   is   not   quite complete. Preliminary ordering analyses   of   the   difficulty levels of the four tasks, of the
search   strategies adopted at different stages in development   by the two groups, and of patterns of errors (in the
case   of   the   DS children, of errors made both before and
after   acquisition) exist between the two groups. Some of
these   results   will be presented here but in general, the
account   given   below   will concentrate on the qualitative
rather   than   quantitative   differences   in   developmental
processes which emerged from the study. These qualitative
differences   in learning patterns have proved to be sufficiently   consistent   both   within   and across the children
with   DS   studied   to justify confidence that they reflect
an   approach   to learning which is very distinct from that
seen   in   normal   development. Results from the older subjects will be presented first.

Results From Older Subjects

To   some   extent, performance patterns in the children
aged   between   3   and   5   years   fell out of the immediate
range   of   interest of this particular study (see Wishart,
1987). While   it   was   expected   that the non-handicapped
control   children   would   be well beyond the stages in ob-

Table 1
Success   rates   in   older   subjects   over six testing sessions

Tasks 2, 3, and 4.
(maximum N = 12 in each subject group)

Down Syndrome Group

Testing Session	1	2	3	4	5	6
Task 2:	5	11	12	8(+2)	11(+1)	10(+1)
Task 3:	5	9	10	12	11	11
Task 4:	2	3	4	4	5	7
Combined Total:	12	23	26	24(2+)	27(+1)	28(+1)

Non-handicapped Group:

Testing Session	1	2	3	4	5	6
Task 2:	10(+1)	10(+1)	11(+1)	9(+3)	10(+2)	10(+2)
Task 3:	11(+1)	9(+2)	10(+1)	10(+1)	10(+1)	7(+2)
Task 4:	10	10	5(+1)	6(+1)	6(+1)	5(+1)
Combined Total:	31(+2)	29(+3)	26(+3)	25(+5)	26(+4)	22(+5)

Notes: Number   in   parentheses   represent   the   number of children scored as failing deliberately - see text.

Task   1   was used only as a warm up task with older subjects;   no child in either subjects group refused or was unable to search under one cup.

ject concept development being targeted it was not expected that the majority of children with DS would also
already be able to pass the highest level tasks. This
ability was not immediately made evident (see Table 1);
performance was very poor on all levels in the first
testing session, a finding consistent with results from
previous cross-sectional studies of object concept development in DS children of this age. Scores increased dramatically over sessions, however. Performance of the non-
handicapped children, by contrast, was near perfect at
first but deteriorated significantly over the weeks; by
the sixth testing session scores in the DS group actually
exceeded those in the non-handicapped group.

There appeared to be a number of factors underlying
these opposing trends in performance over sessions in the
two subject groups. It was very clear that "poor" performance in later sessions in the non-handicapped children stemmed from a growing tendency to tease rather than
from some drastic change in ability level. Although initially anxious to demonstrate to the experimenter that
they did indeed understand the tasks, later sessions
tended to degenerate into elaborate social games and "errors" - cajoling and bribery (the introduction of chocolate for correct responding) could often restore error-
less performance, however. Teasing was seldom evident in
the children with DS. Poor levels of language development
to some extent precluded this type of behavior, drawing
attention to the fact that it can be difficult to give
children with mental handicap the same benefit of the
doubt that poor performance could be a case of "wouldn't
do" rather than "couldn't do". Nevertheless, it appeared
that poor performance in the early sessions did reflect
true levels of competence in these children at that time:
neither the introduction of chocolate nor coaxing made
any significant difference to success rates in the DS
group in these - or indeed any - testing session. The
overall improvement in performance shown by this group
over just two months of testing is, however, quite remarkable; this sequence of development, it will be recalled, normally takes two years to unfold in children
without mental handicap.

How then can we interpret this pattern of results in
the DS subjects? Given the extent and rate of improvement found, straightforward acquisition processes seem

unlikely to be at the base of the rapid improvement seen
over this short period. It could perhaps be suggested
that all of the children studied were simply very close
in any case to achieving success on these tasks on entering the study. The age difference between youngest and
oldest subject - over two years - makes this explanation
highly unlikely; even if it were accepted that all children might have been in a transitional stage of object
concept development at time of testing, this could not
possibly have been true for all levels of task, given
their proven hierarchical relationship to each other. It
seems more likely that these children were in fact re-ac-
quiring the object concept, re-tuning earlier learning
which had been inadequately consolidated at the time of
initial acquisition. In the absence of data from earlier
periods in these particular children's development, any
such hypothesis can obviously be neither proved nor dis-
proved. The data to be presented below from the younger
DS subjects in the Edinburgh study lend considerable support to a re-learning interpretation, however; with only
one exception, all of these younger children passed the
highest level task by the age of three, many before
reaching two. Since all children in the study were drawn
from the same sources, there is no reason to believe that
older subjects differed from younger subjects on any dimension likely to be of relevance to object concept development. We are left then trying to explain why 3-5
year old children with DS initially have difficulty with
tasks which babies with DS apparently solve easily.
   The simple solution will be to collect data on a group
of 3-5 year olds whose earlier developmental history on
these tasks is already known; this study is presently
underway, with longitudinal testing of subjects from the
younger age group being continued through into these later years. The developmental significance of the data from
the present subjects must, in the meantime, remain uncer-
tain. This part of the original study nevertheless drew
attention to two important issues. The first is that cognitive ability in children with DS may be poorly measured
by single-session testing; had the first testing session
of this longitudinal study been the only testing session
given, cognitive ability in these 3-5 year old children
would have been seriously underestimated (see also Morss,

1985). This finding obviously has important implications for assessment procedures. Secondly, these results make it clear that in the absence of normative data from non-handicapped children, there is a need for caution in evaluating the performance of children with mental handicap on tests designed for and validated on younger, non-retarded subjects; such tests may simply not engage older children adequately, whether handicapped or non-handicap-capped. Results from the older subjects studied here suggest that the role of motivational factors in both developmental processes and in the expression of these proces-cesses in performance require our much closer attention. It cannot simply be assumed that the relationship between underlying competence and performance is equivalent in handicapped and non-handicapped children. Evidence of occasional reversals in competence with increasing age - U-shaped curves in cognitive development - also suggest caution in assuming that competence demonstrated at earlier ages will always be present at later ages (Strauss, 1982; Emde & Harmon, 1986); this would appear to be true of development in both handicapped and non-handicapped children, although the reasons for apparent reversals in competence may differ in the two populations.

Results From Younger Subjects

Age on entry to the study of the remaining younger subjects ranged from 4 months to 2 years 9 months. By the end of data collection, 30 subjects will have completed this part of the study, each having provided pre- and post-acquisition data on a minimum of at least two stages in object concept development. As with older subjects, younger subjects were tested on all four tasks every two weeks. Development was monitored over periods ranging from 9 months to 3 years, length of monitoring period being determined by age/developmental stage on entry to the study.

Contrary to expectations, all first-level analyses of the results show developmental progress in these younger subjects to lag surprisingly little behind the norms for achievement of success on each of the four levels of task under study (Table 2). Despite the poor showing of older

Table 2
Interim results for younger subjects.
Age of achievement of success on hiding tasks 1-4.

DS subjects:

	Task 1	Task 2	Task 3	Task 4
Mean age of achievement	7.75	10.50	19.25	18
Range of age of Achievement	6.25-10.75	7.25-14	14.5-26.75	11-25.25

Non-handicapped subjects:

	Task 1	Task 2	Task 3	Task 4
Age at which 75% of Ss passed	5	10	15	22+

Longitudinal data (Edinburgh control group):

	Task 1	Task 2	Task 3	Task 4
	4.75	7.75	12.25	14.5
Range of ages of achievement	4-5.75	4.75-8.5	9.25-14.15	10.25-17

Note: All ages are expressed in months, and have been rounded up to nearest .25

children with DS in previous cross-sectional studies of object concept development and in sharp contrast to the low scores registered in early testing sessions by the 3-5 year old subjects tested here, age of success on most tasks was within the normal range for many of the younger subjects; in a few cases, normal rates of development were even bettered. If these results are representative of average ability levels in infants with DS, it would seem that early learning in children with DS may not be as severely impaired as previously believed.

In evaluating these results, it should be borne in mind that these babies were being tested regularly on these tasks, at fortnightly intervals. We already know from studies with non-handicapped children that regular exposure to these tasks can in itself accelerate the learning process (Bower & Paterson, 1972). Nonetheless, the results from the DS group are encouraging. The first set of ages given in the Table for non-handicapped children are from a large, cross-sectional normative study in which the babies - 228 of them - were tested only once (Wishart & Bower, 1984). The second set are interim results from a large, cross-sectional normative group of non-handicapped subjects used in this longitudinal study. Not surprisingly, the DS group did not perform as well as the control subjects. With the exception of Task 1, however, mean age of success in the DS children was very similar to that of non-handicapped children tested cross-sectionally; mean performance on Task 4 was actually better than in normal children. It would have been surprising if success on Task 1 had not been delayed, given the poor initial motor ability in young DS babies. Once reaching was established, however, cognitive development seemed capable of proceeding at more or less the normal rate. While it is important to remember the extra experience that these DS babies had had with these tasks, it still remains that they showed themselves capable of achieving these mental milestones at ages similar to - and, in several cases, earlier than - non-handicapped children.

Lack of consolidation of early learning

Less encouraging, however, was the subsequent develop-

mental history of these acquisitions. Although the infants with DS we tested would work enthusiastically at
acquiring the next cognitive step, it seemed that this
may have been at the expense of consolidation of the most
recently acquired step. Many infants tested in later,
post-acquisition months showed little interest in recent-
ly-mastered tasks, often "switching out" when they were
presented (see below and Wishart, 1986); many errors were
made and infants showed little evidence of ever having
understood tasks which had been mastered only a few
months previously (see also Sloper, Glenn & Cunningham,
1986; Morss, 1983). The unsuccessful search strategies
applied in these post-acquisition months were typically
either random or of a low-level (always, say, picking the
side corresponding to the preferred hand); the higher-
level, "thoughtful" strategies of earlier months were no
longer in evidence. Given that previous research has
shown that the developmental progression underlying success on these hiding tasks is normally both closely-inte-
grated and hierarchical (Bower & Paterson, 1972), these
results suggest not only that DS children fail to consol-
idate recently-acquired knowledge but also that they are
put at a further disadvantage by being unable or less
able to build effectively on newly-acquired knowledge.
Together, these deficiencies in learning could help to
explain the increasing gap which appears in developmental
progress in DS and non-handicapped children as they grow
older.

   Non-handicapped infants, by contrast, worked well
throughout the period of study on all levels of task:
once success was achieved on any task, it was reliably
repeated in virtually all subsequent testing sessions
(Table 3). The patterns of post-acquisition behavior seen
in the children with DS, however, proved to be consistent
both across subjects and within individual subjects at
different points in their development. If the typically
poor post-acquisition behavior shown by the Edinburgh
subjects is a pervasive aspect of DS learning patterns,
it might explain the divergence between the ages of a-
chievement of cognitive milestones found in this study
and those reported in cross-sectional studies with a-
dults, unable to solve these search tasks (see above).
If, once learned, a task holds no further interest and

Table 3
Typical pre-and post-acquisition performance in a
non-handicapped infant and in an infant with DS: Task 4.

		Non-handicapped infant Pass/ Fail	Score	DS infant Pass/ Fail	Score
	6	Fail	0/4	Fail	0/4
	5	Fail	2/4	Fail	2/4
Pre-	4	Fail	0/4	Fail	3/4
acquisition	3	Fail	3/4	Fail	2/4
Sessions	2	Fail	2/4	Fail	3/3 (switched out)
	1	Fail	3/4	(Pass)	2/4 (standard trials)
					4/4 (choc. trials)

Session at which success to criterion
achieved (4/4 on two consecutive sessions:

	Pass	4/4	Pass	4/4
	Pass	4/4	Pass	4/4

Post-acquisition Sessions:

		Pass/Fail	Score	Pass/Fail	Score
1		Pass	4/4	Fail	3/3 (switched out)
2		Pass	4/4	Pass	4/4
3		Pass	4/4	(Pass)	1/4 (standard trials)
					4/4 (choc. trials)
4		Pass	4/4	(Pass)	2/4 (standard trials)
					4/4 (extra trials)
5		Pass	4/4	Fail	3/4
6		Pass	4/4	Fail	2/4

Note: See Wishart & Bower (1984) for more detailed
account of developmental trends in error pattern.

little use is made of the recently, hard-won knowledge, it would not be surprising if that knowledge simply deteriorated; some support for the suggestion that early understanding is inadequately consolidated and may require re-learning comes from the pattern of results in the 3-5 year old children with DS reported above. Although, as we have seen, no firm conclusions about developmental processes in DS could be drawn from data alone, one thing <u>was</u> clear; original learning was still intact and the motivation to demonstrate that ability still, within limits, present.

On a more positive note, there was some evidence that in the initial post-acquisition months at least, newly-acquired knowledge was not necessarily irretrievably lost in these infant subjects. Although introduction of a reward for correct responding (chocolate) had little effect on performance in older DS subjects, it often led to a sudden "revival" of both interest and success in infant subjects. Presentation of extra trials of the task frequently had the same effect, a finding again suggestive of a re-tuning process coming into operation. Neither tactic proved to have much effect further into the post-acquisition phase, however, the infant's recently-gained competence apparently having deteriorated beyond retrieval. Poor performance in later post-acquisition sessions seemed to reflect genuine failure, and was unaltered by either changes in reinforcement or presentation of extra trials. This is consistent with the findings from older subjects reported above.

Whether underlying competence still exists and performance is merely poorly-motivated during these developmental periods is currently being investigated. Pilot experimental work suggests that manipulation of motivational factors at specific points in development can play a more important role in learning in DS than in normal infants and that success/failure rates during learning influences the course of that learning differentially in the two populations (see below).

Avoid New Learning

One other finding from the Edinburgh study seems to have important implications both for educational prac-

tice and for assessment methods. All of the children with
DS we studied proved very willing to work hard at learning the immediately-next developmental step. However, the
longitudinal data show that this willingness operated only within a highly prescribed cognitive focus. The infants studied would go to considerable lengths to <u>avoid</u>
learning situations in which the task presented was one
step or more beyond their current developmental status.
As we have seen, tasks previously mastered also seemed to
fall outside the range of interest, with performance on
lower-level tasks typically falling away in the months
following initial acquisition.

Both positive and negative tactics were used by the
subjects to get out of the task being presented if that
task was developmentally too difficult (see Wishart,
1986, op. cit.). A form of "cognitive avoidance" seemed
to come into play: before all four trials could be presented, the infant would "switch out" into some form of
either protest (younger infants) or diversionary social
interaction (older infants). In many cases, the infant
would attempt to divert the experimenter by resorting to
charm, smiling hopefully at her or producing some sort of
"party trick" such as clapping hands or "dancing" when
required to attend to the hiding sequence or to retrieve
the hidden object.

This cognitive avoidance behavior proved to be highly
specific to the level of difficulty of the task presented, and occurred irrespective of whether the immediately
preceding trials of that task had been successful or not.
In general, it was total and irreversible; no amount of
coaxing or enthusiasm on the part of the experimenter
could persuade the infant to search again. Cooperation
resumed immediately, however, if the experimenter moved
on to a more developmentally-appropriate task. Non-handicapped infants, as we have already seen, will generally
work well at all of the tasks under study, regardless of
whether any given task is above, equal to or below their
current ability level; they engage quickly and fully in
all levels of task, anxious to demonstrate, even to a
stranger, their willingness and ability to "play the
game".

Obviously, this "switching out" behavior produces all
sorts of problems in assessing the infant's true stage in

development. The success/failure criteria used in object concept testing are based on four trials; any infant who does not complete the trials, even if all the trials attempted are successful, must by definition fail. Conveniently for the developmental psychologist, the number of trials the average, non-handicapped infant is willing to perform generally coincides with this statistically-determined number of trials. It may be, however, that for the child with DS, that statistically-convenient number is in excess of the number considered cognitively or motivationally relevant. The cognitive style - and motivational framework - of the child with DS may simply not match our methods of assessment. Often a child who refuses to complete a testing session is recorded as "untestable", a description which, while technically accurate, is not particularly helpful either to the child or to our understanding of the child. It is important to note that it was not simply the case that the DS infants tested here would not cooperate in testing. Cooperation would be readily and enthusiastically given on other tasks presented either before or after the task being avoided, even though these tasks involved searching for the same object under the same cups. The counter-productive avoidance behavior could not therefore simply be attributed to either poor attentional capacity, fatigue or a generalized low level of motivation being characteristic of learning in children with DS. Patterns of avoidance behavior were highly specific to the developmental stage, tightly tied to the level of task being presented in relation to the infant's current cognitive status.

Mis-use of Social Skills in Learning Contexts

What should we make of this "switching out" behavior and more specifically, of methods used by these children to get out of difficult learning situations? As we have seen, the most common methods of opting out involved attempting to divert the experimenter away from the task in hand; the "social" behaviors involved were often highly stereotyped and inflexible, and could not in any way be described as being truly interactive. A frequent ploy, for example, was to attempt to catch the experimenter's eye and then simply stare at her, refusing to watch any of the hiding actions or to interact with her in any productive way. Children with DS are commonly described as being "highly social", "affectionate" and "outgoing". Little objective evidence to support this stereotype actually exists. Previous research into early social development has shown that, in infancy at least, the DS children are if anything <u>less</u> socially interactive than the non-handicapped age- or stage-matched children (Rogers-Warren et al., 1981; Gunn & Berry, 1985). It may be, however, that children with DS learn to use - or, rather, misuse - social skills to avoid learning situations. Parents expecting the child to have difficulties in any case in such situations, may unwittingly reinforce this behavior, setting aside the teaching attempt for the moment and engaging instead in social interaction. To some extent then, this type of behavior in the DS child can be seen as adding to his or her already existing handicap.

One last aspect of the data from the Edinburgh Longitudinal study is relevant here. From Table 2, it can be seen that ages of achieving success on Tasks 3 and 4 (the inference and switching tasks, respectively) were very similar in the DS group but differed markedly in the non-handicapped groups, Task 3 proving to be considerable easier than Task 4 for these subjects. Tasks 3 and 4 are alternate forms of the Stage V-VI task; in both, the hiding sequence involves an invisible displacement of the object. Although mean ages for success on the two tasks were very similar in the DS group, ordering analyses show that in individual subjects, success on these tasks was achieved in reverse order to that seen in normal development, with Task 3 proving to be a major hurdle for the children with DS.

Of all of the object concept tasks used here, Task 3 is the only one with any interpersonal element: the actions of the experimenter rather than simply the laws of physics dictate where the object can be found. Non-handicapped children patently enjoy the "trick" element in this task and rise willingly and enthusiastically to the challenge it presents. With increasing age and competence, search patterns graduate from search in one location (the hand), through search in two locations (not necessarily the correct two), then to exhaustive search in all three locations, followed finally by the direct hand - correct cup search sequence required for a pass to be credited (Wishart & Bower, 1984 op.cit.). Developmental patterns of search in the children with DS were quite different, however, and many seemed to find this task led frequently to a total collapse of search of the experimenter's hand although minutes earlier, the same child had shown himself both willing and able to search in more than one location in one of the other two-cup tasks. The children with DS seemed unable to accept the experimenter's role in this task and were neither able to solve it nor to engage the experimenter's help in solving it together. In real-life learning situations, learning frequently derives from the actions of others; in many instances, its success depends on the support of others. The lowered interpersonal motivation revealed by this particular task, when considered in conjunction with the non-responsiveness of these same infants to attempts to engage or reengage their interest in tasks which fall outside the developmentally-defined cognitive focus described above, highlights the possibility that the motivation for learning in children with DS may differ significantly from that of non-handicapped children. If this is the case, much of our hard-won understanding of normal processes of development may turn out to be of limited usefulness and relevance to our aim of understanding developmental processes in handicap to better effect.

In Conclusion

The results from the Edinburgh study suggest strongly that while early learning ability in DS is not as severely impaired as previous cross-sectional studies have suggested, poor consolidation of newly-acquired understanding plus a tendency to underuse the ability that is present combine to limit achievement of developmental potential in DS. It is obvious from the results that important differences exist in the ways that the DS child approaches learning. To have any chance of effecting long-term amelioration in development, intervention programs will need to take these differences into account and to be more responsive to the needs, skills and learning style of the infant with DS. Teaching strategies which work with normal children may have little effect on progress in handicapped children. Overemphasis on the development of compensatory social skills may be both inappropriate and, in the long run, counter-productive.

The Edinburgh study emphasizes the need for more longitudinal studies of early cognitive development in handicap. Both observational and experimental data will be required if we are to understand fully the nature and the course of early development in children with DS and identify the extent to which that development is open to modification. A new project is now underway in Edinburgh which intends to investigate early patterns of learning in greater detail; this will include infants much younger than those who took part in the study described here. We aim to identify the conditions under which the DS infants learn most easily and to investigate any developmental changes in response to the parameters of a number of different learning tasks. From these studies, we hope to gain some insight into why the early ability evidenced in the study reported here is not put to better long-term effect.

Our new project will use operant learning techniques to determine which particular schedules of reinforcement are likely to best promote learning effort in infants with DS and to identify the schedules most likely to encourage better consolidation of that learning once it is achieved. Learning the relationship between one's actions and events - operant learning - is paradigmatic of almost all human learning. Few situations in real life, however, allow perfect contingency between one's actions and surrounding events; the same effect, moreover, can often be caused by someone else, quite independently of one's own activity. The amount of control that the infant has over the situation will therefore by varied in our studies and small percentages of "free" reinforcement will also be included in the schedules.

Pilot operant work has suggested that young DS infants, like normal infants, will respond well when given less than perfect control in a learning task. Older DS infants, however, seemed to make little attempt to explore and master this kind of task. They settled happily for a

small percentage of free reward, even though a much higher rate was potentially available if they exerted their
own control over the situation. Older non-handicapped infants, by contrast, seemed to be even more highly motivated in this situation, intrigued by the occurrence of the
rewarding events in the absence of any activity on their
part.

Our project intends to investigate whether the counter-
productive learning patterns observed in this pilot operant work and in the study of object concept development
are in themselves learned. Avoiding difficult learning
situations and settling for low success rates rather than
risking errors is perhaps an understandable response to
the adverse success/failure rates which must typically be
experienced by the DS infant in early learning situations. An increasing awareness of low personal efficacy
may lead to secondary, "iatrogenic retardation" or to
"learned helplessness" (see above). In the earliest
months of development, the mental handicap associated
with DS is compounded by the very poor muscle tone generally present. This deficiency in motor skill must inevitably restrict the opportunities to make use of whatever
learning ability is present in these early months. The
operant tasks being used in our new project have been designed to encourage exploratory learning activity but
have minimal motor requirements. This makes them suitable
for us with even very young DS infants, thereby allowing
us to investigate any effects of early positive learning
experience on subsequent developmental progress.

Acknowledgments

This research was funded by Project Grants Nos. G8314998N
and G8703875N from the Medical Research Council and by
the Lothian branch of the Scottish Down Syndrome Association. I would like to acknowledge, with many thanks, the
help of all of the mothers and children who took part in
the project. I am also grateful to the Scottish Down Syndrome Association, to the Department of Child Life and
Health (University of Edinburgh), to Ms. Patricia Ellis
(Cytogenetics Lab, Royal Hospital for Sick Children,
Edinburgh) and to Dr. Sandy Raeburn (Human Genetics De-

partment, Western General Hospital, Edinburgh) for their invaluable help throughout the period of this research. Thanks are also extended to Drs. Brigid Daniel and Tom Pitcairn for helpful and constructive comments on the draft manuscript of this paper.

Paper presented at the Scientific Symposium of the National Down Syndrome Society, New York, December, 1987.

REFERENCES

Abroms, K. I., & Bennett, J. W. (1983). Current findings in Down syndrome. Exceptional Children, 49, 449-450.
Anderson, M. (1986). Understanding the cognitive deficit in mental retardation. Journal of Child Psychology and Psychiatry, 27, 297-306.
Bayley, N. (1969). Bayley Scales of Infant Development. New York: Psychological Corporation.
Benda, C. E. (1954). Psychopathology of Childhood. In: L. E. Carmichael (ed.), Manual of Child Psychology (2nd edit.). New York: Wiley.
Birns, B., & Golden, M. (1972). Prediction of intellectual performance at 3 years from infant tests and personality measures. Merrill-Palmer Quarterly, 18, 53-58.
Bower, T. G. R. (1982). Development in Infancy (2nd ed.). San Francisco: Freeman.
Bower, T. G. R., & Paterson, J. G. (1972). Stages in the development of the object concept. Cognition, 1, 47-55.
Breg, W. R. (1977). A review of recent progress in research. Pathobiological Annuals, 7, 257-303.
Carr, J. (1975). Young Children with Down's syndrome. London: Butterworth.
Carr, J. (1985). The development of intelligence. In: D. Ane and B. Stratford (eds.), Current Approaches to Down's syndrome. London: Holt, Rinehart & Winston.
Centerwall, D. J. & Centerwall, W. R. (1960). A study of children with mongolism reared in the home compared to those reared away from home. Pediatrics, 25, 678-685.
Cherkes-Julkowski, M., Gertner, R., & Norlander, K. (1986). Differences in cognitive processes among handicapped and average children: a group learning approach. Journal of Learning Disabilities, 19, 438-455.
Cunningham, C. C. (1986). Patterns of development in

Down's syndrome. Paper read at International Down's syndrome Congress, Brighton, April (Proceedings to be published by Wiley, London, 1988).

Duffy, L., & Wishart, J. G. (1987). A comparison of two procedures for teaching discrimination to Down's syndrome and normal children. British Journal of Educational Psychology, 57, 265-278.

Emde, R. E., & Harmon, R. J. (Eds.) (1984). Continuities and Discontinuities in Development, New York: Plenum.

Fagan, J. F. (1984). The relationship of novelty preferences during infancy to later intelligence and later recognition memory. Intelligence, 8, 339-346.

Fagan, J. F. (1985). Early novelty preferences and later intelligence. Paper presented at Society for Research into Child Development Annual Conference, Toronto, April.

Fagan, J. F., & Singer, L. T. (1981). Intervention during infancy: general considerations. In: S. L. Friedman & M. Sigman (eds.), Preterm Birth and Psychological Development, New York: Academic Press.

Gibson, D. (1978). Down's syndrome: The Psychology of Mongolism. Cambridge, England: Cambridge University Press.

Gunn, P, & Berry, P. (1985). The temperament of DS toddlers and their siblings. Journal of Child Psychology and Psychiatry, 6, 973-979.

Halpern, R. (1984). Lack of effects for home-based early intervention? Some possible explanations. American Journal of Orthopsychiatry, 54, 33-42.

Harris, S. R. (1981). Relationship of mental and motor development in Down's syndrome infants. Physical and Occupational Therapy, Pediatrics, 1, 13-18.

Harris, P. L. (1986). The development of search. In: P. Salapatek and L. B. Cohen (eds.), Handbook of Infant Perception. New York: Academic Press.

Hayden, A. H., & Haring, N. G. (1977). The acceleration and maintenance of developmental gains in Down's syndrome school-age children. In: P. J. Mittler (ed.), Research to Practice in Mental Retardation, Vol. 1: Care and Intervention. Baltimore: University Park Press.

Heuther, C. A. (1983). Projection of Down's syndrome births in the United States 1979-2000, and the potential effects of prenatal diagnosis. American Journal of

Public Health, 73, 1186-1189.

Hogg, J., & Moss, S. C. (1983). Prehensile development in Down's syndrome and non-handicapped preschool children. British Journal of Developmental Psychology, 1, 189-204.

Hook, E. B. (1982). Epidemiology of Down syndrome. In: S. M. Pueschel and J. E. Rynders (eds.). Advances in biomedicine and the Behavioral Sciences, Cambridge, MA: Ware Press.

Hunt, J. McV., Paraskevopoulus, J., Schickedanz, D., & Uzgiris, I. (1975). Variations in the mean age of achieving object permanence under diverse conditions of rearing. In: J. E. Rynders and J. M. Horrobin (eds.), The Exceptional Infant: Vol. 3. New York: Brunner/ Mazel.

Illingworth, R. S. (1972). The Development of the Infant and Young Child: Abnormal and Normal (5th edit.). Edinburgh: Churchill Livingstone.

Illingworth, R. S. (1980). The Development of the Infant and Young Child: Abnormal and Normal (7th edit.). Edinburgh: Churchill Livingstone.

Kearsley, R. B. (1979). Iatrogenic retardation: a syndrome of learned incompetence. In: R. B. Kearsley and I. E. Sigel (eds.), Infants at Risk: Assessment of Cognitive Functioning. Hillsdale, N.J.: Erlbaum.

Kiernan, C. C. (1984). The development of communication and cognition. In: J. Dobbing et al. (eds.), Scientific Studies in Mental Retardation. London: Macmillan Press.

Krasner, S. M. (1985). Developmental aspects of communication in children with Down's syndrome. Unpublished Ph.D. thesis, University of St. Andrews, Scotland.

Laveck, B., & Laveck, G. D. (1977). Sex differences among young children with Down syndrome. Journal of Pediatrics, 91, 767-769.

MacPherson, F. D. (1984). The structure of sensori-motor intelligence in severely and profoundly mentally handicapped children. Unpublished Ph.D. thesis, University of Southhampton, England.

Mans, L., Cicchetti, D., & Sroufe, L. A. (1978). Mirror reactions of Down's syndrome infants and toddlers: underpinnings of self-confidence. Child Development, 49, 1247-1250.

McConkey, R. (1980). Designing and evaluating toys for the mentally handicapped child. Journal of Practical

Applications in Development and Handicap, 3, 10-15.

Melyn, M. A. & White, D. T. (1973). Mental and developmental milestones of noninstitutionalized Down's syndrome children. Pediatrics, 52, 542-545.

Miller, D. L., & Farmer, R. D. T. (1982). Epidemiology of Diseases. London: Blackwell.

Morgan, S. B. (1979). Development and distribution of intellectual and adaptive skills in Down's Syndrome: implications for early intervention. Mental Retardation, 17, 247-249.

Morss, J. R. (1983). Cognitive development in the Down's Syndrome infant: slow or different? British Journal of Educational Psychology, 53, 40-47.

Morss, J. R. (1984). Enhancement of object-permanence performance in the Down's Syndrome infant. Child: Care, Health and Development, 10, 39-47.

Morss, J. R. (1985). Early cognitive development: difference or delay? In: D. Lane & B. Stratford (eds.), Current Approaches to Down's Syndrome. London: Holt, Rinehart & Winston.

Moss, S., & Hogg, J. (1987). The integration of manipulative movements in children with Down's Syndrome and their non-handicapped peers. Human Movement Science, 6, 67-99.

Patterson, D. (1987). The causes of Down Syndrome. Scientific American, 257, 42-48.

Piaget, J. (1955). The Construction of Reality. London: Routledge & Kegan Paul (original French Edition, 1937).

Piper, M. C., Gosselin, C., Gendron, M., & Mazer, B. (1986). Developmental profile of Down's syndrome infants receiving early intervention. Child: Care, Health and Development, 12, 183-194.

Rogers, S. J. (1977). Characteristics of the cognitive development of profoundly retarded children, Child Development, 48, 837-843.

Rogers-Warren, A. K., Ruggles, T. R., Peterson, N. L., & Cooper, A. Y. (1981). Playing and learning together; patterns of social interaction in handicapped and non-handicapped children. Journal for the Division of Early Childhood, 3, 56-63.

Rondal, J. A. (1984). Linguistic and pre-linguistic development in moderate and severe mental retardation.

In: J. Dobbing et al. (eds.), Scientific Studies in Mental Retardation. London: Macmillan Press.

Rynders, J. E., Spiker, D., & Horrobin, J. M. (1978). Underestimating the educability of Down's Syndrome children. American Journal of Mental Deficiency, 82, 440-448.

Schuberth, R. E. (1982). The infant's search for objects: alternatives to Piaget's theory of object concept development. In: L. P. Lipsett and C. K. Rovee-Collier (eds.), Advances in Infancy Research: Vol. 2. Norwood, New Jersey: Ablex.

Seligman, M. E. P. (1975). Helplessness. San Francisco: W. H. Freeman.

Shapiro, B. L. (1983). Down Syndrome - A disruption of homeostasis. American Journal of Medical Genetics, 14, 241-269.

Sharev, T., Collins, R., & Schlomo, L. (1985). Effect of maternal education on prognosis of development in children with Down's Syndrome. Pediatrics, 76, 387-391.

Silverstein, A. B., Brownlee, L., Hubbell, M., & McLain, R. E. (1975). Comparison of two sets of Piagetian scales with severely and profoundly retarded children. American Journal of Mental Deficiency, 80, 292-297.

Simeonsson, R. J., Cooper, D. H., & Scheiner, A. P. (1982). A review and analysis of the effectiveness of early intervention programmes. Pediatrics, 69, 635-641.

Sloper, P., Glenn, S. M., & Cunningham, C. C. (1986). The effect of intensity of training on sensori-motor development in infants with Down's Syndrome. Journal of Mental Deficiency Research, 30, 149-162.

Smith, G. E. (Ed.) (1985). Molecular Structure of the Number 21 Chromosome and Down Syndrome. Annals of the New York Academy of Science, 450, (entire vol.).

Stratford, B., & Steele, J. (1985). Incidence and prevalence of Down's Syndrome - a discussion and report. Journal of Mental Deficiency Research, 29, 95-107.

Strauss, S. (Ed.) (1982). U-Shaped Behavioral Growth, New York: Academic Press.

Uzgiris, I., & Hunt, J. McV. (1975). Assessment in Infancy: Ordinal Scales of Psychological Development. Urbana, Illinois: University Press.

Wachs, T. D. (1975). Relation of infants' performance on Piaget scales between 12 and 24 months and their Stanford-Binet performance at 31 months. Child Development, 46, 929-935.

Walker, S., & Howard, P. J. (1986). Cytogenetic prenatal diagnosis and its relative effectiveness in the Mersey region and North Wales. Prenatal Diagnosis, 6, 13-23.

Weisz, J. R., & Zigler, E. (1979). Cognitive development in retarded and non-retarded persons: Piagetian tests of the similar sequence hypothesis. Psychological Bulletin, 86, 831-851.

Wishart, J. G. (1979). The development of the object concept in infancy. Unpublished Ph.D. thesis, University of Edinburgh, Scotland.

Wishart, J. G. (1986). The effects of step-by-step training on cognitive performance in infants with Down's Syndrome. Journal of Mental Deficiency Research, 30, 233-250.

Wishart, J. G. (1987). Performance of young non-retarded children and children with Down Syndrome on Piagetian infant search tasks. American Journal of Mental Deficiency, 92, 169-177.

Wishart, J. G., & Bower, T. G. R. (1984). Spatial relations and the object concept: a normative study. In: L. P. Lipsitt and C. K. Rovee-Collier (eds.), Advances in Infancy Research: Vol. 3 (pp.57-123). Norwood, New Jersey: Ablex.

Wishart, J. G., & Bower, T. G. R. (1985). A longitudinal study of the development of the object concept. British Journal of Developmental Psychology, 3, 243-258. (Reprinted in: G. E. Butterworth and P. L. Harris (eds.), Infancy. Leicester: British Psychological Society, 1985).

Wohlheuter, M. J., & Sindberg, R. M. (1975). Longitudinal development of object permanence in mentally retarded children: an exploratory study. American Journal of Mental Deficiency, 79, 513-518.

Zelazo, P. R. (1979). Reactivity to perceptual-cognitive events: application for infant assessment. In: R. B. Kearsley and I. E. Siegel (eds.), Infants at Risk: Assessment of Cognitive Functioning. Hillsdale, New Jersey: Lawrence Erlbaum.

Zigler, E., & Balla, D. (Eds.) (1982). Mental Retardation: The Developmental-Difference Controversy. Hillsdale, New Jersey: Erlbaum.

2

QUALITATIVE DIFFERENCES IN THE WAY DOWN SYNDROME AND NORMAL CHILDREN SOLVE A NOVEL COUNTING PROBLEM

Rochel Gelman and Melissa Cohen
University Of Pennsylvania
Department of Psychology,
3815 Walnut St.,
Philadelphia, PA, 19104.

Introduction

We believe that the roots of human cognition are best understood through the comparison of the performance of different populations of subjects on similar tasks and through the comparison of a given population's performance on a variety of conceptually related tasks. Here we show that comparisons of Down Syndrome and normal children's solutions for a novel counting problem shed light on the nature of counting knowledge.

There are two different accounts of the development of counting knowledge. One of these is based on the assumption that the capacity to form associations underlies all concept learning, no matter what the domain of the concept. The second account is based on the view that conceptual development benefits from an initial, albeit skeletal, set of domain-relevant principles or constraints. In the case of counting, the assumption is that a skeletal set of counting principles serves both to focus children's attention on counting- relevant inputs, and to support the build up in memory of a coherent representation of counting-relevant knowledge.

Cornwall (1974) concluded that Down Syndrome (hereafter DS) children learn to count by using associative, rote learning procedures. This suggestion gains support from some of our own data (Gelman, 1982) as well as the emerging consensus that DS individuals can learn by rote, despite their difficulties when required to use conceptual or rule governed learning strategies (e.g. Edgerton, 1979; Hartley, 1986). If so, the data from the DS children in this study should be best characterized by the first class of learning models. Additionally, if Siegler & Shipley (1987) and Fuson (1988) are correct in their contention that association models apply for the normal child as well, then the data from a normal control group should parallel those of the DS children. However, if our position, that normal preschoolers' knowledge of counting reveals the workings of counting principles (e.g. Gelman & Gallistel, 1978; Gelman & Greeno, in press), is correct, then the solution types of the two groups should be qualitatively different. What these differences might be will be considered in Section III.

Assume we find DS children's counting is better characterized by the association model of learning and that normal preschool children's counting is better characterized by the principle-first model. Obviously, we would not be justified in attributing the difference to the genetic mechanisms underlying the development DS. For the difference could well be mediated by a variety of other variables, and we would want to know how other categories of retarded children do. Despite this, we would be able to go beyond statements of "delayed" or "different" and say something quite specific about the ways in which at least DS children differ from normal children. Further, we would have some reason to conclude that normal children learn to count in a way that differs from at least DS children. The idea that normal children's learning about counting benefits from the availability of implicit principled knowledge of counting would gain weight. Finally, as we shall see, we can offer some suggestions about ways to alter arithmetic instruction for DS, and possibly other retarded, individuals.

Some Details About The Two Classes of Models

The Association-Reinforcement Model - The core of the learn-by-association account of how our young come to share our concepts comes from the British Empiricist theory of knowledge acquisition. The position is that we can explain concept learning if we grant humans but two pertinent capacities: (a) the ability to detect and respond to sense data and (b) the ability to learn according to the laws of association, these being the laws of contiguity and frequency. Associations are formed for the sensory inputs that occur in close (temporal or spatial) contiguity to responses and/or other sensory inputs: The strength of these associations is a function of the frequency with which the pairings are encountered. As these associations build up, it becomes possible to form associations between other inputs and those that are already established in memory. In this fashion one acquires more complicated associative representations of the world. Modern versions of the associative account of knowledge acquisition add further assumptions about the learner. Especially in developmental circles, the learner is granted the ability to imitate others and emphasis is placed on the role of reinforcement. Pairings between stimuli and imitations or other appropriate responses that are reinforced are more likely to be associated than those that are not. How does this kind of theory get applied to the case of counting?

Starting from a point of no knowledge or understanding about counting, acquisition proceeds as a function of opportunity to encounter, and be reinforced for using, examples of conventional counting lists and other response components of counting procedures. In a piece-meal way, children gradually build up a store of counting pertinent procedures, ones like listing the conventional counting string of words, repeating the last word said in a count list, pointing to objects, etc. The pace at which associations between procedures and the counting words are acquired depends on both a child's ability to form associations and a child's opportunity to be reinforced for the use of counting stimuli and responses. Eventually, when enough of these have been learned, the child is in a position to abstract the generalizations common to these. The result should be a principled understanding of counting (e.g. Baroody, 1984; Briars & Siegler, 1984; Fuson & Hall, 1983).

The Principle-First or Rational-Constructivist Model - As Feldman and Gelman (1986) note, the principle-first, or in their terms the rational-constructivist learning mod-

el, belongs to that class of models which grant learners
some innate dispositions to focus selectively on those
inputs that are relevant in a given domain. Whereas the
association model presumes that it is sufficient to pos-
tulate the very general, all-purpose, mental ability to
form associations, this class of models does not. The
position is that it is necessary to grant that the young
bring some implicit, yet organized, knowledge to the task
of learning. The theoretical motivation for such an assumption derives from the fact that very young children
do much to control the nature of their supporting environments. They are known to respond selectively to the
stimuli presented to them. Further, there are times when
the children actively seek out those inputs which foster
their construction of knowledge within a domain (Brown,
Bransford, Ferrara & Campione, 1983; Gelman & Brown,
1986). If young children are granted some skeletal representations, we have a beginning account of such self-initiated activities. The principles serve as enabling tools
for learning. Skeletal sets of principles function to define the class of relevant inputs and therefore help the
learner find those inputs that are relevant to learning
in the domain in question. Similarly, they set the stage
for the fleshing out, and development of, the skeletal
principles themselves.

We prefer the second class of models, in part, because
we see a need to account for how young children know what
are relevant data for learning about counting and number
concepts. Environments do not, by themselves, force themselves on the learners, who are actively involved in con-
structing their knowledge base. Instead learners select
their environments; they determine what serves as relevant inputs. This concern for what we characterize as the
problem of relevance is deeply related to Quine's (1960)
discussion of "gavagai" and a review of it helps clarify
the problem as it applies to number concepts.

Quine wondered how naive language learners come to know
the intended referent of the sound sequence "gavagai",
even if the speaker points in the direction of the target
item, say a rabbit. For, in the absence of any clues to
the contrary, the speaker could mean ear, furry stuff,
space beside the thing, etc. How does the naive listener
choose among these possible hypotheses, especially if the

listener is a beginning language learner? Why should the child presume the speaker means rabbit? Similarly, why should the child presume that the sounds "one", "two", are not labels for objects as a whole? Put differently, what is there within the learner as characterized by association theorists that would bias the learner to treat some speech data as label-relevant and other speech data as counting-tag relevant?

Unless we take the position that children must already share some implicit hypotheses with knowledgeable speakers, for example that a novel "word" uttered in the context of an object probably refers to the object as a whole, our young charges are guaranteed to end up with some unshared interpretations of the environment. In other words they will be at risk with respect to their ability to learn the concepts that adults have and want them to master. To help dispel the reader's doubt that naive learners would have such problems if we did not grant them some shared assumptions about the nature of counting, we turn to a consideration of the association account of how children might learn the English count list.

The learning-by-association account of counting is straight forward. The idea is that a knowledgeable speaker (e.g. a parent) points to each of a set of objects and then says "one, two, three," etc. The more the speaker in question does this, the more likely it is that the child will come to learn that the presented string of words can be used for counting. Let us assume that something like this has to be going on. Yet, it cannot be the complete story. For one, the point-and-label theory should also apply to the learning of color terms. Given the seemingly endless sets of colored preschool toys, picture books, and children's television programs that focus on color, it should be a trivial matter for young children to learn their color terms. But it is not: Surprisingly, the preschoolers have a very hard time learning color terms, this despite clear evidence that even infants perceive colors much as do adults (e.g. Bartlett, 1977; Bornstein, 1985).

Further, the point-label-associate account of how the children acquire the count words predicts that some of the children will think that the acoustic counterparts to

the words "one" and "duck" are interchangeable labels for
ducks. To see why, consider the book-reading ritual that
occurs in this country with many a young child. Over and
over again, one reads the same book. For sake of argument
assume that the book in question has colored pictures of
a duck and a pig on the first page. On one day the adult
points to these depicted objects and says "duck", "pig"
while doing so. On day 2, the same adult points to the
same items in the same order and says "one", "two". On
day 3, pointing occurs to the same items yet again, but
now the adult says "yellow", "pink". Two clear predictions follow about the kind of learning that will take
place if a child learns as outlined in the first model.
A child could conclude that the duck should be labelled
with all three of the words, "duck", "one", and "yellow".
Alternatively, on the assumption that the different associations would interfere with each other, a child could
think none of these terms apply. But neither of these
possibilities fits with either what does happen, or what
we want to happen to young learners.

Very young children keep separate the set of the count
words from the set of object labels; they use them in
their appropriate contexts (Gelman & Meck, 1986). Given
this, we have argued (e.g. Gelman & Greeno, in press)
there must be an alternative account of the way young
children master counting. How it is that the principle-
first account helps children sort out the count words and
labelling words is taken up in Section III below. But for
now, we note that the infants and preverbal toddlers respond in a numerical way to the displays that they could
treat otherwise (Cooper, 1984; Sophian & Adams, 1987;
Starkey, Spelke, & Gelman, 1983; Strauss & Curtis, 1981,
1984). Such data encourage us to think that our young
help themselves determine what counts as numerically relevant input.

It is clear, infants have a great deal to learn about
counting. Should anyone think we mean otherwise, they
miss the fact that the principle-first model of learning
is a model about learning. The next section expands on
this theme.

How the Counting Principles Might Support Learning to Count

The Principles - To start to develop the principle-first account, we consider the one-one counting principle. This principle captures the fact that each and every item in a to-be-counted collection must be tagged once and only once with a unique tag. For the one-one principle to be put into practice, the counter must have available some set of distinct tags that is at least as large as the to-be-counted set. Counters must not skip or repeatedly tag individual items in the set. Put differently, the one-one counting principle yields the counting constraints, e.g. do not double count or skip items, that a plan must reflect for it to be an acceptable plan for counting. If one puts into action a plan that violates the constraints of the one-one principle, one will fail to honor the principle. Should this happen, we can say the counter followed an erroneous plan of action.

There is more to counting than what is captured by the one-one principle. Additionally, there are two further how-to-count principles, the stable-ordering and cardinal principles. These capture the facts that the set of tags must be repeatedly ordered, and that only the last tag used on a particular count can represent the cardinal value of the set.

Note that the counting principles say nothing about the kind of items one can count or the sequence in which items are to be tagged. As long as the how-to-count principles are applied, it matters not what items are collected together for a count. Nor does it matter whether items are counted in a row, one after the other, and so on. These latter two considerations led Gelman and Gallistel (1978) to add item-indifference and order-indifference princi- ples to the core of their proposed list of early counting principles. Their abstraction principle captures the fact that there are no constraints on the kinds of individual items that can make up a counting set. Similarly, their order-irrelevance principle serves to capture the lack of constraints on the item-tagging order.

Note also that the principles do not dictate the kind of tags one must use when counting. One does not have to

use the conventional count words to count. In fact, one
does not even have to use words when counting. Witness
computers. The only constraints on the nature of the tags
are those given by the one-one and stable ordering principles, i.e. that it be possible to treat them as all
different and as an ordered set. Should finger positions,
marks on the sand, short term memory bins, etc, be adapt-
able to his function, then fine. This consideration is
what motivated Gelman and Gallistel (1978) to distinguish
between numerons and numerlogs; they reserve the latter
term for those tags which are count words in a given language.

Principles Help the Learner: Finding count lists in the
environment - The above points regarding the absence of
constraints on the type of items that can be counted, the
source of the tags, and the order in which tagging can
take place, bring us back to the question we raised in
Section II. How do naive learners keep straight what
string of words are or are not used for counting; how do
children come to correctly sort their verbal environment
into labels, words, color terms, etc., and do so without
mixing them up at first? We submit they do this by taking
advantage of the domain-specific principles they bring to
the learning task. To expand this theme we contrast the
counting principles with what is known about labelling
principles.
   Markman (1986) and Spelke (1988) each assume that
children are biased to think that words used in the context of a novel object most likely refer to the object as
a whole. Additionally, novices have a tendency to assume
that once an object in a class has been assigned a label,
that label applies to the other same-level members of the
class (Au & Markman, 1987; Waxman, 1985). The idea is
that like us, the young assume once a rose is a "rose"; a
rose is a "rose" - despite differences in color, breed,
size, number of petals, and so on, of the exemplars. Add
to this our variant of Markman's mutual exclusivity principle, this being that each same-level class of natural
objects or artifacts shares but one name, and we end up
with the following proposal: Very young children's principles for labelling objects lead to their implicit hypotheses that: (1) Categories of objects share the same

unique label; (2) once an item is labelled, it cannot be assigned another label if it is treated as a member of the same category; and (3) once assigned, that label must be assigned to other exemplars of the same-level category. If children make these implicit assumptions, they then have some clues as to what to expect over time as they continue to hear those words that serve labelling functions. For the words they have begun to assimilate to their lexicon should continue to follow the use rules that are dictated by the principles.

Now contrast the one-label-for-classes-of-like-objects constraints with the use rules that could operate given implicit knowledge of the counting principles: One way, although by no means the only way, to satisfy the stable order principle is to use a list of words to tag items. Therefore, on the assumption that this principle is available to structure the environment for children, ordered lists of words should be salient to them. But this principle cannot by itself tell the children how to use these lists. This depends on the availability of further principles. These principles indicate that, when counting, the same words can be used with different objects over trials, and, in contrast, that the same words cannot be used within a trial -- even if items are alike. Such constraints follow from the abstraction or item-indifference principle. In the absence of the stable-order and item-indifference principles then, the above list of the children's assumptions about labels could well lead them to think the count words are in fact labels for objects.

Thus, it is a combined consideration of the stable order and item-irrelevance principles that leads to the conclusion that number words are not names for objects but instead are tags for counting. Add to this Shipley and Shepperson's (1987) finding that young children will count any separably identifiable entities, including broken pieces of the same toy, and we see how they can know counting terms are not object classification terms -- at least not in the sense that labels or nouns are. The bottom line then, is that a child who is granted principles for organizing the verbal environment and its use over time, is given good reason to assume that labels and count words serve different linguistic roles and cognitive functions.

The counting principles enable a toddler to recognize when words are being used as count words and start to learn them as such. But it still remains a question as to how the child knows what to do with these words.

Principles Help the Learner: Finding counting relevant behaviors - When counting a set, one does not have to point to each item, start at the beginning of a row, arrange items in a row, count anything in particular, etc. There are multiple ways to keep track of the number of items used in a count-on strategy (Fuson, 1982). So are there multiple count strategies for solving a variety of arithmetic problems (Resnick, 1986). All of these count strategies are united by their common function: Solving the problem of determining the cardinality of a set. They do not serve to determine the cause of an object's acceleration, improve one's memory for places, learn the name of an object, or any of an infinite number of alternative goals.

How are we able to determine that these disparate events are in the equivalence class of possible procedures of counting? What gives us license to say of a variety of distinct behaviors that they are all instances of the class of counting behaviors? Again, our answer is that the availability of counting principles serves this function. For, if the constraints of these principles are reflected in procedure, then that procedure is an example of counting. Hence, the principles and their consequent constraints underlie our ability to define and identify members of the equivalence class of counting behaviors. Just as principles of counting help define the class of acceptable instances of counting.

Principles Help the Learner: Transferring or devising novel solutions to novel problems - The fact that principles make it possible to define the equivalence class of counting behaviors is related to another characteristic they possess. They serve as the basis from which the novel instances can be generated. This is because their constraints are ones that a planner must honor when generating a plan for counting (Greeno et al., 1984). Whatever else the requirements of a novel setting, the planner must honor the constraints of the principles if the

setting calls for a counting solution. Otherwise, the solution cannot be considered an example of counting.

Should the planner have such a constraint list available, it can at least "monitor" the output of a solution
with respect to whether or not it has met the constraint.
Further, it can recognize inputs that signal failures to
do so. Hence, there is the potential for generating an
improved plan the next time round and doing so without
explicit external feedback as to what to do in order to
improve. We return to the issue of generality when we
consider the kind of evidence one can use to attribute
implicit knowledge of the counting principles to an individual.

A Caveat - To be sure, it is necessary to focus on that
part of the input that is in fact relevant to the task of
learning more about the domain. Still, it is not sufficient to do so. It is one thing to know what it is that
one must master and quite another thing to do so. Knowing
that the count words are the kinds of words one has to
master in order to use symbols as tags does not guarantee
that the learning will take place automatically. Indeed,
in the case of the count words of English, everything we
know about serial learning points to a protracted period
of learning. So, although we can explain the fact that
the young children and infants respond to the environment
in numerical ways before they could have been given explicit instruction to do so (e.g. Cooper, 1984; Strauss &
Curtis, 1984), this does not imply the patently false
conclusion that the infants know all there is to know
about counting. Nor does it mean that none of the learning that has to be accomplished will be done by rote. It
simply means that children will get started on the right
course, a course that is likely to be very protracted.
For, given that they have to memorize, by rote, a long
count list in English, and given that serial learning
tasks are hard for college students, ultimate mastery of
the count list itself should take a long time. For a discussion of the further complexity involved in acquiring
understanding of the mathematical symbol system, see
Gelman & Greeno (in press).

A Point of Contact - The idea that principles serve to

direct attention to the relevant inputs that can foster knowledge acquisition in a given domain is consistent with various constructivist theories of mind. Cognitive scientists' contentions that prior knowledge in a domain determines what and how other materials are interpreted and learned (Bransford, 1979; Mandler, 1984; Schank & Abelson, 1977) represent a similar class argument. So does the Piagetian view that stimuli can serve as food for a particular cognitive activity only when there is a requisite structure with which to assimilate that stimulus. The Piagetian proposal that preschoolers cannot help but fail seriation tasks, this because they lack the requisite seriation structures, is but one illustration of the general position that mental structures are what support the interpretation and use of environments. From this perspective, when preschoolers invent counting algorithms to solve simple addition problems we give them, it follows that they must be using a knowledge structure that is characterizable in terms of counting principles.

Focus on Novelty

The above considerations of the way a principle-first model could help a child solve novel tasks led us to focus on how DS and preschool children negotiated a novel counting task. We wanted to know whether both groups of children would deal with the same task in different ways and, if so, whether the differences could be attributed to differences in the way counting was understood by the children in the two different groups.

The Constrained Counting or the "Doesn't Matter" Task - In order to assess young children's understanding of the abstraction principles, Gelman and Gallistel (1978) asked the preschool children to solve what amounts to a novel counting task which we will call the Constrained Counting Task. In the Gelman and Gallistel study, children started out simply counting a row of 5 heterogeneous items. The constrained counting task began when the children were asked to count the same display in a special (or different, or trick) way, this being to count all of the items by tagging the second item from the left "the one". That trial complete, children were next asked to count again in the same special way, this time so that the designated target item was tagged "the two". Subsequent trials involved requests that the target item end up "the three", "the four" and "the five". There are a variety of solutions that one can use on this task. Some of the successful ones we have seen the children use are illustrated in Fig. 1.

Each row of Fig. 1 schematizes a heterogeneous set of 5 objects. The X inside a given circle indicates the posi-

Figure 1. The schemata of possible solutions to the Constrained Counting Task. Take X = n to mean "make this, the target item, the 1, 2, ...or n". The numbers over the schematized items indicate the count word used; the arrows indicate the flow of points made by a child as she pointed to items.

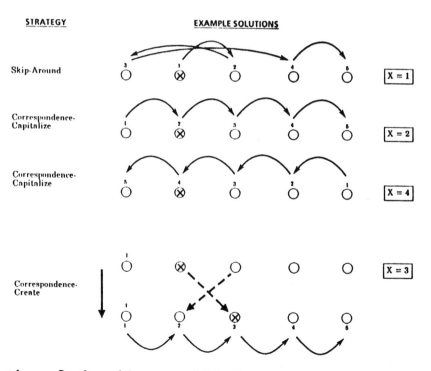

tion of the object to which the tagging constraint applied on that trial. The values in the right hand column give the numeral that was to be used for the targeted object. The actual observed pointing and tagging assignment orders are represented by the flow of arrows.

The solutions depicted in Fig. 1 are examples of ones generated by normal preschool children (Gelman et al. 1986). Row 1 shows that one way to succeed on the task is to start counting at one end, skip X if one has not yet gotten to the appropriate point in the count list, and then return to X when the tag in question is reached in the list. Hence, the label "Skip-Around" for this kind of solution. Another solution type involves recognizing that the target item is in the same relative linear spatial position from an end of the display as is the to-be-assigned tag in the count list. When this is the case, one can then count from the left or right. Hence, our choice of the label "Correspondence-Capitalize" for solutions shown in the second and third rows. (Note that such solutions cannot be used on all trials, including the kind shown in the first and last rows. Children who do not realize this, will "pass" some trials if they simply count as usual. For this reason, the reader should bear in mind that upcoming analyses of strategy use required that children used this solution selectively).

A final example of a possible correct solution, Correspondence-Create, is shown in the bottom row of Fig. 1. This solution involved moving items in the display to create a correspondence between the spatial position of the target item and list position of the to-be-assigned count word.

Down Syndrome Children Might Have Trouble with a Novel Task - Our account of how availability of counting principles might feed the generation of novel solutions involved several components. The first was that the principle-determined constraints serve to define the class of acceptable performances. So should a response be inappropriate, the child could recognize this was the case and at least start again. Second, if such constraints are operative, they can serve in the selection of possible responses in the first place. That is they can lead to the assembly of an appropriate plan. Third, if one is sensitive to the constraints on an acceptable plan, then one might well benefit from an experimenter's hints or reminders when one's solution failed to honor such constraints.

All of the preceding regarding the role of principles in the ability to solve a novel problem are variants on a common theme: That principle-governed searches for novel solutions can work to encourage children to monitor their own performance, to try out solutions, and to generate a plan that honors the counting constraints. Still, even if children have implicit knowledge of the counting principles, there is no guarantee that they will succeed on all novel problems. For, the children might know the counting principles but not have a sufficiently developed planning capacity -- no matter what the domain. In Greeno et al's (1984) terms, children might possess the relevant conceptual competence but be limited with respect to their procedural competence.

The Gelman and Greeno (in press) treatment of potential sources of error that contribute to variable performance highlights yet another reason why all of our subjects may fail. The generation of a competent plan of action is dependent on the planner's ability to monitor two sets of constraints: Those that pertain to the conceptual competence being assessed and those that are dictated by the task and the setting of the task. To deal with the latter a variety of interpretative competencies need to be well enough developed. These include ones that bear on understanding what to focus on in the instructions, the domain-relevant terms that are used in the instructions, as well as the rules of question-answering for the experimental setting (see also Donaldson, 1978; Siegal, Water, & Dinwiddy, in press; Gelman, et al. 1986). So limits on the ability to understand the instructions and rules of the setting could serve as a systematic error source, again even if children have implicit knowledge of the counting principles.

Fortunately, there are some clues in the literature as to how to proceed. Consider the following: Toddlers will systematically alter their search for missing objects (DeLoache, 1984); young children alter their approach to balancing blocks as a function of whether they generate a "theory" of balance or not (Karmiloff-Smith and Inhelder, 1974/75); as toddlers persist at playing with stacking cups they become better at applying an ordering schema (DeLoache, Sugarman, & Brown, 1985). Together these find-

ings   suggest that children who possess the requisite competence   but   nevertheless   fail   their first attempt on a
novel   problem, can come to succeed <u>if they are allowed to
persist   at   the   problem</u>. Without explicit feedback, performance   improves   over   trials.   Surely,   self-generated
trials   could   not   lead   to   success unless some implicit
knowledge   of   the   principles   in the domains in question
were   available   to help children constrain, and therefore
develop their successive efforts.

The   foregoing   considerations   led   us to a design that
allowed   children   to repeat a trial, either on their own,
or   in   response   to hints from us. Children who are given
hints   or   opportunities to start again cannot improve unless   they have some way to interpret the hints or monitor
the output of a new effort (Wilkinson, 1984).

Our   design   varied   the way we built in the plan to repeat   instructions,   and   give hints, depending on whether
the   subjects   were   from preschool or DS samples. The experimenters   who   worked   with the preschool children were
told   that   they   could paraphrase instructions, or repeat
crucial   features   of   the instructions, or ask a child to
do   a   trial   again. The experimenters working with the DS
children   were   allowed   more options. In particular, they
were   allowed to introduce more explicit hints if the less
specific   ones failed to lead to improved performance. For
this   allowed   us   to see if the children that did not improve   on   their   own   could nevertheless recognize sample
solutions   and   other   explicit   hints for what they were,
that   is   relevant   inputs   to their problem at hand. They
should   if   they have some implicit knowledge of the principles   (See   the   Section   - Principles Help the Learner:
<u>Finding   counting relevant behaviors</u>). But if the proposal
that   the   DS   children   learn to count by rote is correct
(Cornwall,   1974),   such explicit hints should do little to
improve   performance   (Campione, Brown, Ferrara, & Bryant,
1984).

Details of the Study

The   Children: The   Down   Syndrome   Children - The ten DS
children   who contributed the data presented here attended
the   Catholic   day-school for retarded children. The Arch-

diocese of Philadelphia runs the school for free and although most of the children at the school come from Catholic families, applicants of all faiths are considered and accepted. The school is in a modern, well-equipped building, with a large, attractive setting in a quiet neighborhood in an upper middle class suburb of Philadelphia. It has a dedicated and talented staff, a fact that is validated by its receipt of major awards for teaching excellence.

The population served by the school is predominantly white and represents a lower-middle to middle-middle socioeconomic class. All children attending the school live at home with their families. They are bused to and from the school on a daily basis. The DS children in our study were so classified by the school staff who used a combination of diagnostic tools and medical records when first interviewing possible admittees. Details from these records were not available to us; still we had no reason to doubt the information we were given as to which of the children at the school were DS children.

The DS children who contributed the results presented below were all but one of the 11 DS children in a class of 21. (Equipment failures account for the need to drop the other DS child). The children in the class as a whole ranged in CA from 9 to 13 years (Median = 11 years); and MA from 3-6 to 6-8 (Median = 5.6). Their I.Q.'s (as measured in 19 cases with the Stanford-Binet, and two cases with the WISC) varied from 43-73. The range and medians for the DS children in the study were 10-13 CA years (Median = 10.6); 4-0 to 6-10 MA (Median = 5.8).

Some, or all, of our sample of children participated, along with other children at the school, in one or more of a wide range of studies conducted by a group at the University of Pennsylvania.[1] These included studies of language production and comprehension skills (such as the ones that Ann Fowler present in another chapter in this volume); causal reasoning; information processing styles; social cognition; and arithmetic skills. The data we present below come from the latter set of tasks. The focus is on the way children negotiated the Gelman & Gallistel constrained counting task and what the pretests revealed about their counting skills. On occasion we consider some additional data available to us, this because they inform the presentation.[2]

The Children: The Preschool Children - The preschool sample consisted of 16 4-year-olds (Range, 48-59 mos., Median = 53 mos.) and 16 5-year-olds (Range, 60-71 mos, Median = 63.5). About half of all of these children were recruited for participation in the study in our laboratory at the University of Pennsylvania. The rest attended a large, well-appointed and well-staffed Day Care Center in the Northeast of Philadelphia. The center is sponsored by the Philadelphia Federation of Jewish Agencies and favors children from homes with a single working mother or two working parents. Overall, the preschool sample served was predominantly white, and tended toward the middle-middle class.

We do not have MA levels for these children but given our information about a variety of pertinent socioeconomics factors, we think these would be slightly higher than their CA's. If so, all the 4-year olds and some of the 5-year-old children represent a sample that overlaps the DS sample with respect to MA. Some children have participated in studies other than the pretest assessment of their counting levels and the constrained counting task. But none of these involved arithmetic related stimuli.

The Children: Counting in the DS School Curriculum - We have worked in two schools that serve retarded children in the Greater Philadelphia Area. In both, counting instruction is a featured part of the school day. Children get daily practice reciting the count list, counting sets of objects, naming written numerals, and learning simple addition facts. In addition, they encounter counting experience at circle time, in the gym, on the playground, etc. In short, theirs is a learning environment that is inundated with counting-relevant inputs. Our preschool children were clearly exposed to a variety of counting opportunities, either at their preschool setting or in their homes; we have no reason to doubt that the Saxe, Guberman & Gearhardt (in press) observations of such inputs applies to the children in our study. Nothing in the study or our own observations of preschoolers in a variety of settings suggests that the exposure of normal preschoolers to explicit instruction in counting is as intense and pervasive as it is in the curricula at the DS children's school.

Procedures - The DS and preschool children reported on below are best thought of as participants in two different studies that have overlapping conditions. Both the studies included pretests of counting levels and a common constrained counting condition. The common constrained task in the experiment proper was the one that was introduced above: all the children were shown a heterogeneous, five-item linear display and asked to count this row. Next they were asked to make a target item "the one", while counting all items; then they were asked to make a target item "the two"; next they were asked to make the target item "the three"' then "the four"; and finally "the five". For half the preschool children the target item was always the second one from the left; for the other half of the preschool children, the target item varied. In the DS study, the target item could occur in the second, third, or fourth position in a row.

   In both studies, two experimenters worked with each child in a quiet setting out of the classroom. During the pretests for counting, one kept track of the children's responses, including whether they pointed as they were counted. During the experiment proper, one experimenter interviewed the child, and the other video-recorded the session. The experimenters in each study were told that they could repeat or paraphrase the instructions. The experimenters for the Preschool study were told they could not give their charges any explicit hints.

   As indicated in Section IV, the experimenters who were working with the DS children had no prohibitions regarding explicit clues. As we will see, they often did offer very explicit help. This is perhaps not too surprising. For, the same experimental team found it necessary to add a demonstration phase to our counting pretests after we noticed that many of the children failed to coordinate their recitation of count words with their points. Since our goal during the pretest was to determine what the children could do in the way of counting, the fact that never before had we run a demonstration test phase with preschoolers did not seem reason enough to avoid doing so with the DS children. (For further details, see below).

In both the DS and Preschool studies, the children were given additional variations of the "doesn't matter" task, ones introduced to provide data on whether the children could be flexible in their choice of solutions. The DS children were given an 8-item version of the task after they completed the 5-item version. When the set size increases, there is a greater chance of forgetting which item is the targeted one. Therefore, one must either remember its position in the row or do something to make the item distinctive, e.g., move it up above the row a bit, rearrange the order of items in the row. Failure to do these and to instead persist at using developed solutions could index a lack of flexibility.

Preschool children were also tested with <u>circular</u> arrangements of a 5-item heterogeneous display. When items are in a row, what is the beginning and end are given by the arrangement itself. In the case of a circle, children have to monitor the items if they are to avoid violating the constraints of the one-one principle. They cannot simply do what they are used to doing, which is to keep counting until they reach the end of the row. There is no "end" unless one constructs one oneself. So again, children who use the same solutions for both kinds of displays could be characterized as inflexible.

Thus, in both studies we have data from a common condition as well as data from variations on this condition, variations that might shed light on the extent to which the children in each sample can be flexible and change plans given a change in the setting.

Assessments of Basic Counting Abilities - We were able to assess the children's counting levels in the two ways summarized in Table 1. The first relied on the regular counting trial that occurred just before the children had been introduced to the requirements of the constrained counting task. The pertinent summary statistics for this trial are shown in the top half of Table 1. The other measures of group levels of counting prowess are summarized in the bottom half of the table and were based on pretests designed for this purpose. Note that the children were tested more than once on a given set size so that we could determine whether they counted reliably.

Also note that the DS children were given a second counting test. Like the preschool children they were first tested without any demonstrations. Following that session they were tested in a Demonstration condition. Now the

Table 1
Down Syndrome And Preschool Samples Counting Skill

	Source Of Data And Index Of Counting Skill			
Data Source & Counting Principle(s)@	4 YRS	5 YRS	DOWN (NO DEMO)	DOWN (DEMO)
Constrained Count Trial to Start Experimental Task				
1-1 and Stable Principles				
X=5	94	100	100	- - - -
X=8	- - - -	- - - -	90	- - - -
Pretests				
1-1 and Stable Principles				
X=5	86	100	60	90
X=8	81	88	70	80
Cardinal Principle				
X=5	86	94	40	90
X=8	38	69	20	70

@ DS children had 3 count trials per set size and had to get 2 of 3 correct to be credited with the one-one and stable principles; at least one correct to be credited with the cardinal principle. Preschool children only had 1 counting trial per set size, unless they erred in which case a further trial was administered. If correct by the time the trial ended, they were scored as having the one-one and stable principles. See the text for a description of the separate cardinal task they received.

experimenter first counted, and while doing so, made sure to point to and/or move each item as it was tagged.

As can be seen in the top half of Table 1, the two pre-school and the DS groups of children counted equally well when tested with the row of five heterogeneous items that would serve as the stimulus set for the constrained counting tasks. This means that they all started the con-strained counting tasks from a common performance level. Unfortunately, it is not clear that children in the dif-ferent groups were in fact all equally good counters. Our reason for saying this is presented in the bottom half of Table 1.

If, for the moment, we ignore the DS children's Demon-stration scores, we can see that both groups of pre-schoolers outperformed the DS children. It is only after the experimenter had herself counted the set and as she did, touched each item and counted aloud, that DS child-ren could perform as well as either preschool group. Even still it is not clear that the DS children were as good as the preschool children at applying a principled under-standing of cardinality. For the preschool children had a harder cardinal task. They had to produce sets of 5 and 8 items, and do so by drawing the target number from a bag. In contrast, the DS children simply had to answer the "How Many?" question that followed their counting of a set. Some researchers have contended that this question can be answered solely on the basis of a rotely learned tendency to repeat the last tag said when counting, and hence, not on the basis of a principled understanding of cardinality (e.g., Fuson, Pergament & Lyons, 1986). The preschool children could not pass our assessment of their use of the cardinal principle by simply repeating the last count word used on a given trial. They had to keep the target value in mind and then generate that value by drawing N items from a bag. In other words, they had to understand the role that counting played in the genera-tion of the cardinal value. The DS children did not nec-essarily have to use the same level of understanding since they did not have to perform a task that required it.

In sum, the data on how well the DS and preschool children count suggest that they are comparable when it comes to meeting the requirement for participation in the

novel   task.   However,   there is a suggestion that the preschool   children,   especially the 5-year-olds, had a better
understanding   of   the   nature of counting. Composite pretest   scores,   ones that take into account the tendency of
each   child   to   be   consistent,   (that is, never err in applying   the one-one and stable principles), and to be able
to   give   some indication of the cardinal value of sets as
large   as   8, fit well with this suggestion. The DS children   were   tested   three times on each set size. If we ask
how   many   of   them   honored   the one-one and stable order
principle   on   at   least   two of these trials and for both
set   sizes   5   and   8, we find that only two of the ten DS
children   met   these   criteria and hence got classified as
Excellent   counters.   One   was 12 years old, the other one
was   10   years   old.   Their   respective MA's were 6.10 and
5.9,   both   of which exceed the Median MA for the DS group
as   a   whole. In contrast, 37.5 and 62.5 percent of the 4-
year-old,   and 5-year-old children met the criteria set to
classify them as Excellent counters.

Additional   data   on   the DS children's numerical abilities   suggested   to   us that the two excellent counters in
this   group   might differ qualitatively from the remaining
DS   children   in   our sample. As a check on this possibility,   we   often will treat them as a subgroup (DS Group A)
and   therefore   analyze   their   data separately from those
for   the rest of the group (Hereafter DS Group B). For the
constrained   counting   task could well pick up differences
in   principal   understanding as well as the ability to take
advantage   of   these   when problem solving. Before turning
to   the   data from the experiment proper, some details regarding data reduction need be discussed.

Transcriptions   of the videotapes - Transcriptions of videotapes   from   the   constrained counting trials were built
up   around   the format shown in Fig. 1. Such diagrams were
placed   alongside   column entries described below. But for
one   case,   every attempt at a solution, no matter whether
it   was correct or not, was displayed on the transcription
sheets   in   a   manner   like that shown in Fig. 1. The only
time   this   was not done was when a child started to count
the   first item, stopped, and started again. In this case,
the   self-generated   restart   of   the trial was noted in a
Comments   column.   Thus,   for every initial test trial and

every repeat of that trial, we ended up with transcripts that showed the children's sequence of points and count words. In addition, the separate columns to the right of these diagrams were used to enter transcripts of all comments and questions, as well as comments on the source of these (child or experimenter). These comments were entered so as to indicate when (before, during, after) the talk occured relative to the counting behaviors diagrammed for the trial. If the experimenter demonstrated anything, this too was described in detail. Further columns on the transcription sheets, and again for each diagrammed entry, were used by two transcribers who together coded whether and when the children hesitated, counted slow or fast, paused, or made eye contact with the experimenter.

An independent observer was trained to read our transcripts and then used 17 of these to see if she agreed with a computer printout of summaries that were generated from these. These summaries included rates of success per trial, the number of times a child encountered a trial, whether children hesitated, restarted a trial (with or without a probe), the amount of speech produced by the experimenter between repeats of a trial, etc. In all, excluding the diagrams and the details on these, the second observer checked our transcripts against 4060 separate sheet entries and agreed with them on all but twenty-nine occasions. Further, she only needed to return to three of the actual videotapes themselves to make sense of an entry on the transcript. This indicates that we succeeded at developing an interpretable transcription of the tapes and that summaries based on these were reliable. Hence, the coded data served as the source of input to the subsequent analyses.

What the Study Reveals About the Nature of Counting Knowledge

Overall differences in the Ability to Deal with Novelty - Our first pass at finding answers to our questions involved a consideration of overall levels of success on the constrained counting task. Fig. 2 plots the overall tendencies of children to generate successful solutions

on their very first encounter with the question or by the
time the trial had ended. (Recall our plan to allow the
children to repeat a trial, either on their own or after
receiving hints). Three salient results are shown here.

First, if we focus on the two DS groups of children (A
and B), there is a clear difference favoring those DS
children we identified as excellent counters (Group A).
In fact, the two DS children performed at ceiling levels.
Second, although both preschool groups outperform the remaining DS children, the two DS children in the A Group
did best of all. Finally, the preschool children, especially the 4-year-old, improved much more than did the DS

Figure 2. The overall performance levels of success for
each group of children tested on the Constrained Counting
Task.

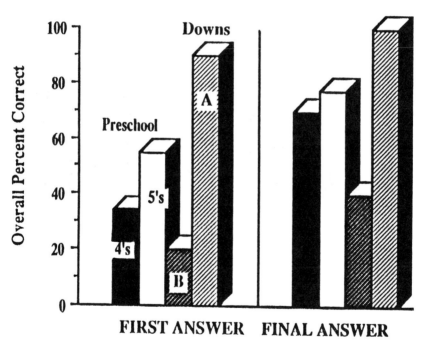

B group of children as they went from their first to final effort with the trial. This is our first clue that
the bulk of the DS sample might not have benefitted from
hints or self-corrected their initial efforts. A more de-

Figure 3. The Percent correct responses on the Constrained Counting Task shown as function of trial kind, group, and whether the response was the first one for a trial or not.

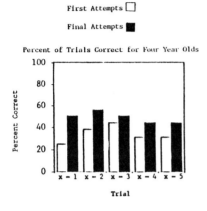

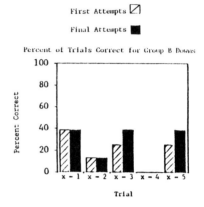

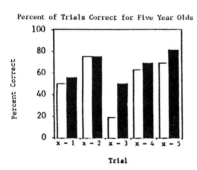

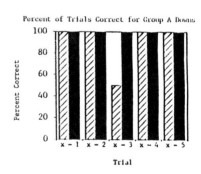

tailed consideration of these results begins to support the hypothesis that the B group of DS children represent a qualitatively different sample with respect to counting knowledge.

Differences in Across-Trial Profiles - Figure 3 presents a trial by trial summary of success levels, again as a function of whether success occurred on the first attempt with a trial or not. Recall that each of the trials varied in terms of which tag (1, 2, 3, 4, or 5) children were asked to assign to a target item. The data for the preschool children are shown on the left; those for the DS children are presented on the right. Again we see a persistent and positive effect of allowing preschool children to attempt a solution more than once. More importantly, a consideration of each bar graph suggests how children in each group differed.

The 4-year-old children generated what is becoming a familiar pattern for us. As in other studies, children of this age improve both as a function of the opportunity to retake a trial and as they moved from X = 1 to X = 3 (See Gelman et al, 1986 for another example). So although they did not do especially well when they first confronted the novel task (X = 1), they clearly "caught-on", despite the fact that they never were told explicitly what to do. The fall-off for X = 4 or 5 most likely reflects the working of fatigue and difficulty factors (cf. Gelman et al., 1986). Contrast these youngsters' performance with that of the majority of the DS children (Group B in the upper right hand corner). It is clear that there was no effect of repeating the trial for either X=1 experience to the X = 2. In fact, there seems to have been negative transfer from the X = 1 experience to the X = 2 trial. And although there appears to have been some learning effects by the X = 3 trial, these dissipated [See Wishart's chapter in this volume for a similar unsteady pattern of responding in DS infants and toddlers.]

The bottom panels in Fig. 3 show that both the 5-year-olds and Group A DS children benefitted from the opportunity to repeat trials and did so just where one might expect this to have happened -- on trials that presented some difficulty. In this regard the X = 3 trial results are especially salient. To understand what might have

happened on the X = 3 trial, it helps to refer first to
Fig. 4 which illustrates one possible set of solutions
across all values of X, given that X is always in the second position.

From Fig. 4, one can see that the X = 3 trial places
the greatest number of demands on the child. In the given
example, it is the only trial which requires the child to
skip an item more than once. A little reflection makes it
clear that this is also the trial where a child would

Figure 4. Schematized solutions to a set of trials where
the target item was always the same across trials with
differing values of X.

EXAMPLE TRIALS

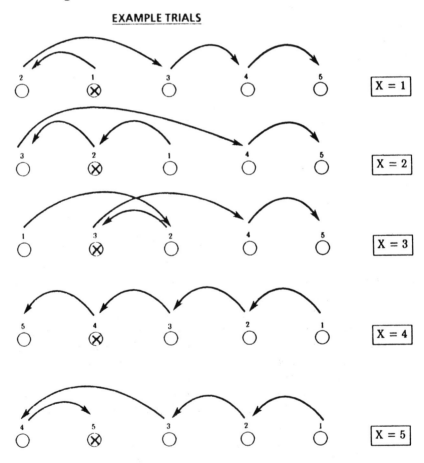

benefit most should she use a Create-Correspondence solution. Yet the Create-Correspondence solution is hardly
one that the child is likely to have encountered before.
So there should be a temporary fall off in performance.
Such considerations help explain why the drop in performance on the X = 3 trial. (Although not all of our Ss were
run in the exact condition shown in Fig. 4, many were.)

The data summarized in Fig. 3 add support to the hypothesis that even our youngest normal subjects generated
solutions that benefitted from their implicit knowledge
of the counting principles. For, just as the 5-year-olds
benefitted from time on task, so did they. And just as
the 5-year-olds then improved on subsequent trials, so
did they. In fact, they turned to trying to generate
correct solutions as soon as they got their instructions.

It begins to look like children's answers on the constrained counting task were determined by two qualitatively different paths. The preschoolers as well as two
of the DS children responded as if they were using principled knowledge. The same does not seem to be the case
for the remaining eight DS children in our study. To see
whether this is a reasonable conclusion, we turn to yet
more detailed considerations of the ways children negoti-

Figure 5. Source of a child's repeat of a given trial:
the child or the experimenter.

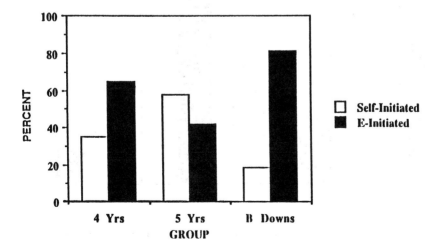

ated the constrained counting task as a given trial proceeded.

Differences in Follow-ups to an Initial Unsuccessful Attempt - We have argued that the children who have implicit counting principles as a problem-solving resource are
also in a position to self-initiate a second attempt. The
following presents 2 lines of evidence that indicate that
the preschool children, but not the Group B DS children,
did just this.
    In Fig. 5 we plot the extent to which a child's tenden-
cy to repeat a trial was self-initiated as opposed to ex-
perimenter-initiated. Since the two Group A DS children
made so few mistakes to start, they are not represented
in this or related analyses.

Figure 6. Mean number of experimenter's utterances between a child's first and final attempt to assign a given
item the target counting tag.

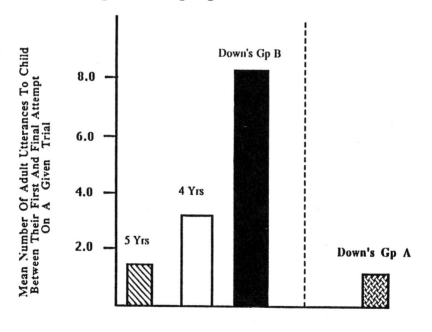

Notice that the DS children seldom repeated a trial on their own. In fact, 80% of the time that the DS children did repeat a trial they did so because of something the experimenter did first. Further, we can show that the experimenter had to work much harder to get DS children to initiate a repeat of the trial. This is clear even if we simply consider the amount of talk an experimenter produced between a child's first and final effort.

Fig. 6 shows that Group B DS children heard an average of about eight adult utterances per target trial. No oth-

Figure 7. Kinds and effectiveness of hints given between a child's first and final attempt on a given trial of the task. Very explicit hints could take the form of instructions or demonstrations. Neutral hints were ones like "Do you want to try that again?".

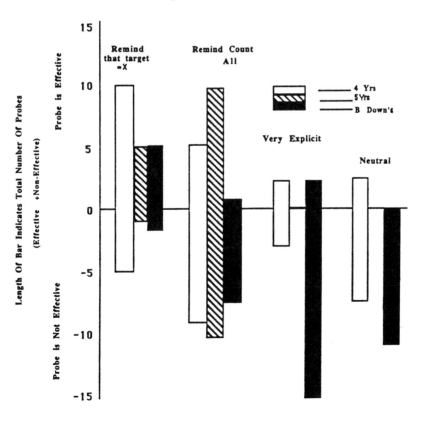

er group heard even half this much talk! Additionally, as
can be seen in Fig. 7, none of the other groups received
as much explicit help. Fig. 7 summarizes the kinds of
hints children received and the extent to which a given
kind of hint was used effectively. The rate at which the
kinds of hints shown in Fig. 7 were offered is reflected
in the total length of a given bar. For example, 5-year-
olds encountered relatively few reminders that they were
to assign a given tag to a given object.

It is important to realize that we scored a child as
receiving a hint no matter how long the utterance. This
means that Fig. 7 is a conservative way of illustrating
the amount of help we gave the DS children. Yet, it is
clear that it was the preschool children who were most
likely to benefit from our hints. The effectiveness of a
particular kind of hint is captured by the height of that
bar. The extent to which the same kind of hint was or was
not effective is captured by the length of portion of the
bar that is above or below the horizontal axis.

Since most of the bars of the DS children are below the
horizontal axis, we can conclude that they benefitted the
least from the tendency of the experimenters to lend a
helping hand. This overall effect supports the idea that
these children were not working with a principled understanding of counting. Not only is it the case that these
children did not self-initiate their follow-up efforts,
even when given hints as to what to do, they failed to
benefit from these hints, -- even when they were extremely explicit. The following protocol excerpts illustrate
both kinds of explicit help they received and how little
effect it had.

[Subject A, DS Group B]
    (x = 4 trial)

    Experimenter: Make the scissors the 4. (Scissors are
    in the middle position.)
    Child: (Starts by tagging the target item.) 4, 5. (He
    pauses at length after saying 5 and puts his hand on
    his head.)
    Experimenter: What's wrong?
    Child: I don't know.
    Experimenter: Okay, let me show you another way to do

it, okay? You can go like this. (The experimenter demonstrates.)
Child: (Counts along with experimenter who points to the objects.) 3, 4, 5.
Experimenter: You don't have to count them all in order. Okay, and another thing, if you want to move these scissors (points to target), you can do that. You can move them anywhere you want. Okay? So do you want to make it number 4 now?
Child: (He counts slowly across the array from left to right, hesitating slightly before saying 4.) 1, 2, 3, 4, 5.
Experimenter: Okay, now this time make them (the scissors) number 4. The last time you made them number 3. Make them number 4.
Child: (Counts from 1 to 5 skipping over the target but returns to tag the target as 5 rather than 4.)
[Experimenter goes to x = 5 trial]

(x = 5 trial)

Experimenter: Make the scissors the 5. (Scissors are in the middle position.)
Child: (Starting with the leftmost item, the subject counts.) 1, 2, 5. (He pauses before saying 5, then holds his head in his hand.) Oh boy.
Experimenter: You want to start over?
Child: Yeah.
Experimenter: Let's see you make them number 5.
Child: (He proceeds to count again from the left) 1, 2, 3. (He pauses after 3 and again holds his head with his hand.)
Experimenter: Okay, you can skip it. Do you want to just skip it? Okay, number 5 (points to target) and when you get to 3 you just jump to the purse. Okay, let's start over.
Child: 1, 2, 3, 4, 5. (He proceeds correctly, following the explicit instructions of the experimenter.)

[Subject B. DS Group B]
    (x = 3 trial)

Experimenter: Make the candle the 3. (The candle is

the second item from the left.)
Child: (Pause) What? (Starts to count from the
candle, the target item, tagging it 1 and continues)
2, 3. That's 3. (The item tagged 3 is actually in
fourth position.)
Experimenter: Okay. This time make the candle be num-
ber three. When you get to number three, call the
candle number three.
Child: (Nods yes. Pause.)
Experimenter: Okay, try that.
Child: Three?
Experimenter: Uh huh.
Child: Okay. (Child produces an exact repeat of the
first attempt.)
Experimenter: Okay. Can you make the candle be number
three this time?
Child: Yes. (No response.)
Experimenter: You made the mirror be three; I want
you to make the candle be three.
Child: (Pause.) One?
Experimenter: Make the candle be number three okay?
Start somewhere and start counting. Then when you
come to number three (Experimenter points to the
target while saying three.) point to the candle. You
can move the candle around if you want. You can move
the candle out (Experimenter demonstrates.)
Child: (No response.)
Experimenter: However you want to do it, okay, you
try it.
Child: Me?
Experimenter: Yeah.
Child: I try it?
Experimenter: Uh, huh. Go on.
Child: What?
Experimenter: (Points to the candle) Make the candle
be number three. [Eight further exchanges like these
occurred before the child finally tried to deal with
the task, again unsuccessfully.]

The above interactions between an experimenter and a
given DS child contrast dramatically with the kind that
occurred between an experimenter and a preschool child.
This is illustrated in the following transcript excerpts

of the protocols from the preschool study. Note the absence of both explicit hints as to what to do and any of
the kind of modelling of solution types that is part of
the above interaction between an experimenter and the DS
child.

[Subject #4 (4 years, 2 months)]
    (x = 4 trial)

> Experimenter: Make the strawberry the 4. (The straw-
> berry is in the second position from the left.)
> Child: 1, 2, 3, 4, 5. (He counts across from left to
> right.)
> Experimenter: You just made the strawberry be number
> 2. Can you make it be number 4?
> Child: (He counts starting with the leftmost item,
> skips over the target, and continues counting to the
> end of the row. He then skips back to tag the target
> as 5.)
> Experimenter: Can you make the strawberry be number
> 4?
> Child: (He now starts again with the leftmost item,
> skips over the target to tag the next two items (in
> the third and fourth positions) as 2 and 3, and re-
> turns to the target, tagging it as 4.)
> Experimenter: Did you get everything?
> Child: I didn't get that. (He now self-corrects but
> just repeats what he did on his second attempt at
> this trial.)

[Subject #6 (4 years, 3 months)]
    (x = 1 trial)

> Experimenter: Make the bee the number 1. (The bee is
> in the second position from the left.)
> Child: (she counts from right to left from 1 to 4,
> stopping after tagging the target as 4.)
> Experimenter: I said to make the bee the number 1.
> Child: (She now performs perfectly on this trial by
> skipping among the items.)

[Subject #7 (4 years, 5 months)]
   (x = 5 trial)

   Experimenter: Make the balloon the number 5. (The
   balloon is in the middle position.)
   Child: (He tags the second item from the left as 1
   and pauses. He then repeats himself but continues by
   tagging the leftmost item as 2, and then the target
   item as 3.)
   Experimenter: (Interrupts the child.) I wanted the
   balloon to be number 5.
   Child: (He now performs perfectly on this trial by
   skipping the target item and returning to it to tag
   it as 5.)
[Subject #11 (4 years, 7 months)]
   (x = 3 trial)

   Experimenter: Make the (target item) the 3. (The
   target is in the second position from the left.)
   Child: Can this be number 2? (Points to the middle
   item.)
   Experimenter: Whatever you want.
   Child: (She starts by tagging the leftmost item as 1,
   skips over the target tagging the middle item as 2,
   and returns to the target to tag it as 3. She then
   pauses.)
   Experimenter: Did you get them all?
   Child: (She continues her count, tagging the remaining two items as 4 and 5. The trial is thus completed
   correctly.)

[Subject #27 (5 years, 6 months)]
   (x = 4 trial)

   Experimenter: Make the bone the 4. (The bone is in
   the rightmost position.)
   Child: I'm thinking about how to do his. (He hesitates for a long time then counts the items to himself.) I can do it if I move the bone to where the
   strawberry is (Second position from the right). (He
   then switches the two items creating a correspondence
   between the items in the array and the words in his
   count list. He counts, beginning with the leftmost

item and counting across to the right tagging the items from 1 to 4.)
Experimenter: Did you get everything?
Child: (He points to the rightmost item which has not
yet been tagged and says 5, thus correctly completing
the trial.)

[Subject #28 (5 years, 7 months)]
   (x = 5 trial)

Experimenter: Make the (target item) the 5. (The target is in the middle position.)
Child: (She hesitates before starting, tags the
rightmost item as 1 and stops.)
Experimenter: We want this one (points to the target)
to be number 5.
Child: (She now performs perfectly on this trial by
starting to count from the rightmost item, skipping
over the target when she gets to it, and returning to
the target to tag it as 5.)

[Subject #31 (5 years, 9 months)]
   (x = 3 trial)

Experimenter: Now, make it (target item) the 3. (The
target is in the leftmost position.)
Child: (He starts with the second item from the left
and tags as 1. He continues to the right with 2, 3,
4, and returns to the leftmost item to tag it as 5.)
Experimenter: Can you count them and make this be
number 3?
Child: (He begins again with the second item from the
left and tags it as 1. He next tags the middle item 2
and returns to tag the leftmost item 3. The trial
continues with the child tagging the rightmost item
as 4 and the item to its left as 5. The result is a
perfect performance on this trial.)

The preceding protocols help illustrate another feature of the results plotted in Fig. 7. Normal preschool
children received the kind of input our design called
for, that is neutral statements or reminders regarding
the constraints of the task. As regards the latter, these

children, especially the 4-year-olds, had a tendency to ignore the task constraint that they use a particular count word for a particular object. Hence, they received a total of 15 reminders about this. Similarly, the preschoolers had a tendency to forget that they were to do this **and** yet count all of the set. So they heard the experimenter say things like "Did you count all of them?"

Overall then, the results graphed in Fig. 7 indicate that DS and normal children were likely to receive different kinds of hints. Normal preschool children were typically reminded about some constraint of the task or simply encouraged to start over. Often as not, these hints led to improved performance levels, despite the fact that the experimenter did not provide explicit suggestions as to how to improve. In contrast, DS children were most likely to receive very explicit hints, which included demonstrations of what to do. Nevertheless, such feedback was not especially effective. This is exactly the pattern of results we indicated one should see if normal children were able to benefit from implicit principles and DS children were not. To repeat, we pointed out that children who already have some implicit knowledge of the counting principles have the wherewithal to recognize -- on their own -- their mistakes, to start over, and to benefit from subtle hints. Children who are not able to take advantage of such a supporting mental structure have no resources other than those provided by others (cf. Brown & Reeve, 1987). Worse yet, even when those resources are presented to them, they are at risk because they may fail to recognize the resources for what they are worth -- just as some of the DS children failed to benefit from explicit clues regarding a solution path.

Further Evidence: Differences in Error Types and Flexibility - Recall that one need not use the conventional count words of a given language in order to honor the counting principles. But one cannot double tag items or omit items in a set and still honor the principles. Given these considerations, children who do have implicit understanding of counting principles might be more willing to alter the nature of the tags they use than to violate basic constraints of the one-one principle. Our first hint that this is indeed what some preschool children did came from our observation that some of them solved the constrained counting problem by tampering with the conventional order of the count list. For example, one child met our request to make the second item from the left end of a row "the three", by tagging the items left to right while saying "1, 3, 2, 4, 5". To be sure, this solution does violate the stable order principle. However, it honors the one-one principle, a principle that one may want to grant a special status given its mathematical import (See Greeno et al., 1984, for a discussion of the mathematical significance of the one-one principle). If so, children might be expected to tolerate errorful plans that violate their rote knowledge of the conventional counting list if it means that they will still honor the one-one principle -- assuming of course that they know they should honor this principle.

To assess the merit of the foregoing line of reasoning, we reviewed the transcripts of individual children to see whether they had inclinations to alter the conventional count list order and if so, what sorts. For this analysis we considered the expanded "doesn't matter" data base we had for the children. We did this in part because the analysis depends on children making errors. Therefore we looked at the responses the DS children made with heterogeneous displays of either five or eight items. In the case of the preschool children, we also looked at their answers when the displays were arranged in circles.

None of the DS children in Group B varied the conventional order of the counting words. Most of the time, this means that they made one-one errors instead. The only way to avoid making one-one errors and still stick to the conventional order is to start a tagging sequence with the target and it's requisite tag. Thus, for example, a child who was asked to make a given item "the three" did just that. She pointed to the item in question and said "3" and then continued to count, thereby producing the count word string "3, 4, 5, 6, 7, 8" while tagging the items. In fact this same child continued on the next trial to make the same item "the four" by counting "4, 5, 6, 7, 8, 9", an outcome which means her successive counts could not serve as evidence that the cardinal value of a set is conserved over count trials.

Both groups of preschool children were less inclined

than were DS children to adhere strictly to the conventional count-list order. Although the preschoolers did make some effort to honor the conventional count list order on their error trials, they also were willing to alter the order, and thereby avoid violating the one-one principle. Of the 16 and 14 4- and 5-year-olds, respectively, who made any errors at all, 44% in each age group showed at least some inclination to alter the conventional counting order.

It is especially interesting that there is no age difference here. For the 5-year-olds surely had more reinforcement for using the conventional list than did the younger children. On a strict associationist account, they should have been more inclined to stick to the conventional count list order. That they did not is consistent with our hypothesis that our preschoolers, unlike Group B DS subjects, were able to put principle ahead of habit -- at least some of the time. So is the fact that some of these young children laughed, or made it clear they were "fooling" or joking when they made errors that seemed to serve the purpose of meeting task constraints. (The extensive counting training offered to our DS subjects might account for the fact that even our two excellent counters maintained a consistent sound word order when they started to make errors, especially on their trials with 8 items.)

The preceding results add weight to our conclusion that the majority of DS children actually did learn to count by rote and that, despite the benefit of a curriculum that is designed to give them a great deal of counting experience, they did not induce the principles that govern counting. Indeed, if anything, this kind of rote learning seems to have produced less flexibility, a conjecture that is supported by the kinds of data Wishart (this volume) presented on the way DS infants deal with the object concept task. It also gains support from one further consideration of the preschoolers' performances.

As discussed in the Section - Procedures, circular displays present a special problem to children should they think they are to recite a list of count words until they come to the end of a row. Unless they are able to take into account their initial starting position and then use this to signal when to stop reciting count words, they run the risk of continuing on and on and on. One clear sign that our preschoolers did not do this comes from the fact that they did better on their circle trials than their line trials! Whereas five children in each of the age groups turned in perfect performances on their circle trials, only 3 of the 5-year-olds did as well on their linear displays. This is hardly what one would expect if the children who are used to counting items in rows have learned to do so without considering the demands of the one-one principle. Indeed, given that children did somewhat better with the circular arrays, we can conclude that they were able to honor the one-one principle in a flexible way.

Summary of Differences - We have presented a variety of findings that all converge on the conclusion that normal preschool children are not only better able to deal with a novel counting task; they approach the task of generating novel solutions in ways that are qualitatively different than those used by all but two of our Down Syndrome children. They are much more inclined to self-correct their false starts, to understand subtle hints, and to vary their solution types as their target instructions and stimulus conditions vary on them. Further, when they do make errors, they are willing to alter the order of the tags in the standard count sequence, a fact which makes them less likely to violate fundamental counting principles, as compared to the majority of the DS children. The DS children seem not able to benefit from hints as to how to solve their novel problem, even when these hints include explicit instructions or demonstrations of possible solutions. Their patterns of responding are consistent with the hypothesis that their learning to count was controlled by a rote, associative learning process. Since the normal children's patterns of responding are so different and fit well with the predictions made by a principle-first learning model, we conclude that qualitative differences in their favor are due to their being able to take advantage of a skeletal set of the counting principles, ones which enabled their novel generation of counting solutions for the Constrained Counting Task.

On Inferring Causality: Proceed with Caution

We have shown that most of the DS children in this
study fit the associative learning model: In contrast,
the responses of the normal preschool children to our
novel counting task are better described by the princi-
ple-guided learning model of counting knowledge. Given
this, we can say that normal children are privileged in-
sofar as they are able to take advantage of a set of
counting-relevant principles in order to generate acceptable responses even when confronted with a novel task.
They are also able to make sense out of subtle hints, the
ones that offer little, if any, guidance as to how to
correct an errorful plan. Also, they seem motivated to
stick with a problem until they find a way to solve it.
These results are buttressed by the findings that show
that, all over the world, individuals invent counting solutions to solve arithmetic problems confronted in their
everyday lives, whether or not they have had any formal
schooling (e.g., Carraher, Carraher, & Schliemann, 1985;
Lave, 1977; Posner, 1982; Scribner & Cole, 1973). Together, these findings converge on two clear conclusions:
First, normal individuals are able to assimilate whatever
mathematically meaningful inputs they encounter, and can
do so, as it were, on the fly. Second, they can generate
solutions to some problems, even if they have not been
given guidance on the matter, in either a hinting or more
direct fashion. These conclusions fit very well with the
rational constructivist account of the acquisition of
counting knowledge. They are not so obviously consistent
with the associationist account.

Although we are able to reach the foregoing conclusions
for normal children, we cannot conclude that DS children
lack an initial skeletal base of counting principles by
dint of their genetic history. Indeed, it is not clear
that we can conclude they totally lack the initial benefit of some skeletal set of counting principles. When we
introduced our research plan we were careful to point out
that should we find that DS children actually produced
qualitatively different solutions than normal preschool
children, we would not have license to attribute the difference to the genetic variables known to contribute to

Down Syndrome. As has been discussed elsewhere in this volume, there is a wide range of variables that need to be considered even if we should find that it is only DS children who differ as described here from normal children. And, of course, it is necessary to determine whether similar results would obtain for children who suffer from other kinds of mental retardation. Baroody's (1986) study of counting abilities in mildly retarded children highlights this possibility. It is also necessary to consider whether the same findings would hold were the DS children offered a different curriculum.

Are the Results Counting Principle Specific? - Assuming that we could determine the range of variables that control the described differences, we still must ask whether we can ascribe the differences to the presence or absence of an initial base of implicit counting principles. One clear possibility is that the difference is due more to the DS child's difficulty in learning to map mathematical symbols to underlying principles. The evidence is mounting that a variety of nonverbal organisms can count in a principled way (Gallistel, in press, for a review). An obvious way in which the human ability to count differs from that of animals has to do with their ability to master a mathematical symbol system that captures the nature of these principles. Given that DS children's ability to master another symbol system, that described by linguistic principles, is limited, we must consider the possibility that they are at risk in general when it comes to mastering symbolic material in a principled way. It is therefore entirely possible that DS children do have some early, implicit understanding of some counting principles but fail to develop them because of limits on their abilities to master the mathematical meanings of count words and other mathematical symbols, a task that we are beginning to see is exceedingly complex and difficult for all (e.g. Gelman & Greeno, in press; Resnick, 1987).

A Return to the Two Models and Some Pedagogical Considerations - We began with the idea that comparative research can offer insights about the nature of human cognition. Our comparisons of the ways the DS and normal preschool children solved the constrained counting task support the conclusion that normal individuals benefit from the availability of counting principles from the outset, ones that support the acquisition of counting knowledge and the generation of novel solutions. Surely the reader is wondering whether it is impossible to arrive at a principled understanding of counting without having started with some skeletal outline of it. We think not. Instead, we prefer to say that the path to such knowledge is ever so much more treacherous when one cannot take advantage of such principled help. With such principles on hand, children can find their way through ambiguous environments for they have guidelines as to which inputs fit the equivalence class that is relevant to the learning. Even if we as teachers fail to present the data base in a way that would best nurture development, children have going for them an inclination to both use and extend their existing knowledge structures. These in turn provide ways of both collecting and storing a coherent set of relevant inputs. So even if these inputs are few and far between, disorganized, and dressed up with irrelevant details, the mental structures can serve to filter the good from the bad. Children who learn only as associationist theorists say they do, are at a disadvantage because they are especially dependent on others to structure their inputs. Put differently, it becomes especially important to develop teaching methods that package inputs in ways that might be expected to support mathematical inductions. From our perspective, there is one clear educational implication of this consequence. We must arrange our teaching materials so that they are congruent with mathematical principles. Instead of drilling children in the count word sequence, we might better turn our efforts to teaching them that count words are only tags, that count words acquire their meaning when they are used in ways that are consistent with the counting principles, that it is not necessary to count from one end of a row to the other, and it does not matter what items are collected together for a count. It is a tall order for sure, but one we might try before deciding it cannot be met. To those who counter that the children should not be asked to deal with matters pertaining to the counting principles unless they have mastered the conventional count list, we respond: What about the 4-year-old children in our study who probably were less practiced on the count list?

Acknowledgments

The research presented in this chapter was supported by NICHHD Program Project Grant No. P01 HD-10965 to David Premack; Deborah Kemler and Rochel Gelman and NSF Grant BNS 85-19575 to Rochel Gelman. It is based in part on Melissa Cohen's senior honors thesis and in part on a paper presented by the first author at the conference reported in this book. We are especially grateful to the parents and children who came to our lab and the children, parents and staff affiliated with St. Katherine's Day School, the Paley Day Care Center, and the Bankcroft School for offering their cooperative participation in our work. Thanks also to Michael Siegel and C.R. Gallistel who read and made comments on earlier versions of this paper.

Footnotes

1. David Premack organized a group of us to do comparative studies with chimpanzees, normal and/or retarded children. In addition to Gelman and Fowler, the group has included Lila Gleitman and Deborah Kemler and students or visitors working with one or more of us.

2. We included sessions with 5 and 8 homogeneous items because we thought children would be forced to move the target item so as to mark its special status. Given they did even more poorly under these conditions, there will be no further mention of them.

REFERENCES

Au T. K. & Markman, E. M. (1987). Acquiring word meanings via linguistic contrast. <u>Cognitive Development</u>, 2, 217-236.
Baroody, A. J. (1986). Counting ability of moderately and mildly handicapped children. <u>Education and Training of</u>

the Mentally Retarded, 21, 289-300.

Baroody, A. J. (1984). More precisely defining and measuring the order-irrelevance principle. Journal of Experimental Child Psychology, 38, 33-41.

Bartlett, E. J. (1977). The acquisition of the meaning of color terms: A Study of lexical development. In R. Campbell & P. Smith (Eds.), Recent advances in the psychology of language, IVa (pp. 89-108). New York: Plenum Press.

Bornstein, M. H. (1985). Colour naming versus shape naming. Journal of Child Language, 12, 387-393.

Bransford, J. D. (1979). Human cognition: Learning, understanding and remembering. Belmont, CA: Wadsworth.

Briars, D., & Siegler, R. S. (1984). A featural analysis of preschoolers' counting knowledge. Developmental Psychology, 20, 607-618.

Brown, A. L., Bransford, J. D., Ferrara, R. A., & Campione, J. C. (1983). Learning, remembering, and understanding. In J. H. Flavell and E. M. Markman (Eds.), Handbook of Child Psychology (4th ed.), Vol. 3, Cognitive Development. New York: John Wiley and Sons.

Brown, A. L., & Reeve, R. A. (1987). Bandwidths of competence: The role of supportive contexts in learning and development. In L. S. Liben & D. H. Feldman (Eds.). Development and learning: Conflict or congruence. Hillsdale, NJ: Erlbaum.

Campione, J. C., Brown, A. L., Ferrara, R. A., & Bryant, N. R. (1984). The zone of proximal development: Implications for individual differences and learning. In B. Rogoff & J. V. Wertsch (Eds.). New directions for child development: Children's learning in the "Zone of Proximal Development". San Francisco, Jossey-Bass.

Carraher, T. N., Carraher, D. W. & Schliemann, A. D. (1985). Mathematics in the streets and in schools. British Journal of Developmental Psychology, 3, 21-29.

Cooper, R. G., Jr. (1984). Early number development: Discovering number space with addition and subtraction. In C. Sophian (Ed.), Origins of cognitive skills. Hillsdale, NJ: Erlbaum.

Cornwall, A. C. (1974). Development of language, abstraction, and numerical concepts in Down's Syndrome children. American Journal of Mental Deficiency, 79, 179-190.

DeLoache, J. S. (1984). On where or where: Memory-based searching by very young children. In C. Sophian. (Ed.), Origins of cognitive skills. Hillsdale, NJ: Erlbaum.

DeLoache, J. S., Sugarman, S., & Brown, A. L. (1985). The development of error correction strategies in young children's manipulative play. Child Development, 56, 928-939.

Donaldson, M. (1978). Children's minds. New York: W. W. Norton.

Edgerton, R. B. (1979). Mental retardation. Cambridge, MA: Harvard University Press.

Feldman, H. & Gelman, R. (1986). Otitis media and cognitive development. In J. F. Kavanagh (Ed.), Otitis media and child development, Parkton, Maryland: York Press.

Fuson, K. C. (1982). Analysis of the counting on solution procedure in addition. In T. P. Carpenter, J. M. Moser, & T. A. Romberg (Eds.). Addition and subtraction: A cognitive perspective, Hillsdale, NJ: Erlbaum Associates.

Fuson, K. C. (1988). Children's counting and concepts of number. New York: Springer-Verlag.

Fuson, K. C., & Hall, J. W. (1983). The acquisition of early number word meanings: A conceptual analysis and review. In H. P. Ginsburg (Ed.), The development of mathematical thinking. New York: Academic.

Fuson, K. C., Pergament, G. G., & Lyons, B. G. (1986). Collection terms and preschoolers' use of the cardinality rule. Cognitive Psychology, 17, 315-323.

Gallistel, C. R. (in press). Animal cognition: The representation of space, time, and number. Annual Review of Psychology, 40.

Gelman, R. (1982). Basic numerical abilities. In R. J. Sternberg (Ed.), Advances in the psychology of intelligence: Vol. 1 (pp. 181-205). Hillsdale, NJ: Erlbaum.

Gelman, R. & Brown, A. L. (1986). Changing views of cognitive competence in the young. In N. Smelser & D. Gerstein (Eds.), Discoveries and trends in behavioral and social sciences, Commission on Behavioral and Social Sciences and Education, Washington, D.C.: NRC Press, 1986. (pp. 175-207).

Gelman, R., & Gallistel, C. R. (1978). The child's understanding of number. Cambridge, MA: Harvard.

Gelman, R. & Greeno, J. G. (in press). On the nature of

competence: Principles for understanding in a domain.
In L. B. Resnick (Ed.), Knowing and learning: Issues
for a cognitive science of instruction. Hillsdale, NJ:
Erlbaum Associates.

Gelman, R., & Meck, E. (1986). The notion of principle:
the case of counting. In J. Hiebert (Ed.), The relationship between procedural and conceptual competence
(pp. 29-57). Hillsdale, NJ: Erlbaum.

Gelman, R., Meck, E., & Merkin, S. (1986). Young children's numerical competence. Cognitive Development, 1,
1-29.

Greeno, J. G., Riley, M. S., & Gelman, R. (1984). Conceptual competence and children's counting. Cognitive Psychology, 16, 94-134.

Hartley, X. Y. (1986). A summary of recent research into
the development of children with Down's Syndrome. Journal of Mental Deficiency Research, 30, 1-14.

Karmiloff-Smith, A., & Inhelder, B. (1974/75). If you
want to get ahead, get a theory. Cognition, 3, 195-212.

Lave, J. (1977). Cognitive consequences of traditional
apprenticeship training in West Africa. Anthropology
and Education Quarterly, 8, 177-180.

Mandler, J. M. (1984). Stories, scripts, and scenes: Aspects of schema theory. Hillsdale, NJ: Erlbaum Associates.

Markman, E. M. (1986). How children constrain the possible meanings of words. In U. Neisser (Ed.) The ecological and intellectual basis of categorization. Cambridge, England: Cambridge University Press.

Posner, J. (1982). The development of mathematical knowledge in two West Africa societies. Child Development,
53, 200-208.

Quine, W. V. O (1960). Word and object. Cambridge, MA:
MIT Press.

Resnick, L. B. (1986). The development of mathematical
intuition. In M. Perlmutter (Ed.) Perspectives on intellectual development: The Minnesota symposium on
child development. Vol. 19 (pp. 159-194). Hillsdale,
NJ: Erlbaum Associates.

Resnick, L. B. (1987). Learning in school and out. Educational Researcher, 16, 13-20.

Saxe, G., Guberman, S., & Gearhart, M. (in press). Social
and developmental processes in children's understanding

of number. Society for Research in Child Development Monographs.

Schank, R. & Abelson, R. (1977). Scripts, plans, goals, and understanding. Hillsdale, NJ: Erlbaum Associates.

Scribner, S. & Cole, M. (1973). Cognitive consequences of formal and informal education. Science, 182, 553-559.

Shipley, E. & Shepperson, B. (1987). Countable entities: Developmental changes. Unpublished manuscript. University of Pennsylvania.

Siegal, M., Waters, L. J., & Dinwiddy, L. S. (in press). Misleading children: Causal attributions for inconsistency under repeated questioning. Journal of Experimental Child Psychology.

Siegler, R. & Shipley, C. (1987). The role of learning in children's strategy choices. In L. S. Liben (Ed.), Development and learning: Conflict or congruence?. Hillsdale, NJ: Lawrence Erlbaum Associates.

Sophian, C. & Adams, N. (1987). Infants' understanding of numerical transformations. British Journal of Developmental Psychology, 5, 257-264.

Spelke, E. S. (1988). In A. Yonas (Ed.), Perceptual development in infancy: The Minnesota symposium on child development: Vol 20. Hillsdale, NJ: Erlbaum Associates.

Starkey, P., Spelke, E. S. & Gelman, R. (1983). Detection of one-to-one correspondences by human infants. Science, 1983, 222, 79-181.

Strauss, M. S., & Curtis, L. E. (1981). Infants perception of numerosity. Child Development. 52, 1146-1152.

Strauss, M. S., & Curtis, L. E. (1984). Development of numerical concepts in infancy. In C. Sophian (Ed.) Origins of cognitive skills. Hillsdale, NJ: Erlbaum.

Waxman, S. R. (1985). Hierarchies in classification and language: Evidence from preschool children. Unpublished Doctoral dissertation. University of Pennsylvania.

Wilkinson, A. C. (1984). Children's partial knowledge of the cognitive skill of counting. Cognitive Psychology. 16, 28-64.

3

EARLY LEXICAL DEVELOPMENT:
THEORY AND APPLICATION

Carolyn B. Mervis
Department of Psychology,
University of Massachusetts, Amherst
Amherst, MA 01003

When is a goose really a duckie, a truck really a car,
and a magazine really a book? When your informant is a
child who recently has begun to acquire language. These
are not isolated examples; the categories to which very
young children assign objects are frequently different
from those adults would choose. Furthermore, these differences are not simply performance errors; similar deviations from the adult standard occur for both comprehension and production (Chapman, Leonard, & Mervis, 1986;
Mervis & Canada, 1983). Eventually, however, young children's categories begin to evolve in order to correspond
more closely to the adult standard. These initial differences and eventual concordance lead to a number of questions. First, why do very young children's categories
often differ from those of adults? Are the differences
principled? Second, what causes young children's categories to begin to evolve in the direction of the adult
standard? Third, what is the role of the child, and what
is the role of adults, in determining the initial structure of the child's categories and the process of evolution of these categories?
  The purpose of this chapter is to consider the early
lexical development of both children who have Down Syndrome and children who are developing normally. I will
focus on the acquisition of names for categories of concrete objects. These words form a substantial part of
children's earliest vocabularies (Gillham, 1979; Nelson,
1973; see also the review by Clark, 1979). The paper is
divided into seven sections. Because most of the data

that will be presented is derived from a longitudinal study of early lexical development, the first section contains a description of the methodology of that study. This study was conducted in collaboration with Claudia Cardoso-Martins and Cindy Mervis. In the second section, the beginnings of a theory of early lexical development are presented. The questions addressed are those raised above concerning the initial differences and eventual concordance between child and adult categories; questions concerning the basis for very young children's choice of labels for their initial categories also are considered. The remaining sections are more descriptive. In the third section, I consider the types of words children learn first, and in the fourth, the relationship between cognitive development and early vocabulary development. In the fifth, the patterns of maternal linguistic input are discussed, and the potential role of this input in determining rate of early vocabulary development is considered. The last two sections consider the value of comparative data concerning early lexical development. The sixth section is focused on the implications of the theory and research presented for development of intervention strategies to facilitate the early lexical development of the children with Down Syndrome. The seventh section concludes with a brief reiteration of the most important of the suggested universals of early lexical development.

Longitudinal Study: Method

Subjects - Six children with Down Syndrome (three boys, three girls) and their mothers and six normally developing children and their mothers participated in this study. The children with Down Syndrome constituted the entire known surviving population of children with Down Syndrome born in two small midwestern cities during a three-month period. The normally developing children were matched to the children with Down Syndrome for sex and birth-order position. All children had hearing and vision within the normal range. All families were middle class, and in all cases the mother was the primary caregiver. At the start of the study, the children with Down Syndrome were between 17 and 19 months old. The normally developing children were 9 months old. None of the children was able to comprehend or produce language referentially. The dyads were visited at home every six weeks between 14 and 21 months.

Procedure - Each visit began with a 30-minute period during which the mother and child played together with a specially chosen set of toys. This play period was audiotaped. In addition, one observer recorded all the nouns and pronouns used by either mother or child, along with their referents. A second observer audiotaped a running commentary describing the nonverbal interaction. For the children with Down Syndrome and their mothers, this commentary included any manual signs produced and the context in which they were used.

After the play period, production testing and comprehension testing were carried out. First, the child was asked to name the toys, if there was any possibility that he or she could produce the names. Such a possibility was considered to exist if the researchers had ever heard the child produce any of the object names, either spontaneously or in imitation, or if the mother thought that her child could produce any of them. Next, the child's comprehension was tested. Four objects were placed in front of the child, and he or she was asked, "Is there an <X>?". The distractor objects were selected according to predetermined rules, to ensure that the objects most similar to members of the target category were used (see Mervis, 1984). If the child appeared tired or fussy, testing was discontinued and then completed within a few days.

Certain visits also included assessments of cognitive development. Four measures were used: the object permanence and means-ends relations subscales of the Uzgiris and Hunt (1975) scales for sensorimotor development, the mental scale of the Bayley Scales of Infant Development (Bayley, 1969), and form L-M of the Stanford-Binet Intelligence Scale (Terman & Merrill, 1960).

The object permanence and the means-ends relations subscales were administered at the first visit and at every second visit thereafter until the child had passed all the items. These scales also were administered at the visit during which referential production first was demonstrated, even if these assessments originally had not been scheduled for those dates. If necessary, the scales were administered at the last visit. The mental scale of the Bayley was administered at the end of the first visit and thereafter at regular intervals of approximately five months. The Stanford-Binet was administered to the normally developing children at the visit closest to their second birthday and to the children with Down Syndrome at the end of the study.

Stimuli - Three basic level categories were studied: ball, car, and kitty. The names for these categories are among the earliest words of both children with Down Syndrome and normally developing children (Gillham, 1979; Nelson, 1973). The objects used included true members of the category (by adult standards), related objects that were predicted to be members of the children's categories (hereafter referred to as child-basic-only objects), and unrelated objects from the same superordinate categories, that were predicted not to be included in either the adult-basic or the child-basic categories.

To predict which items should be included in a child-basic category, the principle that basic level categories are the most general categories whose members share similar overall shapes (forms) and similar functions or characteristic actions was used (see Rosch, Mervis, Johnson, Gray, & Boyes-Braem, 1976). I began with observation of the functions for normally developing 13-month-olds of a prototypical exemplar (in toy form) of the adult-basic category labeled by each target word. Any object that could fulfill these functions (whether or not they were appropriate for that object from an adult perspective) and that had a shape similar to the prototypical exemplar was predicted to be a member of the child-basic category. For example, anything that could be thrown, could roll, and was approximately spherical was predicted to be included in the child-basic ball category. The objects used are listed in Table 1.

Early Categories and Category Evolution

Very young children, like adults, form object cate-

Table 1
Toys Used in the Play Sessions

	Category		
Predicted Membership	Ball	Car	Kitty
Adult-basic and child-basic:	rubber ball whiffle ball soccer ball football[a]	sedan car sports car wooden car[a] jeep[a]	house cat sachet cat[a] beanbag cat[a] potholder cat[a]
Child-basic only:	multisided beads Christmas ornament round candle round owl bank round bell	van bus moving truck fire engine cement truck dump truck	panther cougar cheetah leopard tiger lion
Neither:	wooden blocks frisbee plastic keys	airplane helicopter boat	dog frog parrot zebra squirrel rabbit walrus turtle elephant duck giraffe lobster camel dinosaur

Note. A subset of these toys was used in each of the play sessions. At the start of the study, five objects from each category were included: one predicted neither. By the end of the study, nine objects from each category were included: two predicted adult-basic and child-basic, five predicted child-basic only, and two predicted neither. For many of the names listed, several different exemplars of the category labeled by that name were used over the course of the study. With the exception of some of the potential undergeneralizaation objects, all objects were realistic representations.
a = Potential undergeneralization object.

gories on the basis of similarity among exemplars. But judgments of similarity differ depending on the attributes to which a person attends. For example, consider the triplet robin, canary, lemon. Almost everyone would agree that the robin and the canary were the most similar pair. In this case, similarity is defined according to general form attributes, function attributes, or biological attributes. However, if the attribute "yellow" were given sufficient weight, then the canary and the lemon would be the most similar. Thus, in talking about categorization, the type of similarity which provides the basis for category assignments must by specified. Murphy and Medin (1985) have argued that adults use informal theories or beliefs along with background knowledge about the world as a basis for determining the types of similarity that will be noticed. Informal theories may be either implicit or explicit. Developmental researchers have argued that children as young as 4 years old (see Carey, 1982; 1985; Keil, 1979; 1987), and even toddlers (Mervis, 1982; 1984; 1987) also use informal theories (generally of the implicit type) and background knowledge as the basis for categorization. Differences in adult and child categories often can be accounted for by differences in the theories and background knowledge of persons of different ages or cognitive levels.

In this section, I consider a few of the informal theories that very young children use when they begin to form categories and when they begin to alter these categories to conform more closely to the adult standard. I begin by considering informal theories concerning attribute correlations. Next, I discuss how these informal theories provide the basis for child-basic categories. I then consider one important informal theory concerning the child's categories. I will not discuss the complete evolution of these categories; at the time the longitudinal study was ended, when the children with Down Syndrome were about 3 years old, there were almost no instances of complete category evolution, see Mervis (1987, 1988).

Correlated Attributes - Not surprisingly, infants' first informal theories are derived from sensorimotor knowledge. Piaget's (e.g., 1954) descriptions provide crucial background. During the first four stages of the sensorimotor period, infants tend to treat all objects in the same manner. Infants have available a few general schemas (e.g., looking, grasping, mouthing, banging) which are applied to all objects to which the infant has access. During the fifth stage, however, infants become curious about objects as objects. Infants begin to explore objects for the purpose of learning about their nature -- about specific properties of individual objects or types of objects. One result of these explorations is that infants begin to discover particular functions or characteristic actions of specific types of objects along with form attributes that are correlated with (afford) these activities. For example, infants discover that objects that are spherical generally can roll. These explorations often involve the infant's direct actions on objects. However, infants also can discover function-form correlations by observing other people interacting with objects or by observing the independent actions of animate objects or the seemingly independent actions of certain inanimate objects (e.g., objects with wheels may appear to move on their own). More generally, infants begin to realize that form attributes usually have correlated function attributes, and that function attributes usually have correlated form attributes.

At this point (by a mental age of 10-12 months), infants also have realized that there are correlations among form attributes as well. For example, ducks have a set of correlated form attributes, including webbed feet, bills of particular type, and the attributes contributing to the typical duck form. Normally developing 10-month-olds take such correlations into account when making categorization decisions. That is, these infants weight correlated attributes more heavily than the attributes that occur equally frequently within the category but that are not correlated with one another (Younger & Cohen, 1985; 1986).

Thus, from the beginning of the fifth stage of the sensorimotor period, infants have become sensitive to correlated attributes. Infants are able to use form-function correlations to predict an object's functional attributes on the basis of its form attributes (Mervis, 1985). By this time, infants behave according to an implicit theory that correlated attributes are more important in determining categories than are equally frequent but uncorrelated attributes. This implicit knowledge will be used through adulthood as a basis for categorization. In addition, infants have developed an informal theory that the form and function of objects generally are noticeably correlated, and this correlation should be used as the basis for categorization. Infants expect objects in the same category to have similar clusters of form attributes and fulfill similar functions or characteristic actions, predictable from their forms.

Child-Basic Level Categories - Form-function correlations are most obvious for basic level categories (Rosch, et al., 1976). These categories are the most general categories for which large clusters of correlated form and function attributes are present. Therefore, if young children behave according to an informal theory that form-function correlations should be used as the basis for categorization, one would expect that children's first categories would be basic level categories. Evidence in support of this claim will be presented in a later section (see also Mervis, 1983; Rosch, et al., 1976). Adult categories, particularly basic level ones, also tend to be formed based on such correlations.

However, an object generally affords more than one set of form-function correlations. Therefore, everyone will not necessarily attend to the same set of correlations for a given object. The actual categories formed on the basis of the form-function principle will vary because different groups notice or emphasize different attributes of the same object as a function of different experiences or different degrees of expertise. Very young children often do not share adults' knowledge of culturally appropriate functions of objects and the correlated form attributes, leading children to de-emphasize attributes of an object that are important from an adult perspective (e.g., Mervis, 1982, 1984, 1987; see Carey, 1982, for a similar position concerning verb concepts). At the same time, children often notice a form-function correlation that adults ignore for that object. In such cases, children would emphasize attributes that are irrelevant to adults. Therefore, children's initial basic level categories often do not correspond to the adult-basic level category labeled by the same word (Mervis, 1982, 1984, 1987). These differences represent differences in compe-

tence,   rather than simply performance errors, as was suggested by Fremgen and Fay (1980) and Chapman and Thomson
(1980), among others. (An extended discussion of this
point is provided in Mervis and Canada, 1983.) The principles governing the determination of basic level categories are universal (e.g, Dougherty, 1978; Mervis, 1984;
Rosch, et al., 1976), but these principles lead to different categories, depending on which attributes are noticed.
   The effect of differences between the attributes to
which the young children and adults attend may be made
clearer by an example. Consider the case of a spherical
bank. Very young children do not have a concept of money
or of saving money. When confronted with a spherical
bank, these children ignore the slot and the keyhole --
two attributes that are important to the adult assignment
of the object to a bank category. At the same time, very
young children do have a concept of balls. Therefore,
these children notice that the object is round and rolls.
Accordingly, they consider it to be a ball (e.g., Mervis,
1982, 1984, 1987). Tversky and Hemenway (1984) have suggested that children often ignore small attributes that
have functional significance for an adult, in favor of
large attributes of the same object that afford an alternative function. In the spherical bank example, the child
would ignore the slot and keyhole in favor of the spherical shape. Thus, both children and adults use the form-
function principle to form basic level categories. However, attention to different attributes leads to different category assignments for many objects. Therefore, the
child-basic categories often differ from the adult-basic
categories labeled by the same word.

Ineffectiveness of linguistic input as a basis for initial categories - I have just argued that differences
between a child-basic category and the adult-basic category labeled by the same name derive from application of
the form-function principle to different sets of attributes. At the same time, however, mothers of very young
normally developing children often label objects with
their child-basic names, rather than their adult-basic
names (Mervis, 1984; Mervis & Mervis, 1982). Therefore,
the possibility that children's initial categories are

based on linguistic input cannot yet be ruled out.
To eliminate this possibility, the initial categories of children whose mothers rarely label objects with their child-basic names must be considered. In a cross sectional study of maternal speech to prelinguistic children with Down Syndrome, Cardoso-Martins and Mervis (1985) found that these mothers almost never used child-basic labels. In contrast, the mothers of normally developing children matched for linguistic level or cognitive level often used child-basic labels. In this study, no data on the children's categories were collected. However, the obtained differences in maternal speech provided the impetus for a longitudinal study, in which both maternal linguistic input and child comprehen- sion and production of object labels were considered.

The results of the longitudinal study replicated those of the cross-sectional study, with regard to maternal labeling patterns during the period just prior to the child's comprehension of the relevant object names. The most relevant analysis involved whether or not mothers labeled at least one of the child-basic-only objects with its child-basic name during the play period on the day that the child first demonstrated comprehension of that name. The mothers of the normally developing children used this type of labeling in 67% of the test cases. In contrast, the mothers of the children with Down Syndrome did so in 31% of the test cases. Thus, in most cases for the children with Down Syndrome and in several cases for the normally developing children, maternal labeling pat- terns provided no indication of the existence of a child-basic category that was not identical to the adult-basic category that was labeled by the same name.

With these results in mind, the data from the children must be considered. The composition of the three categor- ies being studied (ball, car, kitty) was measured by com- prehension of the category name on the day that compre- hension of this word first was demonstrated. The initial composition was identical to the predicted child-basic categories in 88% of the cases for the children with Down Syndrome and in 94% for the normally developing children. The deviations in the remaining cases were minor and were not consistent with the linguistic input.

The persistence of the children with Down Syndrome despite conflicting input is well illustrated by one child on the day she first comprehended "kitty". When I asked Suzanne (a pseudonym) if there was a kitty, she handed me a stuffed tiger. Her mother immediately told her that it was not a kitty and then asked me to repeat the trial. I did so, with the same result. This time, Suzanne's mother told her loudly and firmly that the object was not a kitty, and again asked me to repeat the trial. By now, Suzanne was upset enough to have tears in her eyes, but she still handed me the tiger. Suzanne clearly considered it to be a kitty. In sum, the combined results from the maternal language analyses and the child comprehension analyses provided strong support for the claim that the children's initial categories are based on the form-function principle, rather than on linguistic input.

Initial Category Evolution

Child-basic categories that differ from the correspond-ponding adult-basic categories eventually must evolve to conform to the adult standard. As a first step, there are three general possibilities which are based on two factors. The first factor involves whether or not the appropriate category for the to-be-assigned object already is included in the child's repertoire. The second factor involves whether or not the to-be-assigned object already is assigned to a different category.

To illustrate these possibilities, consider the situation of a spherical candle that a child is about to assign to a candle category. In the first case, the child does not yet have a candle category, and spherical candles already are included in another category (presumably ball). In this case, the child's ball category is overextended relative to the adult ball category. In the second case, the child already has a candle category, but spherical candles are not included in this category or in any other one. In this case, the child's candle category is underextended relative to the adult category. In the third case, the child already has a candle category, but spherical candles are not included. Instead, spherical candles are included in ball. In this case the child's candle category is both underextended and overextended relative to the adult category.[1] Because the first case is by far the most likely to obtain (Mervis, 1984), only this case will be considered in the present chapter. (For consideration of the other two cases, see Mervis, 1984, 1987, 1988).

The evolution process depends on the child noticing new form-function correlations.[2] Thus, during the initial category evolution phase, the child acts according to an informal theory derived from the form-function principle. In particular, the child assigns a child-basic-only object to an additional newly formed category only if he or she is given concrete evidence of a new form-function attribute correlation.

Identification of New Form-Function Correlations - Indications of the presence of a new (i.e., previously unnoticed) correlation may occur in several different ways; as part of all of these, the adult generally provides the adult-appropriate name for the object. As one possibility, the important attribute might be indicated by the child. The adult would be likely to respond by acknowledging the attribute that the child had indicated and then labeling the object with its adult-basic name. For example, if the child pointed out the wick of a spherical candle to an adult, the adult probably would respond by commenting on the wick and its function and then labeling the object, "candle."

Alternatively, an adult may point out the important attributes. This may be accomplished in three ways. First, the adult can show the child a critical form attribute and/or demonstrate a critical function attribute of the object, that serve to make it a member of its adult-basic category. At the same time, the adult may provide a verbal description of these attributes. For an example, the adult might run a finger along the slot of a round bank, drop in a coin, and tell the child that this is a slot into which you put money. Second, the adult may show and/or demonstrate critical attributes to the child, without a verbal description. Third, the adult may provide only a verbal description. In all cases, the adult also provides the adult-basic name for the object.

Finally, the adult may label the object with its adult-basic name without either an implied request from the child or some form of explanation. The use of an adult-basic label alone constitutes an implicit statement of the existence of attributes that make the object a member of the named category.

Effectiveness of Adult Category Introduction Strategies - Given the informal theory which governs the early stages of category evolution, one would expect that the most effective methods of introduction of the adult-basic name would involve a clear indication of the form-function correlation on which the new category should be based. Among the methods of adult indication, the most explicit indication involves a concrete illustration of relevant form attributes and the correlated function attributes, accompanied by a verbal description. Use of a concrete illustration without a verbal description or a verbal description without a concrete illustration should be less effective, because the correlation is not made as explicit. The concrete illustration method should be more effective than the verbal description method for very young children, because these children are more oriented to objects and action than to language. Finally, use of the adult-basic name alone is extremely unlikely to be effective. The metacognition necessary to realize that the use of a new label implies the existence of a new form-function correlation is relatively sophisticated. As children's cognitive and linguistic skills increase, the effectiveness of the verbal description and label-only strategies should increase; see Mervis (1984, 1987) for a discussion.

The results of the longitudinal study support this position in its broad outlines. A summary of these results is presented here; for a more detailed description, see Mervis and Mervis (in press). Because relatively few cases of certain strategies occur, the four strategies were combined into two more general strategies, according to whether or not a concrete illustration was provided. For the children with Down Syndrome, virtually all of the cases in which new labels for the child-basic-only objects were learned involved objects initially included in the child-basic ball category. In every case, initial comprehension of the new label followed a maternal illustration of attributes crucial to the object's adult-appropriate category assignment. In most cases, a verbal description accompanied the illustration. For the normally developing children, new labels generally were learned for child-basic-only members from all three child-basic categories. In 74% of the cases, the mother had provided an appropriate illustration during the play session immediately prior to the child's comprehension of the adult-basic label. In almost all cases of illustration, the mother also provided a verbal description of the relevant attributes. Furthermore, examination of the transcripts from prior sessions, beginning when the child demonstrated referential comprehension, indicated that illustrations were rare. For the normally developing children, the first case of comprehension following an illustration occurred four months before the first case without an illustration. The mean age at comprehension following an illustration was more than three months less than the mean age at comprehension without an illustration.

These results indicate that maternal illustration of crucial attributes that make an object a member of its adult-basic category generally provides a sufficient basis for comprehension of adult-basic name for a child-basic-only object. This evidence, however, is correlational; no manipulation of the input to the child was possible. To provide direct experimental evidence concerning the relative effectiveness of various maternal strategies for introduction of the adult-basic label for a child-basic-only object, Banigan and Mervis (in press) conducted a cross-sectional study with normally developing 24-month-olds as subjects. The children first were pretested to ensure that they included the relevant objects in the predicted child-basic categories and did not comprehend or produce the adult-basic labels for these objects. Each child was then assigned to one of four conditions, corresponding to the four strategies outlined above. Children were given input regarding six adult-basic labels. After training, comprehension and production testing of both the child-basic and the adult-basic names occurred, using objects that differed from those in the pretest and training phases. The results of the comprehension tests indicated that the illustration-description condition was significantly more effective than any of the other conditions, that the illustration condition was more effective than either of the other two conditions, and that there was no difference in performance between the description condition and the label-only condition. Performance in the last two was quite poor. Results for production were virtually identical. Thus, the results provide strong support for the importance of illustrations, optimally accompanied by verbal descriptions, in helping very young children to learn the adult-basic label and begin to form a new category for an object previously included only in its child-basic category.

Initial Nonexclusivity of Basic Level Categories - The informal theory governing initial category evolution allows for the simultaneous assignment of an object to two or more categories that are mutually exclusive by adult standards. In fact, objects can belong to as many basic level categories as meet the requirements of the form-function principle. For example, a young child could consider a spherical candle to be both a candle and a ball.

This simultaneous assignment provision contrasts with principles proposed by other researchers. For example, both Markman's (1987) exclusivity principle and Tversky and Hemenway's (1984) mutual exclusivity principle for basic level categories have been proposed to hold from the time categorization begins. In addition, Clark's (1983, 1987) contrast principle often is considered to preclude simultaneous assignment. This principle does not need to; Clark has argued only that two words should not have identical meanings, not that there can be no overlap between them. However, the examples cited in support of this principle include instances of mutual exclusivity taken from early diary studies.

The available systematically collected data are consistent with the informal initial evolution theory. The data from the longitudinal study provide strong support, based on the comprehension tests administered on the day a child first comprehended the adult-basic name for a child-basic-only object. Membership in the old and new categories initially overlapped in 93% of the test cases for the normally developing children with Down Syndrome and in 96% of the test cases for the normally developing children (Mervis, 1984). Banigan and Mervis (in press) also found initial overlap in 96% of the test cases for normally developing 24-year-olds. Preliminary analyses of the diary data from my son Ari indicate further support (Mervis, 1987). Furthermore, Merriman (1987) has reanalyzed the diary data formerly considered to support mutual exclusivity (e.g., Clark, 1973) and has found several cases of nonexclusivity. Finally, Merriman and Bowman (1987) have completed a series of experiments which indicate that 2-year-olds do not yet honor the mutual exclusivity principle, although 3 1/2-year-olds do.

Informal Theories of Category Labels - As I have indicated above, very young children ignore linguistic input that is contradictory to their cognitively established categories. However, these children must attend to the linguistic input enough to assign names to their already established categories. Two informal theories are particularly useful for determining labels.

Words Refer to Object Categories - An important assumption underlying all theories of early lexical development is that very young children initially behave according to the informal theory that when a new word is used in reference to an object whose name is unknown, that word refers to the object as a whole rather than to a part or attribute of that object or an action performed by the object. Furthermore, these children assume that the new name refers to all the members of the category to which that object has been assigned (Mervis, 1987, 1988; for related proposals, see Dockrell & Campbell, 1986; Markman & Hutchinson, 1984).

Several examples consistent with this informal theory were reported, illustrating the use of adjectives, interjections, and verbs as object labels. Velleman (1987) reported several instances from her longitudinal study of mother-child interaction. One of these was produced by a child with Down Syndrome. When Jane (a pseudonym) initially learned the word "hi," she assumed it meant "telephone." One of the normally developing children who participated in the study made the same assumption. Hoffman (1968; cited in Macnamara, 1982) reported that when his son first learned the word "hot," he assumed it meant "stove." My son Ari's early vocabulary development also provided several instances (Mervis, 1987). For example, Ari initially believed "hot" meant "cup," "more" meant "juice," and "tickle" meant "fish." There was no evidence in any of these reports that object names ever were misinterpreted to refer to anything other than whole objects.

Laurel Long and I conducted an experimental test of this assumption, using specially designed artificial stimuli (Long & Mervis, 1987). In this study the experimenter pointed directly at a part of an object at the same time as she provided a nonsense word as a label. She then removed the original object and placed three additional objects in front of the child. One object had the same overall shape as the initial object but did not have the part that was labeled, one object had a different overall shape but had the labeled part in the same position as in the original object, and one object had neither the original overall shape nor the original part. The child was asked to show the experimenter the [label]. The results indicated that 18-month-olds, 24-month-olds, and 4-year-olds all behaved according to the informal object category as the referent theory; the label was treated as the name for the category to which the whole object belonged, rather than for the indicated part.

Salient Units are Object Names - The second informal theory relevant to the behavior of very young children when trying to determine the names for already established categories is that the most salient unit in an utterance probably is the name of the object referred to. This informal theory is superordinate to a series of principles proposed by Peters (1985) and Slobin (1973, 1985) for extracting linguistic units from the speech stream. For example, some of the principles which Peters has proposed to guide the young child's determination of which parts of an utterance are salient include attending to units that are bounded by silence, attending to units that have separate intonation contours, attending to units that are stressed, and attending to units that are at the end of utterances. To the extent that these principles converge on the same unit, the saliency of that unit is greatly increased. In English motherese, these principles tend to converge on the last word in an utterance. This convergence is appropriate for English; in speech to children who are just beginning to talk, object names tend to occur in utterance-final position.

The convergence of these principles on the last word in an utterance is most noticeable in the cases in which the last word is not actually an object name, but the child nevertheless adopts the word as the name for the object. Peters (1985) cites an example from R. Clark (1977) in which an adult produced the sentence, "That's an elephant, isn't it?" and the child then called elephants "intit" for several weeks, despite numerous attempts by adults to correct him. The data from Ari's early vocabulary acquisition provide several additional instances (see Mervis, 1987). The examples cited above in support of the informal object category as referent theory also fit the informal salient unit theory; in all cases, the word that was mistaken for an object name consistently occurred in utterance-final position. Several other instances that fit the salient unit principle also were noted. For example, Ari initially called all animals whose names were introduced in utterances that included their characteristic sounds in utterance-final position by their sounds, rather than by their names. However, in cases in which the sounds were introduced along with the label, but the label occurred in the utterance-final position, Ari called the object by its label, rather than its sound.

First Words

In the previous section, I discussed a few of the informal theories that ultimately will serve as basic components of an explanatory theory of early lexical development. These informal theories have direct implications for the development of intervention programs concerned with early language development. From the perspective of intervention, several other aspects of early lexical development also deserve attention. In the next three, relatively brief, sections, the focus will be on those aspects for which the data from the longitudinal study are

available. The present section is concerned with children's first object names. The next is concerned with the
relationship between cognitive development and early language development. The third is concerned with maternal
language input and early lexical development.

Choice of Initial Objects to Name - When children begin
to talk, the words they produce are remarkably consistent. These words are not a random sample of those used
in child-addressed speech. Initial object names, whether
produced by children with Down Syndrome or normally developing children, are concentrated on a limited subset
of categories: food, clothing, animals, people, vehicles,
toys, household items used in daily routines, and eventually body parts (Clark, 1979; Gillham, 1979; Nelson,
1973). Even within this subset, the particular exemplars
chosen are consistent for the two groups. For example,
within the clothing category, both groups of children
produced "shoe" and "sockie" well before "shirt" and
"pants." In Gillham's (1979) longitudinal study, 83% of
the object words produced by at least half of the children with Down Syndrome in their first 50 words were also
included in the first 50 words of the normally developing
children. The basis for these similarities in choice of
early words is children's interest in objects that either
move independently or can be manipulated by the child
(see Nelson, 1973).

Priority of Basic Level Names - Basic level categories
are more fundamental than categories at other hierarchical levels (Rosch, el al., 1976). The basic level is the
most cognitively efficient level; it is the most general
level at which the category members have similar overall
shapes and at which a person uses similar motor actions
for interacting with category members. Attribute correlations are most apparent at the basic level. Therefore,
children would be expected to acquire basic level categories prior to categories at other hierarchical levels.
    The available data from both normally developing child-
ren and children with Down Syndrome support the primacy
of the basic level. The object names included in early
vocabularies of 47 normally developing children described
in turn-of-the-century diary studies almost all corre-

spond to basic level categories (Mervis, 1983). All of the object names listed by Gillham (1979) for his subjects who had Down Syndrome are names for basic level categories. In our longitudinal study, all object names produced by the children with Down Syndrome were at the basic level. There was little evidence of comprehension of subordinate level categories, and in all cases, the child previously had comprehended the object's basic level name. (Superordinate level names were not tested.) Even after the children know more than one name for an object, the basic level name is preferred by both children with Down Syndrome (Tager-Flusberg, 1986)[3] and normally developing children (Rosch, et al., 1976).

Relationship between Cognitive Development and Early Vocabulary Development

The results of several studies of older children and adults with Down Syndrome indicated that their level of language development, for both vocabulary and syntax, was less than would be expected based on their cognitive level (e.g., Evans & Hampson, 1969, Lyle, 1959; 1960; Share, 1975; Thompson, 1963). The only available data regarding very young children with Down Syndrome derive from our longitudinal study. Below, I summarize these data; for a more detailed description, see Cardoso-Martins, Mervis, and Mervis (1985).

Cognitive Level at the Emergence of Language - To determine the children's cognitive levels at the emergence of referential comprehension and production, two sets of measures were used. The first was estimated mental age, derived from the child's score on the mental scale of the Bayley (1969) test. The second was level of sensorimotor cognitive development. This level was determined separately for object permanence and means-ends relations, based on the stage which is represented by the most advanced item passed on the relevant Uzgiris and Hunt (1975) subscale. Dunst's (1980) stage assignments were used.

For both measures, the cognitive abilities of the two groups of children at the emergence of language were very similar. The mean mental age at the onset of referential comprehension was 14.5 months for the children with Down Syndrome and 13.8 months for normally developing children. At the onset of referential production, the mean mental ages were 18.9 months and 19.5 months. At the onset of referential comprehension, there were about half of the children in each group that were in stage 5 of object permanence development; the remaining children were in stage 6. All children were in stage 5 of means-ends relations development. At the onset of referential production, all children were in stage 6 of object permanence development. All but one child in each group was in stage 5 of means-ends relations development; the remaining children were in stage 6. These sensorimotor stages are consistent with those previously reported for these language landmarks (e.g., Chapman, 1978; Corrigan, 1978; Folger & Leonard, 1978; Ingram, 1978; Ramsey, 1978).

Vocabulary Sizes at Different Levels of Cognitive Development - When the vocabulary sizes of the children at different levels of cognitive development were compared, differences between the two groups emerged. For object permanence, the children with Down Syndrome comprehended significantly fewer object names than normally developing children upon complete attainment of stage 5 and complete attainment of stage 6. Upon completion of stage 6, the children with Down Syndrome also produced significantly fewer object names than the normally developing children. For means-ends relations, the children with Down Syndrome comprehended significantly fewer object names than the normally developing children upon complete attainment of stage 5. Comparisons for complete attainment of stage 6 could not be made because several of the children with Down Syndrome did not reach this landmark during the study.

No differences between the two groups of children were apparent when vocabulary sizes at various mental ages were compared. However, comparisons were possible only to about age 20 months. The data from a larger study of 81 children with Down Syndrome (Schnell, 1984; Strominger, Winkler, & Cohen, 1984), when compared to available norms for normally developing children (Smith, 1926), suggest that dramatic differences may exist at a mental age of 21

months. (The analyses leading to this conclusion are reported in detail in Mervis, in press.) Normally developing children generally begin their vocabulary spurt by
age 21 months (Anisfeld, 1984). Age at complete attainment of object permanence and the onset of the vocabulary
spurt are very strongly correlated for normally developing children (Gopnik & Meltzoff, 1987). Thus, it appears
that an important reason for the large discrepancy in vocabulary size between the two groups, even when they are
equated on mental age or sensorimotor cognitive development, is that normally developing children begin their
vocabulary spurt at a younger mental age and cognitive
level than the children with Down Syndrome.

The difference between the two groups of children in
rate of vocabulary development probably is due in part to
specific cognitive deficits that children with Down Syndrome may have. Learning vocabulary necessarily requires
use of memory. Thus, problems in storing and retrieving
information, which individuals with Down Syndrome appear
to have (Bilovsky & Share, 1975; Dodd, 1975; McDade &
Adler, 1980), would be likely to hinder vocabulary acquisition. At the same time, differences in maternal speech
may contribute to the differences in rate of vocabulary
acquisition. Several such potential differences are considered in the next section. An additional important potential difference concerns the likelihood that the mother will use the most effective strategies for teaching
new vocabulary. The data from our longitudinal study suggest that mothers of children with Down Syndrome may be
less likely than mothers of normally developing children
to provide concrete illustrations when introducing new
labels to their child.

Linguistic Input and Early Lexical Development

In this section, I consider the similarities and differences in maternal linguistic input to children with
Down Syndrome and normally developing children, regarding both maternal labeling practices and responses to
child labels and also general features that often are
considered in studies of motherese. I then consider the
potential role of linguistic input in determining the

child's rate of vocabulary development relative to cognitive development.

Labeling Strategies - In the course of interacting with
their children, mothers have frequent opportunites to
label objects and to respond to the labels their child
uses. In this section, I first consider maternal labels
for the child-basic-only objects. I then consider maternal disagreements with the child's use of child-basic
names for these objects. The results for the normally
developing children are described in more detail in
Mervis and Mervis (in press).

Maternal Labels - As mentioned previously, mothers of the
prelinguistic children with Down Syndrome have been found
to be less likely to use child-basic labels than mothers
of normally developing children matched for mental age or
linguistic level (Cardoso-Martins & Mervis, 1985). In the
longitudinal study, the mothers of the children with Down
Syndrome were much less likely than mothers of normally
developing children to label objects with their child-
basic names on the day that the child first demonstrated
comprehension of the child-basic label (Mervis, 1984). In
this section, I consider patterns of maternal object labeling over time. These patterns contrast with those at
the time of first comprehension of child-basic labels.

Adjustments as a function of child knowledge of relevant
adult-basic label - Maternal use of adult-basic labels
for child-basic-only objects often predominates from the
beginning, even though mothers frequently use child-basic
labels as well (see Mervis & Mervis, in press, for an explanation). However, if mothers are sensitive to their
child's knowledge of the adult-basic names of objects,
mothers would be expected to adjust their labeling strategies as a function of their child's linguistic knowledge. Thus, maternal use of the adult-basic label for a
child-basic-only object should increase once the child
comprehends that label and should increase again after
the child is able to produce it.
    The data from the transcripts of the play sessions in
our longitudinal study are consistent with this pattern.
Both groups of mothers used a significantly greater

proportion of adult-basic labels[4] for child-basic-only
objects after their child had comprehended the relevant
adult-basic label than before its comprehension. The
mothers of the normally developing children again increased this proportion significantly after the child
produced the relevant adult-basic label. This analysis
could not be performed for the mothers of the children
with Down Syndrome because too few of these children produced adult-basic labels for child-basic-only objects.
Further analyses indicated that the significant increases
in proportion of adult-basic labels are not due simply to
increases over time (e.g., as a function of the child's
age), independent of the child's knowledge of the relevant adult-basic labels.

Stimulus effects on maternal use of adult-basic labels -
In deciding how to label a child-basic-only object, the
mothers might be expected to be sensitive to the relationship between the referent object and the adult category named by the child-basic label for the referent. If
so, maternal use of the adult-basic label for a child-
basic-only object should vary as a function of how dissimilar the referent object is to the best examples of
the adult-basic category named by the child-basic label.
For example, mothers should be more likely to call a ce-
ment mixer "truck" (as opposed to "car") than to call a
pickup truck "truck." The child-basic-only objects in
Table 1 are listed from least similar to most similar, as
determined based on judgments by a separate group of
adults.
    The data indicate that both groups of mothers were sen-
sitive to these differences in similarity. The dissimilarity orders and the orders based on proportion of the
maternal use of adult-basic label were identical or virtually identical for all three categories for the mothers
of the normally developing children and for two out of
the three categories for the mothers of the children with
Down Syndrome.

Maternal Disagreements - Analyses parallel to those performed for mothers' spontaneous use of adult-basic labels
also were performed for mothers' disagreements with their
child's use of a child-basic label to name a child-basic-

only object. In these cases, the responses of these two groups of mothers followed different patterns.

Adjustment as a function of a child knowledge of relevant adult-basic label - The probability that mothers would disagree with their child's use of a child-basic name for a child-basic-only object might also be expected to vary as a function of the child's knowledge of the object's adult-basic name. The proportion of disagreements should be very low prior to the child's comprehension of the adult-basic name. Increases in proportion of disagreement should occur following comprehension of the adult-basic name and then again following its production (see Mervis & Mervis, in press).

The data from the longitudinal study are consistent with this pattern only for the mothers of the normally developing children. These mothers disagreed with their child's label slightly less than 10% of the time prior to the child's comprehension of the relevant adult-basic label. The proportion of disagreement increased significantly following comprehension of this label, and then increased again (although not significantly) following its production. Once again, these differences could not be attributed to increases in disagreement over time, independent of child knowledge of the relevant labels. The mothers of the children with Down Syndrome disagreed with their child 25% of the time prior to comprehension of the relevant adult-basic label. The proportion increased, but not significantly, following first comprehension. Overall, the mothers of the children with Down Syndrome disagreed with their labels 35% of the time. In contrast, despite their children's greater knowledge of adult-basic labels, the mothers of the normally developing children disagreed only 16% of the time.

Stimulus effects on maternal disagreement - In deciding whether or not to disagree with their child's label, the mothers might be expected to take into account how similar the referent object is to other objects appropriately labeled by the word the child used. If so, maternal disagreement should vary as a function of the dissimilarity of the referent object to the best examples of the adult-basic category named by the child-basic label. The more

dissimilar   the referent object, the more likely the mother   should be to disagree. This pattern was upheld for all
three   categories for the mothers of the normally developing   children but   not   for any of the categories for the
mothers of the children with Down Syndrome.

Maternal   Linguistic Interaction Style - Maternal linguistic   style   often   has been assumed to affect rate of language   development.   In   discussion of rate of acquisition
of   language   in   general (rather than rate of acquisition
of   specific   aspects   of   syntax), two overlapping dimensions   were   hypothesized   to   play   a crucial role. Cross
(1978)   has   suggested   that mothers who adopt a semantically   contingent   style -- who usually comment on what the
child   is   doing   or   has   said -- provide a more adequate
linguistic   environment   than mothers who adopt a non-con-
tingent   strategy.   McDonald   and   Pien (1982) have argued
that   mothers   who   adopt a conversational-eliciting style
provide   a more adequate linguistic environment than mothers   who   adopt a directive style. In this section, I discuss   the   relevant maternal speech data from our longitudinal   study.   I   first   consider the similarities and the
differences   between   the   two   groups   of mothers. I then
consider   the potential effects of maternal speech on rate
of   vocabulary acquisition by children with Down Syndrome.
These   topics   are   discussed   in   more detail in Cardoso-
Martins and Mervis (1984) and Mervis (in press).

Maternal   Linguistic   Style: Correlational   Analyses - To
consider   linguistic   styles of the two groups of mothers,
their   language   was   compared   for each of five different
play   sessions.   At each session, the two groups of children   had   similar estimated mental ages and similar receptive   and   productive   vocabulary sizes. The results indicated   that the mothers of the children with Down Syndrome
were   both more directive and less semantically contingent
than   the mothers of the normally developing children. The
mothers   of   the children with Down Syndrome were significantly   more likely to use several language features characteristic   of both the directive and noncontingent styles
of   interaction: requests   for   an action, prompts for an
action,   and overall use of directives. These mothers also
were   significantly less likely to use several of the fea-

tures characteristic of both the conversational-eliciting and semantically contingent styles: the action-reflective questions, verbalization-reflective questions, low constraint questions, positive feedback for the child's action, positive feedback for the child's verbalization, and overall positive feedback. However, they were significantly more likely to use one feature characteristic of both these styles: vocalization-reflective question. Finally, the mothers of children with Down Syndrome were significantly less likely to ask test questions and significantly more likely to provide negative feedback for vocalization. These features are associated with both the directive style and the semantically contingent style.

Maternal Linguistic Style: Partial Correlation Analyses - The results of the previous analyses indicate that the mothers of the children with Down Syndrome tended to use a noncontingent and generally conversational-eliciting style. In the present context, this difference would be important if early acquisition of vocabulary was affected by maternal use of features associated with a particular style of interaction. The results of time-lag partial correlation analyses suggest that this may well be the case.

Because there are a small number of subjects, the results should be considered suggestive. Nevertheless, a consistent pattern emerged, suggesting that semantic contingency was more important than conversation-eliciting for vocabulary acquisition. Two features were significantly negatively correlated with rate of child receptive or productive vocabulary acquisition: overall use of directives and real questions. Three features were significantly positively correlated with the rate of vocabulary acquisition: positive feedback for the child's verbalization, overall positive feedback, and negative feedback for the child's vocalization.

The basis for the positive impact of language features that generally are semantically contingent and the negative impact of language features that generally are noncontingent is clear. The features associated with semantic contingency include reference to the object of the child's attention, which should facilitate vocabulary acquisition by making the relationship between the object name and its referent particularly salient. In contrast, features associated with noncontingency generally do not make the word-referent relationship clear to the child. The results of two related studies are relevant. Roth (1987) found that mothers of normally developing children who use a noncontingent style also tend to take a relatively long time to respond to their child's vocalizations and verbalizations. Thus, even when semantically contingent responses are provided, the child is more likely to have changed his or her focus of attention, so that the relation between word and referent is not salient. Velleman (1987), using a somewhat different definition of contingency, found a very consistent difference between mothers of children with Down Syndrome and mothers of normally developing children. When the mothers of normally developing children produced contingent responses to vocalizations and verbalizations, these mothers tended to repeat what their child said as part of their response. In contrast, when mothers of children with Down Syndrome produced contingent responses, these mothers tended not to repeat what their child said. In a large number of cases, the utterances to which the mother was responding included phonemes that were part of the name of the object to which the child was attending. This difference points to another potential problem with the style adopted by the mothers of the children with Down Syndrome. Even when their mothers produce contingent responses, these responses often do not include the name of the object to which the child is attending. Input including the label is crucial for vocabulary acquisition.

Basis for Differences in Maternal Linguistic Style - Differences in maternal interactional intent provide a partial explanation for the differences in linguistic style found between the two groups of mothers. Bell (1964; Bell & Harper, 1977) and Jones (1977; 1979; 1980) have found that mothers of young normally developing children tend to follow the child's initiatives when interacting with the child. Thus, these mothers would be expected to use a conversational-eliciting or semantically contingent style of interaction. In contrast, mothers of children with handicaps, including Down Syndrome, are much less likely to follow their child's initiatives, and much more likely to expect the child to follow their initiatives. Jones (1980) has suggested that mothers of handicapped children may believe that their child needs more direction than the normally developing children do. These mothers may, therefore, be more motivated than mothers of normally developing children to direct their child's behavior.

Child factors also are important. The differences between the two groups of mothers reflect, in part, adaptive responses by the mothers of the children with Down Syndrome to their children's handicaps. Children with Down Syndrome often have been described as more passive and less socially responsive than normally developing children (e.g., Buckhalt, Rutherford, & Goldberg, 1978; Jones, 1977; 1979; 1980). In addition, children with Down Syndrome do not use language as often as the normally developing children do (Cardoso-Martins, 1984; Cardoso-Martins, Mervis, & Mervis, 1983; Gillham, 1979). It is possible, therefore, that mothers of children with Down Syndrome feel less motivated than mothers of normally developing children to try to elicit their child's participation in the conversation.

The results of an analysis of the "What's that?" questions asked by the mothers in the longitudinal study support this possibility. When children first begin to talk, the only way that their mothers can elicit "conversation" is to ask this type of question. The "What's that?" questions asked by the mothers of the children with Down Syndrome were significantly less likely than those asked by the mothers of the normally developing children to refer to objects whose labels were included in the child's productive vocabulary. Of the "What's that?" questions that were addressed to the children with Down Syndrome, 54% were asked in reference to an object for which the child could produce an appropriate label; the corresponding figure for the normally developing children was 69%. Interestingly, the percentage of "What's that?" questions that were answered correctly, given that the child could produce an appropriate label, was virtually identical for the two groups: 14% for the children with Down Syndrome and 15% for the normally developing children. Thus, when given the opportunity, the children with Down Syndrome were as likely as the normally developing children to hold up their end of the conversation.

Suggestions for Application

The material presented in this chapter provides the basis for several suggestions for facilitating the conceptual and lexical development of young children with Down
Syndrome. In this section, I outline the most important
of these applications regarding acquisition of concrete
object categories and their referents. Once a variety of
such categories and their names has been acquired, introduction of the verb and attribute categories and their
names can begin, based on the same procedures.

Intervention specifically related to conceptual development probably should begin during late stage 4 or early
stage 5 of the sensorimotor period, when infants become
sensitive to and interested in the properties of objects
that are relevant to category assignment. For example,
infants become interested in the roundness and rollabil-
ity of a ball, whereas previously they were interested in
only its more general properties, such as that it could
be banged or mouthed. It is important that the child have
available a variety of objects that have easily discover-
able functions and corresponding form attributes. The
availability of such objects will facilitate the child's
formation of child-basic categories, consistent with the
informal correlated attributes and the form-function theories. Referential comprehension can be expected to begin
during stage 5 of the sensorimotor period, at a mental
age of about 12-15 months.

The categories initially chosen for intervention should
be categories of whole objects, so they fit the child's
informal object category as referent theory. Basic level
categories of objects that can move independently or can
be manipulated by the child should be used. The best objects to include are realistic representations of good
examples of the category (see Hupp & Mervis, 1982; Mervis
& Pani, 1980).

Intervention should take the form of playing, rather
than teaching, and should take place throughout the day,
during routine family activities as well as special play-
times with the child. The adult should follow the child's
initiatives if the child is actively involved with an object. If the child is not involved with an object, then
the adult should choose a toy that the child is likely to

find interesting and show the child the object's special
form features or its function. It is important to label
the toy while the child is still attending to it (see
also Tomasello & Farrar, 1987). Labels should be included
in phrases or short sentences, in a manner that fits the
child's informal salient unit theory (e.g., in final,
stressed position). Children who are just beginning to
acquire language will need many repetitions of a word,
both within an interaction and across interactions with
relevant objects, before comprehending the object name.
Once the child appears to comprehend the name, then the
child's category corresponding to the word can be determined informally, for example by asking the child for objects within the context of play. Errors that extend beyond the boundaries of the child-basic category (e.g.,
retrieving a car when asked for a ball) should be corrected, but at this stage, errors within boundaries of
the child-basic category (e.g., retrieving a round bead
when asked for a ball) should not. The latter type of
error is expected and quite reasonable, given the attributes the child is likely to notice. An informal determination of whether or not an object would be appropriate
for a child-basic category can be made by deciding what
the function(s) of category members is for the child and
then deciding whether the relevant object can have the
function, even if it is not appropriate by adult standards, and whether the object has a shape quite similar to
other members of the category. Positive feedback for correct comprehension is an important part of semantic contingency and as such is crucial to the success of the intervention.

Referential production can be expected to begin during
late stage 5 or stage 6 of the sensorimotor period, at a
mental age of about 16-20 months. As Gillham (1979) has
pointed out, the most effective way to facilitate production is not to force the child to imitate words, but instead to ensure that comprehension of the word is well
established. Thus, the continuation of the same programs
should facilitate production as well as comprehension.

Eventually, adults should begin to teach the child the
correct names for objects that the child is including incorrectly (by adult standards) in his or her child-basic
categories. The child is ready for this step when he or

she is able to appreciate the attributes that make the object a member of its adult-basic category. The new labels should be introduced using the concrete illustration plus verbal description strategy, to provide the type of input most likely to fit with the child's informal category evolution principles. In addition, the adult should take advantage of situations that arise spontaneously, in which the child appears to notice one of these attributes on his or her own (e.g., the child is fingering the wick on a round candle which is included in his or her _ball_ category). If the child is ready, procedures that fit the child's informal category evolution theory should make it relatively easy to teach adult-basic names to the child. However, even after the child learns these names, he or she will not automatically exclude the object from its previous category. Again, this is expected based on the typical developmental pattern and should not be a source of concern.

Once comprehension of the adult-basic name of an object is well established, the adult may want to begin to correct the child's use of the child-basic name in reference to the object. Correction, if used, should follow the concrete illustration plus verbal description strategy. Correction should not be insisted on if the child indicates disagreement, for example by playing with the object as if it were a member of the child-basic category, by repeating the name of the child-basic category, or by acting upset. Positive feedback for the correct use of the new name is important.

The strategies parents use spontaneously vary widely, as does parental awareness of their own patterns of interaction. The effectiveness of an intervention program of the type outlined would be enhanced if the people planning the intervention were aware of the strategies currently used by individual parents and their awareness of these strategies. In order to facilitate this process, Rae Banigan and I have begun developing a questionnaire concerning parent-child interaction patterns (Banigan & Mervis, 1987). Questions address such topics as decisions concerning what should be talked about, modes of introducing new labels, correction strategies, and enjoyment of interaction with the child. This questionnaire can be filled out both by the parent and a professional (e.g., a speech therapist) who is working with the child. The professional would base his or her responses on observation of interaction patterns of the parent-child dyad. From the results, both the strategies used by the parent and the parent's awareness of the strategies used can be determined. An individualized intervention program that is designed to facilitate parental implementation of the suggestions presented earlier in this section can then be developed.

Conclusion

The comparative study of the early lexical development of children with Down Syndrome and normally developing children has had substantial benefits. First, the detailed knowledge of the process of early lexical development by children with Down Syndrome has provided a basis for intervention guidelines designed to enhance this aspect of development. These guidelines were considered in the previous section. Second, the availability of comparative data has greatly increased our knowledge of universal aspects of early lexical development that transcend differences in intelligence. This paper concludes with a brief reiteration of some of these universals.

In this chapter, I have argued that children's early lexical development is guided by implicit informal theories and by background knowledge, much as categorization by adults is. Informal theories concerning the importance of correlated attributes for categorization and the existence of correlations between form attributes and function attributes are among the earliest informal theories specifically relevant to category formation. I have argued that both children and adults categorize in accordance with these informal theories, although the categories formed may differ as a function of experience or expertise. The data presented support the use of such theories by very young children, whether or not they have Down Syndrome. Data from the children with Down Syndrome were particularly useful in demonstrating that early categories are based on informal theories such as those proposed rather than on the labels used by adults. For these children, the linguistic input at the time of first comprehension of category names almost always was consistent with the adult categorization scheme. Nevertheless, the children formed the predicted child-basic categories. Both groups of children honor the informal object category as referent theory, treating new labels for novel objects as though they refer to the entire object rather than to attributes, parts, or actions of the object. Although more data are needed, both groups of children appear to honor the informal salient unit theory, choosing the most salient word or phrase as the object name. Finally, the initial evolution of child-basic categories to begin to conform to the adult standard fits with the informal theory of early category evolution for both groups of children. As expected based on this informal theory, the mothers play an important role in initiating the evolution process. Children are most likely to acquire an adult-basic label for a child-basic-only object, and then begin to form a new category, following a concrete illustration and verbal description of the attributes crucial to the object's assignment to its adult-basic category. This pattern is especially strong for the children with Down Syndrome. Also in keeping with the informal evolution theory, children initially do not consider basic level categories to be mutually exclusive.

Further research on the early lexical development of children with Down Syndrome is needed, with particular focus on children at a slightly later point in development than the children who participated in the longitudinal study described in this chapter. This research will provide tests of later informal theories (e.g., Mervis, 1988), as well as a basis for revising and expanding the scope of the theory. Additional suggestions for intervention should result as well. The presently available theory and data, however, seem to provide a good start.

Acknowledgements

I thank the children and mothers who participated in the studies discussed in this chapter. I also thank my collaborators: Cindy Mervis, Claudia Cardoso-Martins, Rae Banigan, and Laurel Long. The theory presented in this chapter has been improved by discussions with John Pani.

The research and theorizing described in this paper were supported by the National Science Foundation, grants BNS 81-21169 and BNS 84-19036. Support for the longitudinal study also was provided by the Department of Education, grant DEG 008002485.

Footnotes

1. The fourth possibility formed by the intersection of the two factors does not constitute a case of evolution; the child has not yet assigned spherical candles to any category and does not yet have a candle category, so there is no category available to evolve.

The examples below, and the use of the phrases "adult-basic category" and "appropriate category," suggest that for overextended categories, category evolution involves a two step process: the second assignment for an initially incorrectly assigned object will be the correct assignment. In many cases, there are intermediate steps. For example, most children initially assign leopards to a kitty category, then to a tiger category, and finally to leopard (see Mervis, 1982). For predictions concerning which types of categories will involve a two step evolution process and which will involve intermediate steps, see Chapman and Mervis (1987).

2. In some cases, even though the child is unable to determine a new form-function correlation, the saliency of a new form attribute or a new function attribute may be great enough that the child chooses to begin to form a new category. Because the form information and function information generally are redundant, the adult-appropriate category still may result. However, it will be considerably easier for the child to acquire the adult-basic category if he or she is aware of and has the background knowledge to understand the relevant form-function correlation.

3. Tager-Flusberg's study included a group of mentally retarded children, half of whom had Down Syndrome. The performance of the children with Down Syndrome was the

136 Mervis

same as that of the other children in the group (Tager-Flusberg, personal communication).

4. In the analyses reported in this section, the dependent measure was the proportion of the adult-basic or subordinate labels, relative to all labels used. Subordinate labels were very rare.

REFERENCES

Anisfeld, M. (1984), Language development from birth to three. Hillsdale, NJ: Erlbaum.

Banigan, R. L., & Mervis, C. B. (1987, November). Mothers' perception of their communicative interactions. Paper presented at the annual convention of the American Speech, Language, and Hearing Society, New Orleans, LA.

Banigan, R. L., & Mervis, C. B. (in press). Role of adult input in young children's category evolution. II. An experimental study. Journal of Child Language.

Bayley, N. (1969). Bayley scales of infant development. New York: Psychological Corporation.

Bell, R. Q. (1964). The effect on the family of a limitation in coping ability in the child: A research approach and a finding. Merrill-Palmer Quarterly, 10, 129-142.

Bell, R. Q., & Harper, L. V. (1977). Child effects on adults. Hillsdale, NJ: Erlbaum.

Bilovsky, D., & Share, J. (1965). The ITPA and Down's Syndrome: An exploratory study. American Journal of Mental Deficiency, 70, 78-82.

Buckhalt, T. A., Rutherford, R. B., & Goldberg, K. E. (1978). Verbal and non-verbal interaction of mothers and their Down's syndrome and non-retarded infants. American Journal of Mental Deficiency, 72, 337-343.

Cardoso-Martins, C., & Mervis, C. B. (1984, July). Maternal speech to Down syndrome and normal children: Interaction styles. Paper presented at the Third International Congress for the Study of Child Language, Austin, TX.

Cardoso-Martins, C., & Mervis, C. B. (1985). Maternal speech to prelinguistic children with Down syndrome.

American Journal of Mental Deficiency, 89, 451-458.

Cardoso-Martins, C., Mervis, C. B., & Mervis, C. A. (1983, March). Early vocabulary acquisition by Down syndrome children: The relationship between language development and intellectual development. Paper presented at the Gatlinburg Conference on Research in Mental Retardation/Developmental Disabilities, Gatlinburg, TN.

Cardoso-Martins, C., Mervis, C. B., & Mervis, C. A. (1985). Early vocabulary acquisition by children with Down syndrome. *American Journal of Mental Deficiency*, 90, 177-184.

Carey, S. (1982). Semantic development: The state of the art. In E. Wanner & L. R. Gleitman (Eds.), *Language acquisition: The state of the art* (pp. 347-389). New York: Cambridge University Press.

Carey, S. (1985). *Conceptual Change in childhood*. Cambridge, MA: MIT Press.

Chapman, K., Leonard, L. B., & Mervis, C. B. (1986). The effects of feedback on young children's inappropriate word usage. *Journal of Child Language*, 13, 101-117.

Chapman, K. L., & Mervis, C. B. (1987). *Patterns of object-name extension in production*. Manuscript submitted for review.

Chapman, R. S. (1978). Comprehension strategies in children. In J. Kavanaugh & W. Strange (Eds.), *Speech and language in the laboratory, school, and clinic* (pp. 308-327). Cambridge, MA: MIT Press.

Chapman, R. S., & Thompson, J. (1980). What is the source of overextension errors in comprehension testing of two-year-olds? A response to Fremgen and Fay. *Journal of Child Language*, 7, 575-578.

Clark, E. V. (1973). What's in a word? On the child's acquisition of semantics in his first language. In T. E. Moore (Ed.), *Cognitive development and the acquisition of language*. New York: Academic Press.

Clark, E. V. (1977). First language acquisition. In J. Morton & J. C. Marshall (Eds.), *Psycholinguistics: Developmental and pathological*. Ithaca, NY: Cornell University Press.

Clark, E. V. (1979). Building a vocabulary: Word for objects, actions, and relations. In P. Fletcher & M. Garman (Eds.), *Language acquisition: Studies in first*

138 Mervis

language development (pp. 149-160). New York: Cambridge University Press.

Clark, E. V. (1983). Meaning and concepts. In J. H. Flavell & E. M. Markman (Eds.), *Handbook of child psychology*, vol. 3: *Cognitive development* (pp. 787-840) (gen. ed. P. H. Mussen). New York: Wiley.

Clark, E. V. (1987). The principle of contrast: A constraint on language acquisition. In B. MacWhinney (Ed.), *Mechanisms of language acquisition* (pp. 1-33). Hillsdale, NJ: Erlbaum.

Clark, R. (1977). What's the use of imitation? *Journal of Child Language*, 4, 341-358.

Corrigan, R. (1978). Language development as related to stage 6 object permanence development. *Journal of Child Language*, 5, 173-189.

Cross, T. G. (1978). Mothers' speech and its association with rate of linguistic development in young children. In N. Waterson & C. Snow (Eds.), *The development of communication* (pp. 199-216). New York: Wiley.

Dockrell, J., & Campbell, R. (1986). Lexical acquisition strategies in the preschool child. In S. A. Kuczaj II & M. D. Barrett (Eds.), *The development of word meaning* (pp. 121-154). New York: Springer Verlag.

Dodd, B. J. (1975). Recognition and reproduction of words by Down's syndrome and non-Down's syndrome retarded children. *American Journal of Mental Deficiency*, 80, 306-311.

Dougherty, J. W. D. (1978). Relativity and salience in categorization. *American Ethnologist*, 5, 66-80.

Dunst, C. J. (1980). *A clinical and educational manual for use with the Uzgiris and Hunt scales of infant development*. Baltimore: University Park Press.

Evans, D., & Hampson, M. (1969). The language of mongols. *British Journal of Disorders of Communication*, 3, 171-181.

Folger, M. K., & Leonard, L. B. (1978). Language and sensorimotor development during the early period of referential speech. *Journal of Speech and Hearing Research*, 21, 518-527.

Fremgen, A., & Fay, D. (1980). Overextensions in production and comprehension: A methodological clarification. *Journal of Child Language*, 7, 205-211.

Gillham, B. (1979). *The first words language programme*.

London: George Allen & Unwin.

Gopnik, A., & Meltzoff, A. (1987). The development of categorization in the second year and its relation to other cognitive and linguistic developments. Child Development, 58, 1523-1531.

Hupp, S. C. & Mervis, C. B. (1982). Acquisition of basic object categories by severely handicapped children. Child Development, 53, 760-767.

Ingram, D. (1978). Sensorimotor intelligence and language development. In A. Lock (Ed.), Action, gesture, and symbol: The emergence of language. New York: Academic Press.

Jones, O. H. M. (1977). Mother-child communication with pre-linguistic Down's syndrome and normal infants. In H. R. Schaffer (Ed.), Studies in mother-infant interaction (pp. 379-401). New York: Academic Press.

Jones, O. H. M. (1979). A comparison study of mother-child communication with Down Syndrome and normal infants. In H. R. Schaffer & J. Dunn (Eds.), The first year of life: Psychological and medical implications of early experience (pp. 175-195). New York: Wiley.

Jones, O. H. M. (1980). Prelinguistic communication skills in Down's syndrome and normal infants. In T. Field (Ed.), High risk infants and children: Adult and peer interactions (pp. 205-225). New York: Academic Press.

Keil, F. C. (1979). Semantic and conceptual development: An ontological perspective. Cambridge, MA: Harvard University Press.

Keil, F. C. (1987). Conceptual development and category structure. In U. Neisser (Ed.), Concepts and conceptual development: Ecological and intellectual factors in categorization. (pp. 175-200). London: Cambridge University Press.

Lyle, J. G. (1959). The effect of an institution environment upon the verbal development of imbecile children. I. Verbal intelligence. Journal of Mental Deficiency Research, 3, 122-128.

Lyle, J. G. (1960). The effect of an institution environment upon the verbal development of imbecile children. II. Speech and language. Journal of Mental Deficiency Research, 4, 1-13.

Macnamara, J. (1982). Names for things: A study of human

learning. Cambridge, MA: MIT Press.

Markman, E. M. (1987). How children constrain the possible meanings of words. In U. Neisser (Ed.), Concepts and conceptual development: Ecological and intellectual factors in categorization (pp.255-287). London: Cambridge University Press.

Markman, E. M., & Hutchinson, J. (1984). Children's sensitivity to constraints on word meaning: Taxonomic versus thematic relations. Cognitive Psychology, 16, 1-27.

McDade, H. L. & Adler, S. (1980). Down syndrome and short-term memory impairment: A storage or retrieval deficit? American Journal of Mental Deficiency, 84, 561-567.

McDonald, L., & Pien, D. (1982). Mother conversational behavior as a function of interactional intent. Journal of Child Language, 9, 337-358.

Merriman, W. E. (1987, April). Lexical contrast in toddlers: A reanalysis of the diary evidence. Paper presented at the biennial meeting of the Society for Research in Child Development, Baltimore, MD.

Merriman, W. E., & Bowman, L. L. (1987, April). Development studies of lexical contrast. Paper presented at the biennial meeting of the Society for Research in Child Development, Baltimore, MD.

Mervis, C. B. (1982, May). Mother-child interaction and early lexical development. Paper presented at the annual meeting of the Midwestern Psychological Association, Minneapolis, MN.

Mervis, C. B. (1983). Acquisition of a lexicon. Contemporary Educational Psychology, 8, 210-236.

Mervis, C. B. (1984). Early lexical development: The contributions of mother and child. In C. Sophian (Ed.), Origins of cognitive skills (pp. 339-370). Hillsdale, NJ: Erlbaum.

Mervis, C. B. (1985). On the existence of prelinguistic categories: A case study. Infant Behavior and Development, 8, 293-300.

Mervis, C. B. (1987). Child-basic object categories and early lexical development. In U. Neisser (Ed.), Concepts and conceptual development: Ecological and intellectual factors in categorization (pp.201-233).

Mervis, C. B. (1988). Early lexical development: The role of operating principles. Manuscript in preparation.

Mervis, C. B. (in press). Early conceptual development by children with Down syndrome. In D. Cicchetti & M. Beeghly (Eds.), Down syndrome: The developmental perspective. Cambridge: Cambridge University Press.

Mervis, C. B., & Canada, K. (1983). On the existence of competence errors in early comprehension: A reply to Fremgen & Fay and Chapman & Thomson. Journal of Child Language, 10, 431-440.

Mervis, C. B., & Long, L. M. (1987, April). Words refer to whole objects: Young children's interpretation of the referent of a novel word. Paper to be presented at the biennial meeting of the Society for Research in Child Development, Baltimore, MD.

Mervis, C. B. & Mervis, C. A. (1982). Leopards are kitty-cats: Object labeling by mothers for their 13-month-olds. Child Development, 53, 267-273.

Mervis, C. B., & Mervis, C. A. (in press). Role of adult input in young children's category evolution. I. An observational study. Journal of Child Language.

Mervis, C. B., & Pani, J. R. (1980). Acquisition of basic object categories. Cognitive Psychology, 12, 496-522.

Murphy, G. L. & Medin, D. L. (1985). The role of theories in conceptual coherence. Psychological Review, 92, 289-316.

Nelson, K. (1973). Structure and strategy in learning to talk. Monographs of the Society for Research in Child Development, 38(1-2 Serial No. 149).

Peters, A.M. (1985). Language segmentation: Operating principles for the perception and analysis of language. In D. I. Slobin (Ed.), The crosslinguistic study of language acquisition. Vol. 2: Theoretical issues (pp. 1029-1067). Hillsdale, NJ: Erlbaum.

Piaget, J. (1954). The construction of reality in the child. New York: Basic.

Ramsey, D. (1978). Object word spurt, handedness and object permanence in the infant. (Doctoral Dissertation, University of Denver, 1977). Dissertation Abstracts International, 38, 1147B.

Rosch, E., Mervis, C. B., Gray, W. D., Johnson, D. M., & Boyes-Braem, P. (1976). Basic objects in natural categories. Cognitive Psychology, 8, 382-439.

Roth, P. L. (1987). Temporal characteristics of maternal verbal styles. In K. E. Nelson & A. van K. (Eds.),

Children's Language Vol. 6 (pp.137-158). Hillsdale, NJ: Erlbaum.

Schnell, R. R. (1984). Psychomotor evaluation. In S. M. Pueschel (Ed.), The young child with Down syndrome (pp.207-226). New York: Human Sciences Press.

Share, J. B. (1975). Developmental progress in Down's syndrome. In R. Koch & F. F. de la Cruz (Eds.), Down's syndrome (mongolism): Research, prevention and management (pp. 78-86). New York: Brunner/Mazel.

Slobin, D. I. (1973). Cognitive prerequisites for the development of grammar. In C. A. Ferguson & D. I. Slobin (Eds.), Studies of child language development. New York: Holt, Rinehart and Winston.

Slobin, D. I. (1985). Crosslinguistic evidence for the language making capacity. In D. I. Slobin (Ed.), The crosslinguistic study of language acquisition. Vol. 2: Theoretical issues (pp. 1157-1256). Hillsdale, NJ: Erlbaum.

Smith, M. E. (1926). An investigation of the development of the sentence and the extent of vocabulary in young children. University of Iowa Studies of Child Welfare, 3, No. 5.

Strominger, A. Z., Winkler, M. R., & Cohen, L. T. (1984). Speech and language evaluation. In S. M. Pueschel (Ed.), The young child with Down syndrome (pp. 253-261). New York: Human Sciences Press.

Tager-Flusberg, H. (1986). Constraints on the representation of word meaning: Evidence from autistics and mentally retarded children. In M. Barrett & S. A. Kuczaj II (Eds.), The development of word meaning (pp. 69-81). New York: Springer-Verlag.

Terman, L. M., & Merrill, M. A. (1960). Measuring intelligence. Boston: Houghton-Mifflin.

Thompson, M. M. (1963). Psychological characteristics relevant to the education of the pre-school mongoloid child. Mental Retardation, 1, 148-151.

Tomasello, M., & Farrar, M. (1986). Joint attention and early language. Child Development, 57, 1454-1463.

Tversky, B., & Hemenway, K. (1984). Objects, parts, and categories. Journal of Experimental Psychology: General, 113, 169-193.

Uzgiris, I., & Hunt, J. McV. (1975). Assessment in infancy: Ordinal scales of psychological development.

Urbana: University of Illinois Press.

Velleman, S. (1987, October). Paper presented at the Boston University Language Development Conference, Boston, MA.

Younger, B. A., & Cohen, L. B. (1985). How infants form categories. In G. H. Bower (Ed.), The psychology of learning and motivation: Advances in research and theory (Vol. 19) (pp. 211-247). Orlando, FL: Academic Press.

Younger, B. A. & Cohen, L. B. (1986). Developmental change in infants' perception of correlations among attributes. Child Development, 57, 803-815.

4

THE EMERGENCE OF LANGUAGE SKILLS
IN YOUNG CHILDREN WITH DOWN SYNDROME

Lars Smith, Stephen von Tetzchner,
and Bjorg Michalsen
Institute of Psychology,
University of Oslo, P.O. Box 1094,
Blindern, 0317 Oslo 3, Norway

Down Syndrome is a condition which has often been assumed to affect all developmental processes simultaneously. Lenneberg (1967) suggested that "...in these cases
all (developmental) processes suffer alike, resulting in
a general 'stretching' of the developmental time scale,
... leaving the intercalation of motor and speech milestones intact" (p. 132). He wrote that the preservation
of synchrony between motor development and speech milestones in cases of Down Syndrome, seen against the background of a similar synchrony among normally developing
children, was strong evidence that language acquisition
is regulated by organic maturation. Lenneberg's study,
purporting to show that the onset of speech among children with Down Syndrome is determined by a delayed maturational schedule, has several shortcomings (cf., Evans,
1977). One part of his hypothesis, i.e., that the onset
of language is independent of environmental influence, is
no longer tenable. Even at the time when the maturational
hypothesis was formulated, potentially damaging evidence
existed. Thus, Stedman and Eichorn (1964), in their pioneering study of matched groups of young children with
Down Syndrome, raised at home or in an institutionalized
setting, had demonstrated that use and understanding of
speech were among the abilities that most clearly differ-
entiated between the groups of different background. More
recently, intervention programs have demonstrated that
the language delay typical of infants with Down Syndrome
can be selectively modified (Kysela, Hillyard, McDonald,

& Ahlsten-Taylor, 1981). The second part of Lenneberg's
maturational hypothesis, i.e., the one that deals with
the issue of synchronization between language development
and general motor development, may be harder to evaluate.
Studies demonstrating the role of the caretaking environment in the development of children with Down Syndrome
suggest caution in applying a main-effect maturational
model. Such a model postulates that the growth processes
within the individual, and the caretaking environment
exert independent influences on development (Sameroff &
Chandler, 1975). Usually a general provision is made to
the effect that the individual is raised in an 'adequate
environment', without specifying what is meant by such a
term. More plausibly, when one is going to make a prog-
nostic statement about developmental outcome, one should
try to specify how a given biomedical condition may have
different outcomes depending on differential environmental factors. This is the interactional point of view.
Other kinds of evidence, using repeated measures over
time of child and environmental factors, stress the plastic character of the milieu, and the individual as an
agent active in making its own environment. Accordingly,
one could view an anomaly, such as Down Syndrome, as "a
continuous malfunction in the organism-environment trans-
action across time which prevents the child from organizing his world adaptively" (Sameroff & Chandler, 1975, p.
235). Needless to say, such a transactional model does
not rule out the importance of maturational variance, but
rather stresses that such variance may operate by establishing differential conditions for the child's incidental learning and for the adult's system supporting the
child's acquisition of developmental skills. Actually,
the transactional model provides a clue as to how individual differences among children with a given biomedical
anomaly, such as Down Syndrome, may give rise to the extensive variance at the level of developmental outcome
that is observed for every major handicap. Such a view,
modified after Scarr and McCarthney's (1983) model of
behavioral development, is illustrated in Figure 1. The
diagram purports to show that the correlation between
children's and caregivers' behaviors may be explained by
a third factor, i.e., the children's biomedical "Eigen-
werts". A child's behaviors are to some extent a function

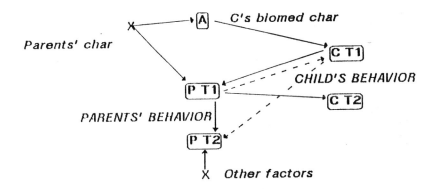

of its biomedical properties. Further, the child's behaviors influence, and are influenced by, the caregiver's behaviors across time. Some distinguishing features of the parents, like their genetic makeup or the prenatal environment which mothers provide, influence the child's characteristics. Similarly, adults' behaviors directed toward the child are to some extent influenced by the child's biomedical properties. The transactions which go on between the child and its caregiver are often simply expressed by the researcher as a set of correlations. But one may well ask what is the origin of such correlations. In the model presented here, behavior of the child and the parent are both influenced by the child's biomedical properties. The child's characteristics partly determine the child's behaviors as well as the adult's caretaking activities, and may thus explain much of the observed correlations. However, the biomedical particulars of the child are conceptually prior to the activities of the persons involved and must therefore be seen as causally related to both.

Evidence supporting such a transactional model in the study of the development of communication and language in the children with Down Syndrome has been hard to come by. This may be surprising, since young children with Down Syndrome are commonly seen as making an atypical contribution to the social interactions that are relevant to language learning. The aim of the present research was to elucidate the communicative and emergent language skills in young children with Down Syndrome while paying attention to aspects of their home environment that probably

interact with such skills in the transactional sense.
   In 1979 to 1980 13 Down Syndrome children were recruited to participate in a longitudinal study carried out in
Oslo, Norway. Ten of these children were followed to age
5 years, losing 3 to follow up after age 3. One of the
subjects was a mosaic, the rest were trisomy 21. Seven of
the children in the original sample had no medical complications. All of the subjects were living at home with
their parents, and most of them were integrated in regular day care centers. For certain purposes the data for
the group of Down Syndrome children and their parents
were compared with the data obtained on a sample of normally developing subjects, who, at the same time, were
followed up to age 3. At 5 years of age half of the
children with Down Syndrome scored at a level below 2.5
years, and half at the 2.5 years level of the McCarthy
scales of children's abilities.
   A first step to language probably takes place at about
nine months of age, when normally developing infants for
the first time seem to be aware of the direction of their
partners' attention (cf., Bates et al., 1979). Communicative skills are preceded by an ability to integrate attention toward object and person. The efforts of the infants to communicate in the last trimester of the first
year of life mainly have two different themes: (1) behaviors which may be seen as attempts to draw the caregiver's attention toward an object which the infant already
possesses and manipulates; or (2) behaviors on the part
of the child which are interpreted by the caregiver as
bids to cooperate in order to gain access to an object
which is beyond the child's reach. The emergence of such
skills will normally be facilitated under circumstances
when the child is accustomed to playing with small manipulable objects in the company of an attending and understanding adult.
   As part of the longitudinal study the stimulating quality of the infants' home environments was assessed at 6.5
months and 17 months, when the infants were observed in
the home in the company of their mothers (Smith & Hagen,
1984). A time sampling method, developed by Yarrow and
his coworkers at NICHHD (Yarrow et al., 1975) for differentiation of the environment of infants at age 6 months
was used, with some modifications of the predefined cate-

gories which make them more appropriate when used for toddlers. As shown in Table 1, among the children with Down Syndrome the amount of focused exploration (i.e., looking at and manipulating an inanimate object) was positively related to how often their mothers were inattentive (i.e., the number of 30 sec periods when "no attention" from the mothers was scored). Among the normally developing children there was a tendency in the opposite

Table 1
Correlations between the children's focused exploration and aspects of the home environment at 6.5 and 17 months (differences between the correlations tested by means of r and z transformations)

| | Focused exploration | | | | | |
| | Down Syndrome | | Nonretarded | | | |
	6.5m	17m	6.5	17m	t	p
No attention scored (6.5m)	.71		-.27		2.96	<.01
Physical stimulation (17m)		-.69		.31	2.87	<.01
Broad Smile (17m)		-.68		.24	2.63	<.02

direction. The difference between the correlations was significant when tested by means of r to z transformations (McNemar, 1962). Furthermore, among the children with Down Syndrome, the amount of focused exploration exhibited at 17 months was negatively related to how much close, or proximal, stimulation (i.e., deliberate, active physical stimulation; and mother smiles broadly while looking at the child who is within arm's reach) their mothers provided. In contrast, this association was in a positive direction among normally developing children. Again the group differences between the correlations were significant. This may imply a deficiency in the instrumental frame (cf., Kaye, 1982) and suggests one way in which young children with Down Syndrome may affect their own environments. It seems that when parents of normally developing youngsters spend time with their offspring, they first tend to wait until the youngsters make object-related acts, and then respond in a contingent manner. Since children with Down Syndrome are deficient in their information processing skills, they probably need more time to organize such object-related acts. In such cases parents may easily lose patience with what they come to regard as a slow learner, and resort to imitation of the child's expressive movements as a final, available resource.

In the second year of life, many of the interactions which occur between parents and their normally developing children consist of discourse related to objects which the youngsters manipulate or pay attention to. Focused exploration of objects, therefore, will sometimes be performed on a parent's lap, and sometimes with the adult a little further away, but usually with a supporting and understanding partner available. However, the parents of children with Down Syndrome seem to realize that interactions are most likely to succeed in the proximal mode, without the intervention of objects. Thus objects are made available to such children mostly when they are left alone. Such differential treatment of the two groups of children may lead to differential language acquisition results.

Parents typically monitor and assign meaning to their infants' activities with objects, and respond to the infants' acts according to such interpretations. In normal cases such behaviors on the parents' part seem to propel the development of communication, shaping the child's acts into more conventional forms (cf., Martinsen & Smith, in press). In contrast, parents of young children with Down Syndrome tend to encourage their babies by means of smiling or active physical stimulation. One may surmise that parents do so because such interventions are rewarding, in the sense that caregivers of children with Down Syndrome discover that proximal stimulation promotes the emotional expressions of their children. In contrast they come to realize that more distal stimulation, in the form of talking with reference to objects, is less rewarding, because children with Down Syndrome are rather

slow and need a lot of sustained effort on the parents'
part in order to pay attention to objects.

In short, normally developing infants tend to be more
attentive to stimulation which their parents give contingent upon the child's object-related acts, as compared to
higher or lower levels of stimulation that actually may
be attempts to elicit emotional expressions but which are
often ill-timed in relation to the infants' behavior. It
is suggested that the same applies to young children with
Down Syndrome, but that these youngsters need more time
in object games that they play with their parents. These
conclusions are in line with Field's (1981) data, which
suggest that infants are more attentive to stimulation
which parents give contingent upon children's acts, as
compared to the higher or lower levels of stimulation.
According to Field's hypothesis of an optimal activation
band of infant arousal, parents of infants with developmental delays or deficits may more easily provide inadequate stimulation to their offspring, stimulation that is
either below their attention threshold or above their
aversion threshold. This may occur because the activation
band is thought to be narrower and the arousal cycles
shorter in developmentally retarded infants.

For such reasons it was hypothesized that parents of
young children with Down Syndrome would prefer to use
proximal stimulation in order to keep their offspring
attentive. In contrast, parents of normally developing
infants were expected to use referential speech as an
optimal strategy in the observed interactions. The data
presented in Table 2 corroborate such a view. Support of
the children's weight, direct physical stimulation, and
broad smile were observed more frequently among mothers
of young children with Down Syndrome. In contrast, forms
of speech, where the mothers were referring to objects of
joint attention or to activities which they would expect
their children to perform, occurred more frequently among
the mothers of normally developing children. The data
analysis showed that these group differences could not be
explained by the parents' socioeconomic status, the presence of medical complications in some of the children
with Down Syndrome, or by maternal age differences. Moreover, the apparent tendency of the mothers of children
with Down Syndrome to exaggerate stimulation in the prox-

imal mode, and to minimize certain forms of speech, was not simply an effect of the mothers responding appropriately to their children's lower developmental ages. The implication is that the mothers of children with Down Syndrome behave differently than do mothers of normally developing youngsters, perhaps responding to qualities in the children aside from developmental level, perhaps for

Table 2
Means and SDs for home observations at 17 months

| Environmental var | Down Syndrome | | Nonretarded | | F | t |
	Mean	SD	Mean	SD		
Mother supports child's weight	12.08	7.29	6.72	4.87	3.05	2.38*
Physical stimulation	7.00	6.88	1.28	1.78	15.01	2.93**
Broad Smile	6.77	4.34	2.44	2.43	3.19	3.24***
Referential speech	15.08	10.32	28.83	8.43	1.50	-2.60**
Referential speech (resp.)	2.15	2.61	7.28	8.14	9.73	-2.50*
Definite directional speech	4.15	4.28	8.06	5.05	1.39	-2.26*
No attention scored	8.77	7.89	3.56	4.03	3.82	2.19*

* p < .05.   ** p< .02.   *** p < .01.

other reasons.

Lenneberg (cf., Lenneberg, Nichols, & Rosenberger, 1962) minimized the importance of communication to the onset of speech in young children with Down Syndrome. If the onset of speech in Down anomaly is determined mainly by maturational factors, as has been suggested, one would expect that speech production would be in general concordance with the child's level of motor competence. Moreover, to the extent that they are dependent on reactions from an interpreting caretaker, the functional level of preverbal communicative skills would be of little relevance to the subsequent emergence of language. In order to throw some light on such questions, further analyses of the present set of data were carried out (Smith & von Tetzchner, 1986.)

According to Lenneberg (1967) the emergence of language skills in man is relatively independent of intellectual factors. Rather he saw the synchrony between motor and language milestones during development as strong evidence that language acquisition is regulated by maturational factors. The present study demonstrated, as predicted from the maturational hypothesis, that gross motor behavior (assessed by means of the Gesell scales, Knobloch & Pasamanick's 1974 revision) at age 24 months was significantly related to language competence at age 36 months (measured by the Norwegian adaptation of the Reynell developmental language scales, Hagtvet & Lillestolen, 1985). However, the simple correlations between gross motor skills and child language performance might have been caused by a third factor, i.e., the child's general

Table 3
Correlations between Gesell subscales and Reynell
(Children with Down Syndrome)

Measure	Gesell 24 months	
	Simple r	Partial r
Reynell Comprehension (36 months)		
Gesell gross motor	.71**	.26
Gesell fine motor	.74**	.69**
Reynell Expression (36 months)		
Gesell gross motor	.55*	.40
Gesell fine motor	.28	-.30

Note: Remaining Gesell subscales were partialled out
* $p < .05$ ** $p < .01$

maturational status. Therefore, partial correlations were computed, in which performance on the Gesell subscales was correlated with Reynell language scores, but with the variance that might be ascribed to the 4 remaining subscales removed. This was done on the assumption that a child's performance on the remaining subscales was a reasonable indicator of his/her general level of maturation.

Table 3 shows that, among the children with Down Syndrome, gross motor behavior was consistently unrelated to emergent language skills, when the contribution from the assumed maturational factor had been removed. However, fine motor behavior at age 24 months was related to comprehension skills 1 year later, independent of general maturation. At this level of development, fine motor behavior probably has an important intellectual component in the form of manipulative exploration. Thus, among the children with Down Syndrome, those who were advanced in fine motor behaviors at 24 months probably possessed skills that were of help when they participated in object-oriented play with their parents, skills such as grasping two cubes with one hand, building a tower of cubes, and placing a small pellet in a bottle. On the hypothesis that children who are interested in using small manipulable objects tend to encourage their parents to refer to such things in their child-directed talk, one would expect that competence in the area of fine motor behavior would be related to later language comprehension. However, fine motor skills at 24 months did not predict language expression. These results support the conclusion that skills on the child's part which support a caregiver's referential and child-directed talk, may be specially important to the development of comprehension. Perhaps the onset of speech is relatively more independent of such support, as Lenneberg suggested.

At the chronological ages of 13 months and 24 months the two groups were matched for an average mental age (Gesell scales) and sensori-motor level (Uzgiris-Hunt scales; Uzgiris & Hunt, 1975). The study was comprised of a comparison of performance on two sets of pragmatic tasks, obtained at 13 months in the case of the normally developing children and at 24 months for children with Down Syndrome. The two sets of tasks that were used, im-

peratives and declaratives, have constituted a major
focus of research on the transition from pre-verbal to
verbal communication (cf., Bates, Camaioni, & Volterra,
1975). In the preverbal stage, acts which one may regard
as imperatives are manifested when children seem to be
using an adult as an agent to achieve some end, in a per-
son-to-object sequence. Imperatives were elicited by
holding a desirable object in front of the child, but
just out of arm's reach or inside a transparent contain-
er. Declaratives were elicited by engaging the child in a
repetitive game with an object, and then handing the
child a substitute object.

Although the two groups were matched for mental age and
sensorimotor stage assignment (Dunst, 1980), the performance of the children with Down Syndrome fell significantly below that of the normally developing children on the
declarative tasks (Table 4). It is of interest that only
one child in each group demonstrated the most advanced
rating category of declarative skills, i.e. picking up an
object and labeling it. Thus the possibility that higher
rating scores had been assigned to the normally developing children because they might have been more proficient

Table 4
Means, SDs, and ranges of communication measures of Down
Syndrome children at 24 months, nonretarded at 13 months

	Means	SD	Range	Mann-Whitney U test
Declaratives				
Down Syndrome	5.5	1.9	4-9	
Nonretarded	6.6	1.7	4-9	76.5
Imperatives				
Down Syndrome	9.2	2.2	6-13	
Nonretarded	9.6	1.9	6-13	97.0

* p < .05

in using verbal responses may be dismissed. The rating
categories which yielded differential results required
only nonverbal responses on the child's part in order to
catch the adult's attention. This suggests a disorder of
communication in children with Down Syndrome rather than
a deficit of speech only. If there were a synchrony between communicative skills and general maturation, as implied by Lenneberg, one would expect communicative competence to be at a level corresponding to the child's mental age or sensorimotor stage of development. This does
not seem to be the case. In contrast, young children with
Down Syndrome seem to make their own deficient learning
environment by performing less of the specific nonverbal
gestures which parents often interpret as communicative
acts. Thus such children may become even more retarded in
developing communicative acts and the subsequent language
skills.

In spite of the fact that the assessment of imperative
behaviors did not yield differential results between the
two matched groups, this type of skill was related to
subsequent expressive language at age 3 years. The predictive association of imperatives to subsequent speech
remained strong after the variance attributable to general development had been partialed out (r = .56). Combined, these results suggest an asymmetry in the importance of the two different areas of pragmatic competence:
The level of declarative performance of children with
Down Syndrome seems to be depressed relative to that of
matched, normally developing children, whereas the individual differences that may be observed with respect to
imperative skills among children with Down Syndrome are
more predictive of later speech.

The relevance of mothers' speech to language acquisition has recently been of much concern (cf., Gleitman,
Newport, & Gleitman, 1984). One question that might be
raised is whether the mothers' speech varies according to
their children's status as normally developing or mentally retarded (Cardoso-Martins & Mervis, 1985). The study
of maternal speech to children with Down Syndrome has an
additional theoretical interest. The hypothesis that language acquisition is advanced if the mothers' linguistic
structures match the child's level of understanding is
based mainly on correlational evidence. One cannot always

comfortably draw conclusions about causes and effects from correlational data. In most studies of nonretarded children, the possibility remains that shared genes will determine both the children's language skills and the mothers' child-directed speech. If one may assume, as has been suggested by Gibson (1967), that the parental geno- type does not survive in cases of Down Syndrome, a study of motherese in these cases may shed new light on the relationship between mothers' speech and their children's language development.

Mothers' speech samples were obtained at home at age 3 years. To make the recording situation as natural as pos- sible, cordless microphones were used, which made it pos- sible for the mothers and the children to move around freely. The audio recordings, which lasted 1 hour, were made without an observer present. The mothers were asked to create an everyday atmosphere and were encouraged to perform activities that they thought would elicit vocal-

Table 5
Mothers' speech categories drawn from 100 sequential utterances

1. Mean length of utterance: Number of words per utterance
2. Frequency of yes-no questions
3. Frequency of Wh-questions
4. Frequeny of positive imperatives
5. Frequency of sound expansions: Mother repeats a vocalization by the child, occurring within the preceding 5 utterances of the mother, where she adds to or completes the child's utterance
6. Frequency of imitations: A whole or a partial imitation of the child's vocalization occurring within the 5 preceding utterances by the mother
7. Answers to the child's utterance: An utterance that is related in topic to the child's preced- ing utterance or vocalization, occurring within 5 maternal utterances

Note. Interobserver reliabilities ranged from .91 to .99

Table 6
Correlations of maternal speech with language skills at 3 years

Maternal speech categories	Maternal measures Mean	SD	Reynell Comprehension	Expression
MLU	3.63	0.65	.35	.17
Yes-no questions	21.70	8.39	.12	.08
Wh-questions	7.90	7.17	.79***	.73***
Pos. imperatives	7.00	6.32	-.60**	-.52*
Sound expansions	2.60	4.06	.81***	.83***
Imitations	3.70	4.11	.60**	.88***
Answers	22.20	10.58	.57**	.80***

* p < .05.   ** p < .025.   *** p < .005.

ization or speech on the children's part. The mothers' speech categories were drawn from 100 sequential utterances, which were written down verbatim, starting after 10 minutes of tape recording. The categories which were used are shown in Table 5.

The correlations between the maternal speech categories and the concurrent child language skills, as measured on the Reynell scales at age 3 years, are shown in Table 6. One sees that the mothers' Wh-questions, sound expansions, imitations, and answers to child utterances were all positively related to the children's language skills. Positive imperatives on the mothers' part correlated negatively with child language skills, whereas the mothers' use of yes-no questions was unrelated to the Reynell performance. It is of interest that the most general measure, mothers' mean length of utterance, also was unrelated to the children's concurrent language skills. These data show that differences in child language skills are related to differences in the linguistic environment. However, the direction of the effect is unknown. Differences in the quality of the mother's speech may have led to differential language development, or, equally likely, individual differences related to the children's understanding and level of competence may have led to differences in the mothers' child-directed talk. However, if one may assume that familial residuals in intelligence are minimal in cases of Down anomaly, these results suggest that child-mother interaction factors must be considered, such as child passiveness, or maternal directiveness. As Cardoso-Martins and Mervis (1985) have pointed out, maternal language may not be adjusted to linguistic level as measured against the nonretarded norm. Mothers may expect their children with Down Syndrome to be markedly delayed in language development and thus may feel that their offspring need more direction. However, the construct of "directiveness" may be too global to be of heuristic value in the study of maternal speech to young children. Elsewhere Smith (in press) has demonstrated that within a narrowly constrained context of object transfer between mothers and their young children, mothers of normally developing infants are more demanding in terms of securing joint attention before they proceed with further action. Conversely, the mothers of children with Down Syndrome, matched on developmental level, appear to be more directive on the level of specifying the actions to be performed. Probably because young children with Down Syndrome are more difficult to arouse, their mothers seem more intent at repeating a small number of activities that are performed with success. This may be more rewarding for the mother, as well as for child, but such practices may put constraints on language learning.

The children with Down Syndrome were observed again when they were 5 years of age (Smith, von Tetzchner, & Michalsen, in preparation). During a visit to the home McCarthy scales of children's abilities (McCarthy, 1972) were administered. This time, too, 1 hour speech samples of mothers and children were obtained, using cordless mi-

crophes   at home with no observer present. For the present
purposes   only the children's speech skills were analyzed.
The   number   of different word forms were computed. Within
one   week   of the home observations the children's Reynell
performances were assessed in an outpatient setting.
As   shown   in   Table   7, the children with Down Syndrome
were   in   the   lower range of language skills, as compared
to what   one   would   expect from their level of cognitive
functioning.   When the 5 children who had a general cognitive   age   equivalent   of   2.5   years were compared to the
Reynell   norms   at age level 2.5, their mean stanine score
on   Reynell   comprehension was 3.8: the mean stanine score
on   Reynell   expression had the same value. The mean of the
stanine   scale, of course, is 5, with a standard deviation
of   1.96. The remaining 5 children could not be assigned a
cognitive   age equivalent on the McCarthy scales, due to a
floor   effect.   The transformations from the composite raw
scores   on   the   McCarthy   scales to general cognitive age
equivalents   were   made   according   to Kaufman and Kaufman
(1977).

Table 7
Language skills of children with Down Syndrome at age 5

| | General cognitive age equivalents | | | | | |
| | <2.5 | | | <2.5 | | |
	Mean	SD	Range	Mean	SD	Range
Reynell Comprehension						
Raw score	20.8	7.3	12-30	31.0	4.7	24-36
Stanine score				3.8		
Reynell Expression						
Raw score	16.0	4.6	10-21	24.8	6.5	16-33
Stanine score				3.8		
Mean length of utterance	1.24	0.2	1-1.49	1.45	0.4	1.06-2.2
Number of word forms	138	73	16-196	207.6	103	48-317

From Table 7 it also appears that the MLUs which were observed were far below the values one would expect for normally developing children at an equivalent cognitive age level. Since the McCarthy scales were not standardized below age 2.5 years, one cannot determine a cognitive age level of the children with Down Syndrome who had the greatest cognitive deficits. However, with one exception, the children with cognitive age equivalents of 2.5 were all in early Stage I speech, i.e., their MLUs were below 1.5 (Brown, 1973). Thus only one child in the present sample had made the transition from early to late Stage I speech which is characterized by the appearance of three-word utterances and by a more prevalent use of the basic stock of semantic relations. Normally developing children have usually proceeded well beyond late Stage I speech at age 2.5.

Finally, it may also be of interest to see how well some of the language skills which had been assessed at age 3 predicted language competence as observed 2 years later, at age 5. These correlations are shown in Table 8.

Table 8
Correlations of language skills at age 3 and 5 years

Language measures at 5 years	Reynell 3 years		3 year
	Comprehension	Expression	Vocabulary
Reynell Comprehension	.35	.27	.35
Reynell Expression	.77*	.82**	.68*
Mean length of utterance	.89**	.86**	.86**
Different word forms	.75*	.90**	.68*

* p < .05,   ** p < .01, one-tailed

One sees that there was a remarkable stability in the present sample of children with Down Syndrome with respect to their language related performances. With the exception of Reynell comprehension, which could not be predicted from the 3 year age level, the other indices of language-related performance at age 5, which were tapping different aspects of speech, were associated with the earlier obtained measures. When one considers that the Reynell test scores at age 3 were strongly related to differences in the linguistic environment, the results lend support to the suggestion that child-parent interaction factors may have longer-term effects on the speech development of children with Down Syndrome.

In conclusion, this paper has taken issue with the maturational hypothesis, which postulates that the emergence of language in children with Down Syndrome is mainly determined by an organic schedule. It appears that young children with Down Syndrome make their own deficient learning environment by giving their parents less opportunities to interpret their behavior as communicative. The emergence of interpretible activities in the child is probably maturationally determined, but the significance of such activities depends upon whether or not contingent reactions are received by an understanding and attentive adult. It is suggested that Lenneberg's hypothesis about the importance of maturation to the onset of language should at least be modified. The child activities which parents tend to subject to "rich interpretation" may well have been under initial maturational control, but the age of onset of language is related to the supportive environment which parents may provide. The present paper has discussed the importance of such relationships during the first stage of language development in children with Down Syndrome.

If there are child-parent social interaction factors involved, one would probably be well advised to maximize the importance of the child's behavioral interpretibility in remedial work. Perhaps this is best done by encouraging skills related to the regulation of joint attention. According to this approach, parents of infants with Down Syndrome should first be trained to monitor and manipulate their children's arousal level. Subsequently they should be asked to react to and to make overinterpretations of their children's manipulative exploration of objects. In such a way one may advance the acquisition of shared meaning between parents and their young children with Down Syndrome and help them to take a first step to language.

Acknowledgments.

The authors give thanks to the parents who allowed their children to participate in this study. We thank Harald Martinsen for helpful comments on earlier drafts of this paper. This research has been partially supported by the Norwegian Research Council for Science and the Humanities, and by the Norwegian Council for Research on Mental Retardation.

REFERENCES

Bates, E., Benigni, L., Bretherton, I., Camaioni, L., & Volterra, V. (1979). The emergence of symbols. Cognition and communication in infancy. New York: Academic Press.
Bates, E., Camaioni, L., & Volterra, V. (1975). The acquisition of perfomatives prior to speech. Merrill-Palmer Quarterly, 21, 205-224.
Brown, R. (1973). A first language. The early stages. London: Allen & Unwin.
Cardoso-Martins, C., & Mervis, C. B. (1985). Maternal speech to prelinguistic children with Down syndrome. American Journal of Mental Deficiency, 89, 451-458.
Dunst, C. J. (1980). A clinical and educational manual for use with the Uzgiris and Hunt Scales of Infant Psychological Development. Baltimore, MD: University Park Press.
Evans, D. (1977). The development of language abilities in mongols: A correlational study. Journal of Mental Deficiency Research, 21, 103-117.
Field, T. (1977). Effects of early separation, interaction deficits, and experimental manipulations on infant-mother face-to-face interaction. Child Development, 48, 763-771.
Field, T. (1981). Infant arousal attention and affect during early interactions. In L.P. Lipsitt & Rovee-Collier, C. K. (Eds.), Advances in infancy research. Vol. 2 (pp. 57-100). Norwood, NJ: Ablex.

164   Smith, von Tetzchner, and Michalsen

Gibson, D. (1967). Intelligence in the mongoloid and his parent. <u>American Journal of Mental Deficiency</u>, <u>71</u>, 1014-1016.

Gleitman, L. R., Newport, E. L., & Gleitman, H. (1974). The current status of the motherese hypothesis. <u>Journal of Child Language</u>, <u>11</u>, 43-79.

Hagtvet, B., & Lillestolen, R. (1985). <u>Reynell developmental language scales</u>. Norwegian standardization. Oslo: University of Oslo Press.

Kaufman, A. S., & Kaufman, N. L. (1977). <u>Clinical evaluation of young children with the McCarthy scales</u>. New York: Grune & Stratton.

Kaye, K. (1982). <u>The mental and social life of babies</u>. Chicago: The University of Chicago Press.

Knobloch, H., & Pasamanick, B. (1974). <u>Gesell and Amatruda's developmental diagnosis</u> (3rd ed.). New York: Harper & Row.

Kysela, G., Hillyard, A., McDonald, L., & Ahlsten-Taylor, J. (1981). Early intervention: Design and evaluation. In R. L. Schiefelbusch & D. D. Bricker (Eds.), <u>Language intervention series: Vol. 6. Early language: Acquisition and intervention</u> (pp. 341-388). Baltimore, MD: University Park Press.

Lenneberg, E. H. (1967). <u>Biological foundations of language</u>. New York: Wiley.

Lenneberg, E. H., Nichols, I., & Rosenberger, E. F. (1962). Primitive stages of language development in mongolism. <u>Proceedings, Association for Research in Nervous and Mental Disease</u>, <u>42</u>, 119-137.

Martinsen, H., & Smith, L. (in press). Studies of vocalization and gesture in the transition to speech. In S. von Tetzchner, L. S. Siegel, & L. Smith (Eds.) (in press). <u>The social and cognitive aspects of normal and atypical language development</u>. New York: Springer Verlag.

McCarthy, D. (1972). <u>McCarthy scales of children's abilities</u>. New York: The Psychological Corporation.

McNemar, Q. (1962). <u>Psychological statistics</u> (3rd ed.). New York: Wiley.

Sameroff, A. J., & Chandler, M. J. (1975). Reproductive risk and the continuum of caretaking casualty. In F. D. Horowitz (Ed.), <u>Review of child development research</u>. Vol. 4 (pp. 187-244). Chicago: University of Chicago

Press.
Scarr, S., & McCartney, K. (1983). How people make their own environments: A theory of genotype -- environment effects. Child Development, 54, 424-435.
Smith, L. (in press). Case studies of maternal speech to prelinguistic children in the format of object transfer. In S. von Tetzchner, L. S. Siegel & L. Smith (Eds.) The social and cognitive aspects of normal and atypical language development. New York: Springer-Verlag.
Smith, L., & Hagen, V. (1984). Relationship between the home environment and sensorimotor development of Down syndrome and nonretarded infants. American Journal of Mental Deficiency, 89, 124-132.
Smith, L., & von Tetzchner, S. (1986) Communicative, sensorimotor, and language skills of young children with Down syndrome. American Journal of Mental Deficiency, 91, 57-66.
Smith, L., von Tetzchner, S., & Michalsen, B. (in preparation). The language of children with Down syndrome from age 3 to 5.
Stedman, D. J., & Eichorn, D. H. (1964). A comparison of the growth and development of institutionalized and home-reared mongoloids during infancy and early childhood. American Journal of Mental Deficiency, 69, 391-401.
Uzgiris, I. C., & Hunt, J. McV. (1975). Assessment in infancy. Ordinal scales of psychological development. Urbana: University of Illinois Press.
Yarrow, L. J., Rubenstein, J. L., & Pedersen, F. A. (1975). Infant and environment. Early cognitive and motivational development. New York: Wiley.

5

THE DEVELOPMENTAL ASYNCHRONY OF LANGUAGE DEVELOPMENT IN CHILDREN WITH DOWN SYNDROME

Jon F. Miller
Department of Communicative Disorders and
The Waisman Center on Mental Retardation and
Human Development
University of Wisconsin-Madison

This paper will examine the early language development of children with Down Syndrome to determine whether there is a distinct pattern of language development associated with this syndrome. A detailed review of the literature on the development of speech, language and communication skills in this population (Miller, 1987) revealed no single pattern or profile of speech and language development that described all children with Down Syndrome. Miller did, however, document two distinct views of language development that appear to be linked to age. Children beyond the age of three to four years exhibited language skills that decreased with increasing age compared to other cognitive skills, while the younger children's rate of language acquisition remained consistent with advancing cognitive skills. This paradox deserves to be studied further in order to determine, first, if the description provided by the literature gives an accurate characterization of the development of language skills through the first five years of life; and second, to explore causal constructs that can be advanced to explain the progress in language development in comprehension and production relative to the rate of cognitive advancement and chronological age.

The data from two recently completed studies (Miller, Streit, Salmon & LaFollette, 1987; Miller, Budde, Bashir & LaFollette, 1987) will be presented. The first study will provide a description of the developmental synchrony of language comprehension and language production rela-

tive to cognitive status throughout the first five years
of life. The second study will document early vocabulary
development and lexical productivity in children with
Down Syndrome as compared to normal controls matched for
mental age and MLU. The transition from single word to
multi-word utterances in language production will be examined with these data.

Background

Children classified as mentally retarded do not develop
language and communication skills at the same rate as
normal children of the same chronological age. However,
despite a variety of methods used to study the various
etiologies resulting in mental retardation, the results
of most studies indicate that retarded children use normal linguistic forms and do not produce bizarre language
patterns, such as unique word combinations, invented word
meanings, or novel discourse characteristics (Duchan &
Erickson, 1976; Graham & Graham, 1971; Kamhi & Johnston,
1982; Lackner, 1968; Miller, Chapman & MacKenzie, 1981;
Naremore & Dever, 1975; Newfield & Schlanger, 1968; Ryan,
1975; Semmel, Barritt, Bennett & Perfetti, 1967; Yoder &
Miller, 1972). Mental retardation is a behavioral classification resulting from a variety of etiologies, including metabolic and genetic syndromes, disease processes,
both pre- and post-natal trauma as well as cultural and
familial influences (Miller et al., 1981). It is impressive that despite a variety of brain syndromes, mentally
retarded children learn the standard form of their native
language. Variation in the rate of language development
and asynchrony of development between comprehension and
production have been reported for retarded populations
(Miller, Chapman & Bedrosian, 1978; Miller et al., 1981).
Effective study of the processes affecting language
growth in mental retardation will require the control of
both biological and environmental characteristics of the
population under study.
    There are two major models of cognitive characteristics
of retarded development; developmental models which are
best described by Zigler (1969; 1973); and difference models described by Milgram (1969; 1973). These models were

originally intended to characterize retarded individuals free from organic impairment. Developmental models propose the same cognitive stage and processes for retarded children as for normal children equated for mental age. Difference models propose that different cognitive processes are operative throughout the developmental period. Cicchetti & Pogge-Hesse (1982) have extended the application of these models to organically impaired mentally retarded individuals to test hypotheses about the cognitive processes of children with Down Syndrome. Across a number of social and affective cognitive domains, Cicchetti and his colleagues have found, like others, delayed attainment of developmental milestones and they have documented a striking similarity of cognitive processes in Down Syndrome and nonretarded infants. Down Syndrome infants displayed similar patterns of cognitive development and similar patterns of organization of cognitive and emotional development as nonretarded children (Cicchetti & Mans, 1985). These data document similar performance for both organic and non-organically impaired children, providing support for studies of organically retarded children where the etiology is known. These studies also provide us with a means to interpret the language status of retarded children. Given the similarity of cognitive processes for Down Syndrome and non-retarded children, measures of nonverbal cognitive status (usually measured as mental age [MA]) can be used to determine the developmental status of language performance.

In a recent review of the literature on language and communication characteristics of children with Down Syndrome, Miller (1987) concludes that language skills are increasingly deviant relative to other cognitive skills with increasing chronological age in this population. The younger children up to about three years to four years of age exhibit similar syntax, semantic and discourse skills as normal children matched on mental age or general language skills (Rondal, 1978; Coggins & Stoel-Gammon, 1982; Coggins, Carpenter & Owings, 1983; Owens & MacDonald, 1982; Coggins, 1979; Scherer & Owings, 1984; Greenwald & Leonard, 1979). Studies of older children report variations in development of syntax (Weigel-Crump, 1981; Rogers, 1975; Leuder, Fraser & Jeeves, 1981; Price-Williams & Sabsay, 1979; Harris, 1983; Rondal, 1978).

There is conflicting evidence in the research literature regarding the time at which these deficits may appear in development, which linguistic features are affected, vocabulary, syntax, semantic or pragmatic aspects, and the extent to which these deficits are exhibited in language comprehension as well as production.

Why should we expect the children with Down Syndrome to have particular difficulty learning language relative to other cognitive skills? Miller (1987) proposes four possible causal constructs. First, there is an increase in the frequency of middle ear infections which are often associated with delayed language acquisition in normal children (Brandes & Elsinger, 1981; Downs, 1980). Frequent middle ear infections can result in a hearing loss which is always associated with language learning problems. Second, the deficits in motor coordination and in timing associated with Down Syndrome adversely affect the speech production system, including respiration, phonation, and articulation of the palate, tongue, lips and jaw (Rosin, Swift & Bless, 1987). Third, environmental variables such as decreased expectation for performance of retarded individuals can result in a learned incompetence or lack of appropriate experience (Coggins & Stoel-Gammon, 1982), inappropriate maternal interaction styles characterized by a lack of responsiveness that originates from early perceptions of Down Syndrome infants as being incompetent (Stevenson, Leavitt & Silverberg, 1984), or the increase in maternal directiveness (Cardoso-Martins, Mervis, & Mervis, 1985). Fourth, in addition to hearing, speech motor and maternal perception and interaction deficits, it can be argued that children with Down Syndrome are organically impaired and therefore may have cognitive deficits which are related to language learning beyond those commonly associated with general cognitive development (Zigler, 1969, 1973; Lincoln, Courchesne, Kilman, & Galambos, 1985; Ellis, Deacon, & Wooldridge, 1985; Miller, Chapman & MacKenzie, 1981; Miller, 1987; Elliot, Weeks & Elliot, 1987).

In considering the general problem of developmental synchrony, each of these explanations makes slightly different predictions of the relationship between language comprehension, language production and cognitive status in the same children as well as the age at which such deficits would be evident.

1. Hearing loss or altered auditory perception would predict both comprehension and production deficits. The timing of these deficits would be variable depending on the frequency and duration of the middle ear infection and the severity of the hearing loss.

2. Speech motor control deficits would predict deficits in language production only, with comprehension developing at the same rate as other cognitive skills. Deficits would be evident by the end of the first year of life when reduplicated sound patterns and word forms are expected.

3. Environmental explanations would predict deficits in both comprehension and production, where language input was deficient or expectation for communication reduced. Deficits in language would be evident early in development but may not be different in rate from other cognitive skills where the environment fails to support general development.

4. Deficits in specific linguistic cognitive skills would predict either comprehension or production deficits depending on the model used. Modularity theory, for example, would predict that both deficits were possible depending upon the modules affected. These deficits would be evident when comprehension and production of the first words were expected.

Do Children With Down Syndrome
Exhibit Asynchronous Language Development
Relative To Non-Verbal Cognitive Skills?

The first problem to solve in evaluating the relative force of perceptual, motor, environmental and cognitive variables on language learning is to describe the development of language skills and cognitive skills in a group of young children with Down Syndrome. The outcome of such a study will inform us about the rate, synchrony and individual variation of development by providing a descrip-

tion of the language strengths and deficits of this population. Miller, Streit, Salmon & LaFollette (1987) addressed the general question of developmental synchrony
of language and cognitive skills. Three specific research
questions were posed.

1. Do language comprehension and language production
develop at the same rate as other cognitive skills
through the first five years of life in children with
Down Syndrome?

2. Can the language and the cognitive skills of these
children be described by a single profile as chronological age increases?

3. Can the profiles of language and cognitive development throughout the first five years of life be logically associated with any perceptual, motor, environmental or cognitive causal construct?

The notion of a profile of language development refers
to the age-related developmental progress of language
comprehension and language production. Where chronological age and cognitive skills diverge, mental age is used
as the metric to predict progress in language development. This view reflects the weak form of the cognition
hypothesis recognizing that cognitive advancement is a
necessary but not sufficient condition for language advancement (Chapman & Miller, 1980). An asynchrony in development, then, can be defined in two ways. First by a
profile which departs from the predicted flat profile
where comprehension and production are equivalent on development to non-verbal cognitive status. We will be particularly concerned with profiles showing production only
deficits vs. profiles documenting comprehension and production deficits. The second definition of developmental
asynchrony is where development among language levels,
vocabulary, syntax, semantics, is not flat. Vocabulary
development may be more advanced in development than syntax in comprehension or production relative to cognitive
status. Asynchronies can exist both within and between
comprehension and production skills.
The subjects were 56 children, 10 months to 5 years of

age, participating in the Waisman Center Down Syndrome Program, a research and service program providing developmental monitoring services for children and families with Down Syndrome. The subjects all came from Wisconsin, distributed across urban and rural residences. Socioeconomic status represented high, middle and low with the majority at a middle SES level.

The children and their families were evaluated at the Waisman Center for speech, language, cognition, motor development, hearing and health status. The experimental protocol used in this study is listed in Table 1. Note that several measurement instruments are listed for each category reflecting the developmental range investigated here. Within each category a baseline task was selected and testing proceeded with subsequent tasks until ceiling performance was reached. The subjects were divided into groups by chronological age at one year intervals. Table 2 lists the age distribution of the subject population along with the mean mental age (MA) for each group.

The developmental age and stage criteria for documenting language production status can be found in Table 3. Similar categories for documenting comprehension can be found in Miller, Chapman, Branston & Reichle (1980). We found that MLU did not discriminate production performance in this period of development. MLU is not appropriate as an index of development at the one word stage of production. A number of investigators have documented the relationship between vocabulary size and advancing language skills in longitudinal diary studies (Benedict, 1979; Nelson, 1973; 1986; Gibson & Ingram, 1983). We explored this construct in cross-sectional data from 88 normal children, 10-21 months of age. Speech samples were 20 minutes in duration taken in a free play context with their mothers. Samples were transcribed orthographically using SALT format (Miller & Chapman, 1983; 1984; 1985; 1986) for computer analysis. The resulting data, ranges reported in Table 3, were reasonably consistent with the longitudinal data relative to rate with expected milestones, e.g., 20 different words, documented at 16-18 months in our data and 15-16 months in Benedict's data. Also note in Figure 1 the expected period of rapid vocabulary acquisition following a vocabulary of 20 different words is evident in these cross-sectional data. The use

Table 1
Experimental   Protocol   for   Study   1:   Developmental
Synchrony in the Language of Children with Down Syndrome

1. Cognition:
    Bayley Mental Scale
    Stanford-Binet Revised Edition, 1986
    Symbolic Play (Lowe & Costello, 1976)
    Piagetian Measures
        Object Permanence
        Means Ends
        Classification
        Seriation
        Drawing
2. Comprehension:
    Miller & Chapman Procedures
    Peabody Picture Vocabulary Test (Dunn, 1981)
    Test   of   Auditory   Comprehension   of   Language
    (Carrow-Woolfolk, 1985)
3. Production
    Free Speech Sample (30 minutes, Play with Parent)
    SALT Analysis (Miller & Chapman, 1986)
        MLU
        Number of Different Words
        Lexical Productivity (Ingram, 1981)
        % Intelligible Utterances
4. Speech
    Speech Sample (IPA Transcription)
    Phonetic Inventory (Stoel-Gammon, 1986; 1987)
    Word and Syllable Shape (Stoel-Gammon, 1986; 1987)
    Percent Consonants Correct
    Weiss Comprehensive Articulation Test (Weiss, 1978)
5. Speech Motor Control (Robbins & Klee, 1987)
6. Hearing Status
7. Family History
    SES
    Health
    Education
8. Genetic Diagnosis

Table 2
Down Syndrome Subjects
Developmental Status of Language Production

Age	No.	MA	No. Delayed	% Delayed
0 - 12 mos.	5	7.4	0	0
13 - 24 mos.	14	11.9	4	.29
25 - 36 mos.	16	18.3	12	.75
37 - 48 mos.	15	26.2	9	.60
49 - 60 mos.	6	23.5	4	.66
Total:	56		29	.52

of these data as criteria for the progress in language
production through the second year of life allows us to
increase the precision of our judgments of progress
relative to mental age expectations.

Two types of analysis were performed on the experimental data. First, in order to examine the individual developmental profiles of language and cognitive development, each child's language comprehension and language
production status was judged as either advanced, delayed
or equivalent to non-verbal cognitive status. The criteria used for these judgments were as follows. For children with MA's at or below 24 months, a criterion of + or
- 3 months was used to classify delayed or accelerated
status. For children functioning above 24 months, + or -
6 months was used. This strategy follows that used by
Miller, Chapman and MacKenzie (1981). They evaluated 42
developmentally disabled children with mixed etiologies
and found three profiles to account for 100% of the data.
Profile 1 was flat with MA, comprehension and production
being equivalent, as predicted by the slow motion view of
retarded development. Fifty percent of the sample had
this profile. Profile 2 was characterized by delayed
comprehension and production relative to MA. Twenty-five

Table 3
Criteria for Establishing Production Age

Level	Activity	Age

Pre-International Period (0-8 months)

I	Reflexive Crying	0-2 mos.
II	Cooing & Laughter	2-5 mos.
III	Vocal Play	4-7 mos.
IV	Re-duplicated Babbling	6-8 mos.
	Non-International	

Intentional Period Pre-Linguistic

V	Intentional Action	8-12 mos.
	Re-duplicated Babbling	
	Communication Games	
	Differentiated Cries	

Linguistic Period

VI	Performatives	12-18 mos.
	Gesture & Vocalization	
	Hi-Bye Routines	
	Request Attention or Object	
	Reject	

VII   First words: Miller & Chapman, 1987

0-5	10-12 mos.
6-10	13-15 mos.
11-20	16-18 mos.
20-50	19-21 mos.

MLU Miller & Chapman, 1981
1-5 years of age (Miller, 1981, p. 26)

Criteria for Establishing Asynchrony

Cognitive Status:
    0-24 months ± 3 months for speech/language measures
        +24 months ± 6 months for language measures

FIGURE 1
Mean Different Words: Normal Sample

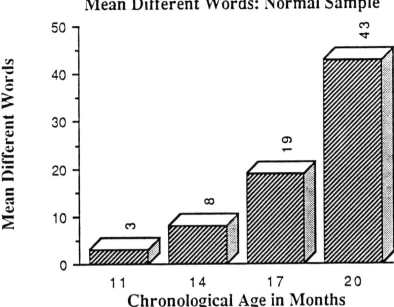

Chronological Age in Months

percent of the sample had this profile. Profile 3 showed delayed productive language relative to MA and language comprehension. Twenty-five percent of the sample had this profile. If we only consider equivalent or delayed status for the three profiles documented by Miller et al. (1981), then by chance 33% of the subjects should fall into each profile type. Or using the Miller et al. 1981 data, 50%, 25% and 25% figures could be used to predict the outcome of this analysis for the children with Down Syndrome.

Profiles Of Language Performance

Table 2 presents the number and percent of the subjects at each age classified as having delayed production, profile type 3. Only 3 subjects had delays in both comprehension and production with the remainder showing a flat profile. Chi-square analyses document significant differences (p < .01) between real and predicted outcomes using

both chance and previous data as criteria. There are two
things to note about these data. First, more than 50% of
the subjects show delays in productive language skills
while only 5% show delays in both comprehension and production. Second, delays are evident within the second
year of life and are frequent (60% +) by the 3rd year of
life.
    The categories for pre-word vocal/verbal speech did not
distinguish rate differences among these children. This
outcome implies that either the categories are too broad
to identify differences with the range of "normal" being
quite variable, or these children manifest generally mental age appropriate speech development until the onset of
word production. The resolution of this issue is confused
by the two different matching strategies used in previous
studies, MA and MLU. This study documents the disassocia-
tion of MA and production measures for the children with
productive language skills between Brown's (1973) Early
Stage I and Stage III. Accordingly, the two matching procedures will yield different results. The MA matches will
produce studies documenting differences between normal
and Down Syndrome samples. MLU matches will likely show
equivalent performance.
    Our success in documenting early developmental deficits
in language production is due in part to the establish-
ment of a new metric to judge progress through the second
year of development.

*Are hearing status, health status, speech motor control
or language input variables associated with the outcome
of this study?*

    Hearing Status: Hearing status was assessed through
measures of middle ear integrity and acuity. Neither of
these measures predicted productive language development
in these children. While a number of children exhibited
middle ear disease, and mild hearing loss, these factors
were not associated in this sample. This should not be
surprising given that these data reflect single day assessments. The impact of otitis media is episodic both in
terms of middle ear integrity and hearing acuity.
    Speech Motor Control Status: Speech motor control was

measured perceptually using the protocol developed by Robbins and Klee (1987). This protocol provides an opportunity to observe the structure of the speech mechanism independently from mechanism function. It provides specific elicitation stimuli to observe mechanism function for each part of the system; larynx-respiration, tongue, teeth, maxilla, mandible, and lips. Coordination speech movements, prosody and voice are also evaluated. Evaluation of the data from this protocol proved to be quite difficult. In general, more of the structural measures could be completed since only minimal cooperation and no specific skills were required. Forty-six of fifty-six subjects exhibited structural differences of some type. These included small or retracted maxilla, occlusion and gaps between teeth, open mouth, hypertrophy of the tongue and deviant tongue carriage, and high palatal vault. Twenty-seven of these children exhibited some type of functional problem. This number is probably an underestimate, as many younger subjects could not be evaluated for coordinated or connected speech movements because they were not talking; others would not imitate the verbal or non-verbal articulatory movements. The better the child's productive language, the more speech motor control measures could be completed. There are both cognitive and motor skills required to complete these tasks. The relationship between the speech motor control measures and productive development has not been satisfactorily established. The relationship between structure and function is complex and the relationship between speech and non-speech movements is not direct. Some aspects of structure seem more related to function than others, the tongue vs. the teeth for example. Our data are insufficient to address the problem of speech motor control deficits in young children with Down Syndrome. They are sufficient, however, to document the difficulty of evaluating the structure and function of the speech mechanism as well as the complexity in formulating an interpretation of the data. It is difficult to assess the motor capacity for speech prior to the onset of first words, and the ability to imitate complex speech movements may not exist for some time after that. You can not test speech without speech. The recent work of Rosin, Swift and Bless (1987) words, and the ability to imitate complex speech move-

ments may not exist for some time after that. You can not
test speech without speech. The recent work of Rosin,
Swift and Bless (1987) confirm that speech motor control
is a significant problem for children with Down Syndrome,
a problem which must be considered seriously in early intervention programs. An assumption of intelligible speech
following language intervention may not be warranted.

Health Status: Children with Down Syndrome suffer from
a number of significant health problems including congenital heart defects and gastro-intestinal problems. Significant health problems may adversely affect development;
directly, by reducing vitality and indirectly, through
prolonged hospital visits. The health status of each of
the children in this study was examined through a health
history questionnaire and a follow-up interview with each
child's parents. Data included a ranking of severity of
the child's health problem(s), corrective measures e.g.,
surgery, the number of hospital visits and the total number of days spent in hospital. Health status -- normal,
mild, moderate and severe -- as well as the number of
hospital days were compared to language status -- delayed
or non-delayed -- using correlation techniques. No significant correlations were found between measures of health
status and productive language development.

Language Input

Maternal input was not examined directly in this study.
Input variables are clearly essential to complete our understanding of the language learning process of children
with Down Syndrome. Several variables identified in the
literature to be deficient in mother-child interaction
patterns can be explored relative to the data reported
here to determine if they may be operative in the families of our children. Miller (1987) found five factors
affecting mother-child interactions, some of which may
have negative consequences for language learning.

1. Both mothers and their infants with Down Syndrome
are less responsive to each other (Stevenson & Leavitt,
1983).

2. Mothers of infants with Down Syndrome talk to their

children more and tend to talk at the same time their infants are vocalizing (Berger & Cunningham, 1983).

3. Mothers of children with Down Syndrome speak at a faster rate, producing more utterances per unit time than mothers of normal children (Buckhalt, Rutherford, & Goldberg, 1978).

4. Mothers of children with Down Syndrome are more directive, intrusive, and controlling (Eheart, 1982; Jones, 1979, 1980).

5. Not all mothers of children with Down Syndrome are alike. Individual differences in patterns of interaction have been documented on dimensions of direction, sensitivity, and elaboration (Crawley & Spiker, 1983). This work establishes maternal sensitivity and direction as independent features of maternal behavior.

None of these five characteristics of language input can logically account for the two patterns of language development found in this study. Where variation in language interaction patterns exists, a flat profile, with language comprehension and production equivalent to nonverbal cognitive status, would be consistent with a rich supportive verbal environment. None of the input deficits, however, would predict deficits in production only. We need to examine more carefully the relationship between the language patterns of individual children and their corresponding verbal environment.

Let us now return to the major findings of this study and review the explanations that can be advanced to account for them.

1. Children with Down Syndrome frequently show asynchronous development of productive language. Deficits in productive language relative to MA were observed in 60 to 75 percent of the subjects older than 18 months of chronological age.

2. The pattern of language development is inconsistent; not all children show the same profile of development.

Two profiles account for 95% of the data: 1) A flat profile where cognition, and language comprehension and production are equivalent, and 2) A profile of delayed language production with language comprehension equal to cognitive status. The first profile accounted for all subjects below 18 months of age and 25 to 40 percent of the subjects in succeeding age groups. Profile two accounted for 60 to 75 percent of the subjects older than 18 months of chronological age.

3. Delayed language production is identifiable within the second year of life and corresponds with the onset of word production.

At this point two explanations can be advanced for the outcome of this study, though neither is satisfactory. One might suggest that there are deficits in cognitive skills specific to language. A model recently proposed to account for all of the data on cerebral specialization in individuals with Down Syndrome by Elliot, Weeks and Elliot (1987) suggests that..."some of the sequential language problems experienced by this population are related to a biological dissociation between cerebral areas responsible for speech perception and the production of complex movements, including speech. Taking a disconnection syndrome position...we propose that it is a breakdown in communication between functional systems that normally overlap that is responsible,...for the language-based problems exhibited by these individuals." This model provides useful direction for hypothesis generation for further research to explore cognitive explanations for language production deficits in these children. The puzzle as to why some children are affected and others are not will be difficult to solve with this explanatory model.

An alternative explanation can be advanced to account for these data. Speech motor control deficits are present in a majority of children with Down Syndrome. These deficits preclude the production of utterances as long and complex as their language skills would allow. Language production would be limited by speech motor deficits. This explanation would account for variations in the profiles observed in this study with some children having more severe motor deficits than others. This explanation, however, fails to account for why production deficits could not be identified prior to the period of single word production. This explanation would predict deficits in pre-speech vocal/verbal behavior.

Two other explanations of deficits in language production can be ruled out. First, environmental factors could play a role in altering the percentages of the profiles found at each age level. We do not believe, however, that language input mechanisms can be argued as the primary mechanism for the deficits in language production documented here. The input deficits would predict deficits in both comprehension and production. Second, hearing deficits would also predict both comprehension and production deficits and therefore are unrelated to the findings of this study. We will need to examine in more detail, the productive language characteristics of young children with Down Syndrome.

Lexical Development And Its
Role In The Transition To Syntax

Concurrent with the first study, we conducted a series of projects exploring the early lexical development of children with Down Syndrome (Miller, Budde, Bashir & LaFollette, 1987). The literature documents conflicting views of lexical development in this population and it became apparent that a resolution of this conflict would have important implications for the development of syntax in these children.

There are two conflicting views of lexical development in children with Down Syndrome. Rondal (1978) found that children with Down Syndrome have advanced vocabulary over normal children with the same MA and linguistic stage. Rondal used the high type-token ratio of Down Syndrome children as evidence for the claim that they use a larger vocabulary when conversing with their mothers in free play than do younger normal children. He concludes that advanced lexical development is present in his subjects because their advanced age permitted more experience, both linguistic and non-linguistic.

Alternately, Cordoso-Martins, Mervis, and Mervis (1985)

claim lexical acquisition proceeds at a slower pace in children with Down Syndrome when compared to normal children matched for language development and MA. They studied 6 normal and 6 Down Syndrome children in a longitudinal study with subjects at a 10 to 12 month developmental level at the onset. Subjects were followed for 14 to 21 months. They found that the acquisition of object names preceded at a significantly slower pace for the Down Syndrome group than the normal group. They argue these results are due to specific cognitive deficits for learning associated with language. Given the delays in vocabulary acquisition, they predict further delays in the onset of syntactic acquisition.

The relationship between lexical and syntactic acquisition has not received much attention, with only one case study reported by Fowler (1984; Fowler, Gleitman & Gelman, 1985) and a recent paper by Cromer (1987) on retarded children in general. These papers suggest that different mechanisms may operate for lexical vs. syntactic learning. Cromer argues that vocabulary learning involves both referential and grammatical aspects. Vocabulary measures, however, tend to focus on the referential aspect of the words which may be acquired gradually over time. Syntax, he argues, requires a reorganization process to accommodate new grammatical data. Fowler suggests that some retarded people may be unable to reorganize their grammar beyond a particular point resulting in a plateauing of their syntactic skills.

Two issues emerge from this discussion: first, do children with Down Syndrome show lexical differences compared to MA matched normal children? And, second, will children with Down Syndrome show differences in early syntactic skills? We addressed these issues by asking the following research questions: 1) Do children with Down Syndrome produce fewer different words in a standard language sample than MA matched control subjects? 2) Do children with Down Syndrome evidence limited lexical productivity compared to MA matched control subjects.

The productivity construct was put forth by Ingram (1981) as an index of the combinational properties of a child's early lexicon. He argued that simple frequency of lexical forms was not sufficient to claim grammatical mastery. The word had to be used with two or more different words preceding it and following it in order to be considered productive on co-occurrence grounds. That is, a word had to be used in at least two different utterances, each with different words preceding and following the target word. Differences in the meanings encoded should also occur. Ingram's productivity index provides us with a mechanism to quantify the combinational properties of early vocabularies allowing us to relate lexical skills to the emergence of syntax. Children with higher percentages of productive words in their lexicon will, therefore, have more advanced grammatical systems.

Three populations of children were examined for this study.

1. A group of 17 children with Down Syndrome from the Boston Children's Hospital Medical Center ranging in age from 24 to 36 months. These subjects were divided into two groups according to MA levels, 5 subjects at 17 months and 12 subjects at 20 months.

2. Seventy-three children with Down Syndrome from the Waisman Center Down Syndrome program ranging from 2 to 12.5 years of age participated in this study. These children were sorted into several MA groups and MLU groups, with some of the children participating in more than one group. Three MLU groups were identified, with 10 subjects each, at mean MLU 1.2, 1.4 and 1.7. Three MA groups were identified with 10 subjects each, at mean MA 24 months, 30 months and 36 months. All of these subjects had speech samples averaging twenty minutes in length. In addition, a group of twelve children with a mean of 36 months of age was identified, each with speech samples containing 100 complete and intelligible utterances.

3. One hundred normal subjects grouped by CA, with 24 subjects each at 11, 14, 17 & 20 months of age and 12 subjects at 36 months of age. From these 100 subjects, 3 MLU control groups were identified with 10 subjects each at mean MLU's of 1.2, 1.4 & 1.7. The 36 month old subjects all had speech samples of 100 complete and intelligible utterances. All other subjects and samples of 20 minutes in length.

Two Year Old Study: Boston Samples

This study attempted to examine the lexical productivity of children with Down Syndrome at what we hoped would be the transition period between single and multi-word utterances. The 17 children with Down Syndrome were compared to 24 normal children, 12 each at 17 and 20 months of age. Language samples of 20 minutes in length were collected from each child in free play with his mother. The samples were transcribed into standard orthographic format following SALT (Miller & Chapman, 1986) conventions. Transcripts were entered into computer files for analysis. SALT provides MLU, number of different words, and Productivity Analysis as a part of its analysis routines.

First we examined the number of different words produced by the four groups and found that the normal children produced significantly more words (p < .01, two way ANOVA) than the MA matched subjects with Down Syndrome. An analysis of the MLU's of the groups confirmed that only the normal children were producing any multi-word utterances. The productivity analysis, therefore, could not be performed. These data confirm, to the extent that the number of different words is a measure of developmental change, that the children with Down Syndrome are significantly delayed in production at the point in cognitive development that we would expect the onset of representational skills with the corresponding rapid acceleration in vocabulary acquisition and the onset of multi-word utterances.

Three Year Old Study: Madison Samples

In order to test the productivity question, we needed to evaluate subjects with more advanced language skills. Given the low level of productive development at twenty months MA, we identified 12 subjects with Down Syndrome and 12 normal children with a group mean for MA at 36 months. All subjects also had language samples, with 100 complete and intelligible utterances to insure we had comparable samples relative to length. All samples were taken in conversational contexts. Down Syndrome children interacted with their mothers and the normal children interacted with an examiner. The samples were transcribed into SALT format for computer analysis. The productivity analysis data based on the percent of the different words in each child's transcript that were productive (two or more different words preceding and following each word) was analyzed with one-way ANOVA. Results revealed a significant difference ($p < .01$) between the Down Syndrome children and normal children, confirming the hypothesis that the early vocabularies of children with Down Syndrome are less productive than normal children. If confirmed, this finding would suggest that children with Down Syndrome exhibit gramatical limitations in the use of their early lexicons. In examining other metrics of productive language use, we found that MLU and the number of different words were also significantly different, again favoring the normal subjects. The mean MLU's were 3.6 for the normal sample and 1.6 for the Down Syndrome subjects. It appeared that the difference in productivity scores could be due to the differences in overall language performance, with normal children significantly more advanced than the Down Syndrome children. Apparently, MA does not predict language production status in children with Down Syndrome.

MLU Study: Madison Samples

To test the hypothesis that differences in productivity scores were due to differences in productive language development, we identified groups of Down Syndrome and normal children at three different MLU levels, 1.2, 1.4 and 1.7. These levels should provide control for overall language learning and provide the proper window in development for Ingram's productivity measure (developed for the early multi-word utterances appearing at the end of the second year of life). Sixty subjects were identified with mean MLU's at the three levels, 10 Down Syndrome and 10 normal subjects in each group. A two-way ANOVA, groups by MLU level, calculated on the percent productive words in each 20 minute sample revealed no significant differences between the groups at any MLU level. The significant finding in the productivity scores at 36 months MA was no

longer evident when overall language level was controlled. Thus, the combinational properties of the
lexicons of the two groups are not different. We did
discover, however, something rather startling when we
examined the number of different words produced by each
group.

An examination of Figure 2 reveals that the children
with Down Syndrome produced significantly more different
words (p < .01 two-way ANOVA) than the normal subjects
matched for MLU. This finding confirms the conclusions of
Rondal (1978) using the Type Token Ratio, suggesting that
children with Down Syndrome with advanced CAs have more
experience to develop their referential skills. However,
we believe that the developmental picture is not quite so
simple. Let us examine the major findings of this last
study.

1. Children with Down Syndrome produce fewer different
words than normal MA matched control subjects.

2. Children with Down Syndrome produce significantly
fewer productive words than MA matched control subjects. When compared to MLU matched subjects the differences no longer exist.

3. Children with Down Syndrome produce significantly
more different words than MLU matched control subjects.

4. MLU and MA are dissociated in children with Down
Syndrome. MA does not predict MLU the way CA predicts
MLU in normal children (Miller & Chapman, 1981).

There appears to be a different relationship between
the number of different words produced and multi-word utterance use in children with Down Syndrome than in normal
children. There are 50 different words associated with
the onset of multi-word speech which occurs at about 19
months of age in normal children (Nelson, 1973). While
these are taken from complete diary accounts of acquisition and ours are cross-sectional samples, the differences are striking: expressive vocabulary and expressive
syntax are diverging in Down Syndrome subjects. The differences in lexical learning that have been demonstrated

FIGURE 2
Mean Different Words by MLU Group

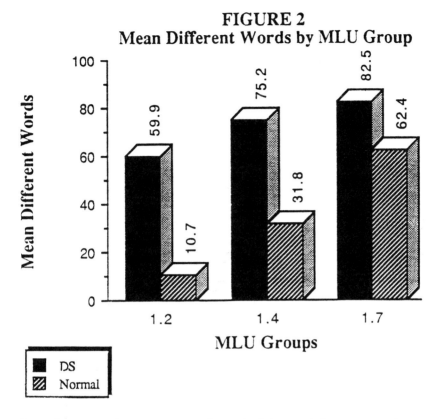

MLU Groups

■ DS
▨ Normal

in these studies suggest that children with Down Syndrome may be demonstrating well-developed referential vocabulary acquisition skills but deficiencies in the grammatical marking of their lexicon.

The studies reported here document that significant numbers of children with Down Syndrome demonstrate delays in productive language development consistent with the Cordoso-Martins et al. (1985) study when matched for MA. These children also show significantly larger vocabularies than normal children at the same MLU levels, which is consistent with the Rondal findings. The apparent paradox can be resolved by understanding that MA does not predict productive language development in the children with Down Syndrome. Productive vocabulary is slower to develop than mental age would predict but faster to develop than syntactic skills as measured by MLU.

Confirmation of this view is found in Figure 1 which

displays the mean number of different words produced by
88 normal subjects 10 to 21 months of age, 24 in each age
group. Contrast Figure 1 with Figure 3, which displays
the mean number of different words produced by children
with Down Syndrome 17 to 36 months of mental age with 5,
12, 10, 10, and 10 children in each group respectively.
These data document the extent of the productive language
delay for the number of different words produced in 20
minute language samples in a cross-sectional study. The
children are delayed on the average 6 months at 20 months
MA and 10 months at 30 months MA. This trend is alarming
because it suggests a progressive deficit. At the same
time, the asynchrony of lexical development with syntax
suggests specific cognitive linguistic deficits may be
associated with the productive language problems of these
children.

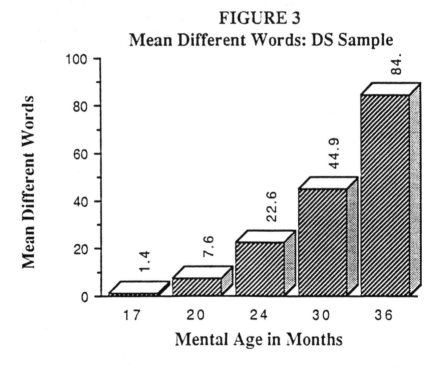

FIGURE 3
Mean Different Words: DS Sample

The results of these studies suggest some reasons for
conflicting outcomes of studies of the language characteristics of children with Down Syndrome. Studies grouping subjects at MA levels would find productive language

status different among normal and Down Syndrome subjects,
a factor which could confound the outcomes of paradigms
assuming equivalent production status. Language input
studies, for example, may be seriously compromised by MA
matching, since maternal language is directed by production status rather than cognition or comprehension status
(Brooks-Gunn & Lewis, 1984). MLU matches, on the other
hand, assume synchrony among language levels, an assumption not supported by the data from Miller, Streit,
Salmon & LaFollette (1987). New grouping strategies will
have to be found using variables relevant to the research
question addressed. Vocabulary size, as measured by the
number of different words produced in a language sample
of standard size, may prove to be a better general index
of early language development than MLU. Clearly, the relationship among language levels assumed in normal children cannot be assumed to hold for biologically distinct
populations.

Conclusion

   Potential explanations have not been developed in sufficient detail to account for the new data presented in
this paper. Asynchronies in language development have
been documented for language production relative to language comprehension and other cognitive skills. Asynchronies were also documented for vocabulary relative to
syntactic skills where vocabulary growth is both slower
in rate relative to mental age and faster in rate relative to advancing syntactic skills measured by MLU. The
90 subjects with Down Syndrome investigated in the two
Miller et al. (1987) studies of individual differences
varied in their profiles of language development. Not all
of these subjects show deficits in the rate of productive
language development. The major findings to be explained
then concern deficits in productive language but not comprehension, onset of productive deficits coinciding with
the onset of word production, an apparent advance in referential skills over grammatical skills and individual
variation in productive language development relative to
other cognitive skills.
   Two avenues of explanation seem plausible to pursue at

this time. The first focuses on further examination of the speech motor control deficits of this population. The second would seek an explanation at the cognitive level, arguing, perhaps, from a modularity point of view or froma cerebral specialization model (Elliot, Weeks & Elliot, 1987). Further elaboration of these explanations have to account for production only deficits, syntax over vocabulary and why some children are adversely affected but not others.

Future Research

Confirmation of the findings of the cross-sectional studies reported here requires longitudinal studies. Such studies would allow the same children to be observed over time and would: 1) Document the differences in children who show productive language deficits compared to those whose language is consistent with the rate of non-verbal cognitive skills, 2) Document the rate of vocabulary acquisition relative to cognitive status, 3) Document lexical productivity over time, 4) Document the relationship between lexical productivity and other measures of syntactic development, and 5) Document the referential vs. grammatical character of the early vocabularies of children with Down Syndrome. It is clear from the studies reported here that 5 to 10 years will be needed to complete the required longitudinal studies. Experimental approaches must be developed to examine the issues raised in this paper.

Acknowledgments

This paper was prepared for the National Down Syndrome Society Symposium entitled "Psychobiology of Down Syndrome" held in New York City, December, 1987. The work reported in this paper was supported, in part, by National March of Dimes research grant #12-197; Mental Retardation Research Center Core support, NIH, NICHD Project #5 P30 HD03352 to the Waisman Center on Mental Retardation and Human Development, University of Wisconsin-Madison; Research Grant #990135 form the Graduate School Research

Committee, University of Wisconsin-Madison. We gratefully acknowledge the support of the Down Syndrome Program of the Waisman Center on Mental Retardation and Human Development.

REFERENCES

Benedict, H. (1979). Early lexical development: Comprehension and production. Journal of Child Language, 6, 183-200.
Berger, J. & Cunningham, C. C. (1983). Development of early vocal behaviors and interactions in Down's syndrome and nonhandicapped infant-mother pairs. Developmental Psychology, 19, 322-331.
Brandes, P. & Elsinger, D. (1981). The effects of early middle ear pathology on auditory perception and academic achievement. Journal of Speech and Hearing Disorders, 46, 301-307.
Brooks-Gunn, J. & Lewis, M. (1984). Maternal responsiveness in interactions with handicapped infants. Child Development, 55, 782-793.
Brown, R. (1973). A First Language. Cambridge: Harvard University Press.
Buckhalt, J. A., Rutherford, R. B., & Goldberg, K. E. (1978). Verbal and nonverbal interaction of mothers with their Down's syndrome and nonretarded infants. American Journal of Mental Deficiency, 82, 337-343.
Cardoso-Martins, C., Mervis, B. B., & Mervis, C. A. (1985). Early vocabulary acquisition by children with Down syndrome. American Journal of Mental Deficiency, 90, 177-184.
Chapman, R., & Miller, J. (1980). Analyzing language and communication in the child. In R. Schiefelbusch (Ed.), Nonspeech Language and Communication: Analysis and Intervention. Baltimore: University Park Press.
Cicchetti, D., & Mans, L. (1985). Stages, sequences and structures in the organization of cognitive development in Down syndrome infants. In I. Uzgiris and J. McV. Hunt (Eds.), Research with Scales of Psychological Development in Infancy. Urbana Champaign: University of Illinois Press.
Cicchetti, D., & Pogge-Hesse, P. (1982). Possible contributions of the study of organically retarded persons to developmental theory. In E. Zigler & D. Balla (Eds.),

Mental retardation: The developmental-difference controversy (pp.277-318). Hillsdale, NJ: Lawrence Erlbaum.

Coggins, T. E. (1979). Relational meaning encoded in the two-word utterances of stage 1 Down's syndrome children. The Journal of Speech and Hearing Research, 22, 166-178.

Coggins, T. E., Carpenter, R. L., & Owings, N. O. (1983). Examining early intentional communication in Down's syndrome and nonretarded children. British Journal of Disorders of Communications, 18, 98-106.

Coggins, T. E., & Stoel-Gammon, C. (1982). Clarification strategies used by four Down's syndrome children for maintaining normal conversational interaction. Education and Training of the Mentally Retarded, 17, 65-67.

Downs, M. (1980). The identification of children at risk for middle ear effusion problems. Annals of Otology, Rhinology and Laryngology, 89 (3. Part 2), 168-171.

Duchan, J., & Erickson, J. (1976). Normal and retarded children's understanding of semantic relations in different verbal contexts. Journal of Speech and Hearing Research, 19, 767-776.

Eheart, B. K. (1982). Mother-child interactions with nonretarded and mentally retarded preschoolers. American Journal of Mental Deficiency, 87, 20-25.

Elliot, D., Weeks, D., & Elliot, C. (1987). Cerebral specialization in individuals with Down syndrome. American Journal of Mental Retardation, 92, 263-271.

Ellis, N. R., Deacon, J. R., & Wooldridge, P. W. (1985). Structural memory deficits of mentally retarded persons. American Journal of Mental Deficiency, 89, 393-402.

Gibson, D., & Ingram, D. (1983). The onset of comprehension and production in a language delayed child. Applied Psycholinguistics, 4, 359-376.

Graham, J., & Graham, L. (1971). Language behavior of the mentally retarded: Syntactic characteristics. American Journal of Mental Deficiency, 75, 623-629.

Greenwald, C. A. & Leonard, L. B. (1979). Communicative and sensorimotor development of Down's syndrome children. American Journal of Mental Deficiency, 84, 296-303.

Harris, J. (1983). What does mean length of utterance mean? Evidence from a comparative study of normal and

Down's syndrome children. British Journal of Disorders of Communication, 18, 153-169.

Jones, O. (1979). A comparative study of mother-child communication with Down syndrome and normal infants. In D. Schaffer & J. Dunn (Eds.), The First Year of Life, New York: John Wiley & Sons, pp. 175-195.

Jones, O. H. M. (1980). Prelinguistic communication skills in Down's syndrome and normal infants. In T. F. Field (Ed.), High-risk infants and children: Adult and peer interactions (pp. 205-225). New York: Academic Press.

Kamhi, A. & Johnston, J. (1982). Towards an understanding of retarded children's linguistic deficiencies. Journal of Speech and Hearing Research, 25, 435-445.

Lackner, J. R. (1968). A developmental study of language behavior in retarded children. Neuropsychologia, 6, 301-320.

Leuder, I., Fraser, W. I., & Jeeves, M. A. (1981). Social familiarity and communication in Down syndrome. Journal of Mental Deficiency Research, 25, 133-142.

Lincoln, A. J., Courchesne, E., Kilman, B. A., & Galambos, R. (1985). Neurophysiological correlates of information-processing by children with Down syndrome. American Journal of Mental Deficiency, 89, 403-414.

Milgram, N. (1969). The rationale and irrationale in Zigler's motivational approach to mental retardation. American Journal of Mental Deficiency, 73, 527-532.

Milgram, N. (1973). Cognition and language in mental re-tardation. Distinction and implications. In D. K. Routh (Ed.), The experimental psychology of mental retarda-tion. Chicago: Aldine.

Miller, J., Budde, M., Bashir, A. & LaFollette, L. (1987, November). Lexical productivity in children with Down syndrome. Paper presented at the annual convention of the American Speech-Language-Hearing Association, New Orleans, LA.

Miller, J., & Chapman, R. (1986). SALT: Systematic Anal-ysis of Language Transcripts: Harris version 4.0. Lan-guage Analysis Laboratory, the Waisman Center on Mental Retardation and Human Development, the University of Wisconsin-Madison.

Miller, J., Chapman, R., & Bedrosian, J. (1978). The relationship between etiology, cognitive development and language and communicative performance. The New Zealand Speech Therapists' Journal, 33, 2-17.

Miller, J., Chapman, R. S., Branston, M. B., & Reichle, J. (1980). Language comprehension in sensorimotor stages V and VI. Journal of Speech and Hearing Research, 23, 284-311.

Miller, J., Chapman, R., & MacKenzie, H. (1981). Individual differences in the language acquisition of mentally retarded children. Paper presented at the 2nd International Congress for the Study of Child Language, Vancouver, B.C. Canada.

Miller, J., Streit, G., Salmon, D., & LaFollette, L. (1987, November). Developmental synchrony in the language of children with Down syndrome. Paper presented at the annual convention of the American Speech-Language-Hearing Association, New Orleans, LA.

Miller, J. F. (1987). Language and communication characteristics of children with Down syndrome. In S. M. Pueschel, C. Tingey, J. E. Rynders, A.C. Crocker, and D. M. Crutcher (Eds.), New Perspectives on Down Syndrome. Baltimore, MD: Brookes, pp. 233-262.

Naremore, R., & Dever, R. (1975). Language performance of educable mentally retarded and normal children at five age levels. Journal of Speech and Hearing Research, 18, 82-96.

Nelson, K. (1973). Structure and strategy in learning to talk. Monograph of The Society for Research in Child Development, 38 (1-2, Serial No. 149).

Nelson, K. (1986). Event knowledge: Structure and function in development. Hillsdale, NJ: Erlbaum.

Newfield, M. & Schlanger, B. (1968). The acquisition of English morphology by normals and educable mentally retarded children. The Journal of Speech and Hearing Research, 11, 693-706.

Owens, R. E., Jr., & MacDonald, J. D. (1982). Communicative uses of the early speech of nondelayed and Down syndrome children. American Journal of Mental Deficiency, 86, 503-510.

Price-Williams, D., & Sabsay, S. (1979). Communicative competence among severely retarded persons. Simiotica, 26, 35-63.

Robbins, J., & Klee, T. (1987). Clinical assessment of oropharyngeal motor development in young children.

Journal _of_ _Speech_ _and_ _Hearing_ _Disorders_, 52(3), 271-277.

Rogers, M. G. H. (1975). A study of language skills in severely subnormal children. Child: Care, Health and Development, 1, 113-126.

Rondal, J. (1978b). Maternal speech to normal and Down's syndrome children matched for mean length of utterance. In C. E. Meyers (Ed.), Quality of life in severely and profoundly mentally retarded people: Research foundations for improvement (pp. 193-266). Washington, D.C.: American Association of Mental Deficiency.

Rosin, M., Swift, E., & Bless, D. (1987, November). Communication profiles of people with Down syndrome. Paper presented at the annual convention of the American Speech-Language-Hearing Association, New Orleans, LA.

Ryan, J. (1975). Mental subnormality and language development. In E. Lenneberg & E. Lenneberg (Eds.), Foundations of language development: A multi-disciplinary approach (Vol. 2) (pp. 269-278). New York: Academic Press.

Semmel, M., Barritt, L., Bennett, S., & Perfetti, C. (1967). The performance of educable mentally retarded and normal children on a modified close task. Studies in Language Learning and Language Behavior, 5, 326-342.

Stevenson, M. B. & Leavitt, L. A. (1983). Mother-infant interaction: A Down's syndrome case study. Paper presented at the 2nd International Workshop on the "At Risk" Infant, Jerusalem.

Stevenson, M. B., Leavitt, L. A., & Silverberg, S. B. (1984). Mother-infant interaction: Down syndrome case studies. In S. Harel and N. J. Anastosiow (Eds.), The "At-Risk" Infant: Psycho/socio/medical Aspects. Baltimore: Brookes, pp. 379-388.

Wiegel-Crump, C. A. (1981). The development of grammar in Down's syndrome children between the mental ages of 2-0 and 6-11 years. Education and Training of the Mentally Retarded, February, 24-30.

Yoder, D., & Miller, J. (1972). What we may know and what we can do: Input toward a system. J. McLean, D. Yoder, & R. Schiefelbusch (Eds.), Language intervention with the retarded: Developing strategies. Baltimore: University Park Press.

Zigler, E. (1969). Developmental vs. difference theories

of mental retardation and the problem of motivation. American Journal of Mental Deficiency, 73, 536-556.

Zigler, E. (1973). The retarded child as a whole person. In D. Routh (Ed.), The Experimental Psychology of Mental Retardation. Chicago: Aldine.

6

VISUAL AND AUDITORY PROCESSING
IN CHILDREN WITH DOWN SYNDROME

Siegfried M. Pueschel
Child Development Center
Department of Pediatrics, Rhode Island Hospital
Brown University Program in Medicine
Providence, Rhode Island

The most compelling inquiries into the way children learn are organized around new findings and new perspectives on learning and knowing. Child study professionals including psychologists and educators have held a fairly stable belief about the nature of perception and learning almost since the turn of the century. During the past few decades, however, a new understanding of these issues has begun to emerge, coming primarily from the fields of neuropsychology, anthropology, developmental psychology, and ethology.

Research into learning has contributed to our understanding of how a young child forms concepts and how the child can make learning become a part of him or her. We know that learning itself is an active and dynamic process. It is dependent upon a rich background of sensory and motor experiences. We know that learning will proceed best under conditions that provide a wealth of diverse sensory and manipulative experiences. Thus, a basic understanding of developmental and maturational processes in early childhood is the foundation upon which concepts of educational programs and learning can be developed.

When we began our research in this area, we soon found that the literature is replete with reports describing various aspects of the intellectual limitations in persons with Down Syndrome. However, there is only very little information available on specific cognitive and learning processes in these children. Since it is assumed that a better understanding of these processes may lead to more appropriate educational planning, our studies were designed to investigate visual and auditory processing in children with Down Syndrome using the newly developed test, the Kaufman Assessment Battery for Children.

Method

The Study population comprised 20 home-reared children with Down Syndrome that were between the ages of 8 years and 12 1/2 years. These children were selected from a group of children with this chromosome disorder who are presently followed at the Child Development Center of Rhode Island Hospital, a University Affiliated Facility. It is of note that the Child Development Center has knowledge of nearly all children born with Down Syndrome in Rhode Island since the vast majority of children with Down Syndrome are referred to the Center for evaluation and follow-up. Thus no known selection bias exists.
Criteria for inclusion in the study sample were:

1) All children should have the chromosomal complement of trisomy 21. Children who have translocation or mosaicism Down Syndrome were excluded since it is well known that children with mosaicism Down Syndrome differ in intellectual functioning significantly from those with trisomy 21 (Fishler, 1975; Rosecrans, 1968; Sachs, 1971; Zellweger & Abbo, 1963) and children with translocation Down Syndrome differ biochemically from those with trisomy 21 (Rosner, Ong, Paine, & Mahanand, 1965).

2) The children with Down Syndrome should be between 8 years and 12 1/2 years of age. This age group had been chosen since younger children with Down Syndrome (< 8 years) usually have marked difficulties with certain test items of the Kaufman test and older children (> 12 1/2 years) were excluded because of the age limitations of the instrument.

3) The intellectual functioning of children in the study group should be in the mild to moderate range of mental retardation. Children with severe and profound

mental retardation were excluded since they usually have difficulties understanding and responding appropriately to the presented test materials.

4) All children with Down Syndrome should be without major medical problems such as severe congenital heart disease, nutritional defiencies, etc. Moreover, children with sensory impairments including hearing deficits and decreased visual acuity were excluded. Children with Down Syndrome who have other identified neurologic or biochemical disorders and those with serious behavioral disturbances were also excluded. The above listed conditions usually affect the overall functioning of the child adversely and hence would limit the validity of the test results.

(5) The children in the experimental group should have had early intervention and preschool nursery experiences and should be enrolled in an appropriate educational program.

(6) The Down Syndrome children should have a younger brother or sister, preferably at a similar mental age.

One control group encompasses 20 younger brothers and sisters of the children with Down Syndrome. Their admission criteria were:

(1) The brother or sister of the child with Down Syndrome should be intellectually normal and be in good physical and mental health.

(2) The brother or sister should be a full sibling since his/her genetic make up will be similar to that of the study subject except that he/she will not have the extra gene doses that originate from the supernumerary 21 chromosome. Any half siblings as well as foster or adoptive brothers and sisters were excluded.

(3) The brother or sister should be from the same home environment and be exposed to similar styles of child-rearing, cultural aspects, nutritional influences and other ecological circumstances as the child with Down

Syndrome.

(4) The brother or sister of the study subject should live with the same biological parents. Thus, parental educational background and socioeconomic factors will be the same in the study and control populations.

(5) The brother or sister of the individual with Down Syndrome should preferably function at approximately the same mental age as the child with Down Syndrome.

Because the latter selection criterion was not uniformly attainable, a second control group was formed of the nonretarded children who had been referred to the Child Development Center because of suspected school difficulties, developmental problems, or medical concerns. Most of these children underwent a comprehensive evaluation at the Child Development Center which, however, indicated that there are no specific neurologic deficits, central nervous system lesions, medical, genetic or chromosomal disorders, and that intellectual functioning is within the average range. They were then matched with children in the experimental group according to sex, mental age, socieconomic status of parents, and ethnic group.

Apparatus

The Kaufman Assessment Battery for Children was used in this study to investigate sequential and simultaneous processing in the children with Down Syndrome (Kaufman & Kaufman, 1983a). The Kaufman test is an individually administered measure of intelligence that has been standardized on a large, representative nationwide sample of more than 2000 normal and exceptional children. The test consists of four areas of functioning: Sequential Processing, Simultaneous Processing, Mental Processing Composite, and Achievement. The latter part of the test battery, which provides information on learned skills, was not used in this investigation. The Kaufman test, particularly the mental processing scales, measures a child's ability to solve problems sequentially and simultaneously with emphasis on the processes used to produce correct solutions. Whereas other intelligence tests tend to be more content-oriented, intelligence, as measured by the Kaufman test is defined in terms of an individual's style of solving problems and processing information. The Mental Processing Scales of the Kaufman test are designed to conform to both the sequential and simultaneous processing paradigm derived from neuropsychological and cognitive theories.

In addition, the Kaufman's built-in teaching component allows the examiner to explain to the child the nature of a task in the first unscored sample item and to use the first two scored items on each subtest as teaching items. Thus, the examiner has a unique opportunity to observe the subject's approach to learning a new task.

Hypothesis

We hypothesized that cognitive and learning processes in children with Down Syndrome differ significantly from those of intellectually normal children of similar mental age. We predicted that children with Down Syndrome would not perform as well in the sequential processing as in simultaneous processing since the former involves short term memory, understanding of chronology, and synthesis of successive events, all of which are impaired in children with Down Syndrome. Moreover, we predicted that the children with Down Syndrome would perform better in areas of visual processing than in areas of auditory processing since their auditory channels of communication are reportedly more adversely affected than are their visual channels of communication (Bilovsky & Share, 1965).

Results

The analysis of specific characteristics of the study population revealed that there was no significant difference of the sex distribution in the three groups (Chi square = 1.2, df = 2, p = .55). As noted in Table 1 the mean chronological age of the Down Syndrome subjects was 10 years and 11 months. Their brothers and sisters as

well as the mental age-matched nonretarded group were significantly younger.
The mean mental age of the children with Down Syndrome was 61.0 months with a standard deviation of 16.4 indicating that the children in the experimental group were functioning in a mild to moderate range of mental retardation. It is apparent from Table 1 that the mean mental age of the children with Down Syndrome (61.0 months) was close to that of children from the second control group (62.7 months), thus matching for mental age was adequate (F = .116, df = 38, p = .735). The siblings of the children with Down Syndrome functioned intellectually above average and the mental age-matched group had average to low average cognitive abilities.

Table 1
Sex Distribution, Means and Standard Deviations of Chronological Age and Mental Age of Children in the Experimental and the Control Groups

Study Group	N			Chronological Age (months)		Mental Age (months)	
				X	SD	X	SD
Down Syndrome	20	11	9	131.4	24.2	61.0	16.4
Siblings	20	8	12	87.3	25.6	105.0	34.1
MA-matched	20	11	9	66.4	10.7	62.7	15.2

In order to test the hypothesis that cognitive and learning processes in children with Down Syndrome differ significantly from those of intellectually normal children of similar mental age means and standard deviations of the Standard Scores were calculated for each group separately (see Table 2).
Since the assumption of homogeneity of variance was met (F max [sequential] = 2.33; F max [simultaneous] = 2.21) two one-way analyses of variance were performed. Comparing the Standard Scores of the Sequential and the Simultaneous Processing Scales of the three groups a highly

Table 2
Means and Standard Deviations of Standard Scores of
Sequential and Simultaneous Processing Scales for child-
ren in the Experimental and the Control Groups

	N	Sequential Processing*		Simultaneous Processing**	
		X	SD	X	SD
Down Syndrome	20	53.6	8.03	54.9	8.74
Siblings	20	108.3	12.26	104.9	12.91
MA-matched	20	90.3	10.67	94.0	13.00

*F = 141.02, df = 57, p<.0001
**F = 100.61, df = 57, p<.0001

significant difference was found (F[sequential] = 141.02,
df = 57, p < .0001; F[simultaneous] = 100.62, df = 57, p
<.001). All follow-up tests indicated that there were
significant differences between the individual groups for
both the Sequential and the Simultaneous Processing Scale
Scores. The Down Syndrome group performed significantly
less well than both siblings and the mental age-matched
nonretarded group. In an analysis of covariance controlling for mental age, Standard Scores of the Sequential
and Simultaneous Processing Scales of children with Down
Syndrome were compared with equivalent scores of their
brothers and sisters. A significant difference was found
for both sequential processing (F = 146.3, df = 38, p <
.001) and for simultaneous processing (F = 111.6, df =
38, p < .001)
     In further analysis of the data, paired t-tests were
performed that contrasted the Standard Scores of the
Sequential Processing Scale with the Standard Scores of
the Simultaneous Processing Scale obtained from children
with Down Syndrome. There was no significant difference
observed (t = .934, df = 19, p = .362). Similar results
were obtained when paired t-tests were done comparing

206   Pueschel

these two scales in the sibling group (t = -.955, df =
19, p = .351) and in the nonretarded mental age-matched
group (t = 1.00, df = 19, p = .329). In order to compare
the performance of children with Down Syndrome in visual
and auditory processing, means and standard deviations of
Scales Scores for a number of subtests were calculated.
These included: Number Recall, which uses auditory-vocal
channels; Word Order, which uses auditory motor channels;
Gestalt Closure, which uses visual-vocal channels; and
Hand Movement, which uses visual-motor channels of communications (Table 3). These subtests were selected because

Table 3
Means and Standard Deviations of Scaled Scores of Subtests Hand Movements, Gestalt Closure, Number Recall, and
Word Order for Children in the Experimental and the Control Groups

	Down Syndrome		Siblings		MA-matched	
	X	SD	X	SD	X	SD
Hand Movement	3.15	1.69	10.60	2.98	7.95	1.90
Gestalt Closure	4.55	2.35	10.25	2.83	8.05	2.33
Number Recall	2.35	1.46	12.25	1.92	9.00	2.60
Word Order	1.70	1.34	11.6	2.72	8.35	1.95

complete data sets were available for them on all children in the experimental and control groups. (Depending on
the child's chronological age, different combinations of
subtests of the Sequential and Simultaneous Processing
Scales are administered. Thus not all children were given
the same subtests.)
   The results of this analysis revealed that the children
with Down Syndrome have more difficulties in their aud-

Figure 1
Test Profile for:

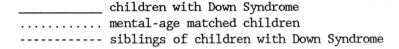

_____ children with Down Syndrome
.... mental-age matched children
------------ siblings of children with Down Syndrome

Scaled Scores:

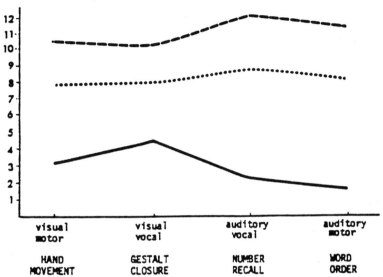

itory-vocal and auditory-motor channels of communication as they performed significantly less well on those two subtests when compared with the other two subtests which primarily employ visual-vocal and visual-motor channels of communication respectively. Highly significant differences were found (Table 4) in the comparison of the following subtests: Hand Movement and Number Recall, Hand Movement and Word Order, Gestalt Closure and Number Recall, and Gestalt Closure and Word and Number Recall, Hand Movement and Word Order, Gestalt Closure and Number Recall, and Gestalt Closure and Word Order. There were no significant differences observed in contrasting Hand Movement and Gestalt Closure, and Number Recall and Word Order.

In the siblings group statistically significant differences were observed for Hand Movement versus Number Recall and for Gestalt Closure versus Number Recall. In

Table 4
T-values and P-values of Paired T-tests Comparing Scaled
Scores of Subtests involving Auditory and Visual Channels
of Communication for Children in the Experimental and the
Control Groups.

Subtests	Down Syndrome		Siblings		MA-matched	
	t	p	t	p	t	p
Hand Movement(T3) vs Gestalt Closure(T4)	1.811	.086	-.418	.681	.172	.865
Hand Movement(T3) vs Number Recall(T5)	-3.263	.004	2.554	.019	1.893	.074
Hand Movement(T3) vs Word Order(T7)	-4.837	.001	1.504	.149	.969	.345
Gestalt Closure(T4) vs Number Recall(T5)	-4.854	.001	2.517	.021	1.235	.232
Gestalt Closure(T4) vs Word Order(T7)	-4.705	.001	1.484	.154	.490	.629
Number Recall(T5) vs Word Order(T7)	-1.228	.234	1.146	.267	-1.378	.184

contrast to the children with Down Syndrome, the brothers
and sisters performed significantly better on the auditory-vocal Number Recall subtest than on subtests that
use visual-vocal and visual-motor channels of communication. The remaining t-tests comparing various subtests in
the siblings group and all the t-tests in the mental age-
matched nonretarded group did not reach statistical significance.

Discussion

    As detailed above, children in the experimental group
differed significanltly in that they performed less well
in sequential and simultaneous processing when compared
with results obtained from their brothers and sisters
(corrected for mental age) and with a mental age-matched
and sex-matched nonretarded group of children. It was
hypothesized that the significantly reduced sequential
and simultaneous processing of children with Down Syndrome resulted primarily from a global neuronal insult
due to such things as genetically determined perturbation
of intraneuronal homeostasis. Although we still lack a
basic understanding of the molecular paradigm that would
assist in the elucidation of the cognitive dysfunction
observed in persons with this chromosomal disorder, the
significant increase of super-oxide dismutase (Sinet,
Lejeune, & Jerome, 1979) that results in lipoperoxidative
neuronal damage, or the prenatal arrest of neuronal proliferation and differentiation may in part explain the
significantly lower cognitive processing abilities in the
children with Down Syndrome. These generalized effects on
the central nervous system integrity may account for the
fact that there were no significant differences be- tween
sequential and simultaneous processing were un- covered
in this investigation.
    Hence, if the main body of this research supports a
"global neuronal insult hypothesis," the question then
arises as to why specific auditory processing dysfunc-
tions were observed in subjects with Down Syndrome. As
noted above, these children had greater difficulties with
auditory-motor and auditory-vocal processing than with
visual-motor and visual-vocal processing. A developmen-
tal-biochemical hypothesis can be advanced in order to
explain this phenomenon: Myelination of nerve fibers
occurs for specific neuronal tissues at different times
in the development of the central nervous system. It is
known that nerve fibers of auditory associations are
myelinated late during development when an increase in
peroxidative damage may occur. Thus selective perturbation of oxygen-free radical metabolism will affect
adversely myelin formation in nerve tracts concerned with
auditory processing. This hypothesis is supported by re-

cent auditory evoked potential studies (Lincoln et al. 1985, Courchesne, this volume).

Also, inner ear dysfunction such as decreased cochlear receptivity or middle ear conditions that lead to conduction deficits may in part explain the observations made in this investigation. It is unlikely, however, that hearing impairments were responsible for the reduction in auditory processing in this study since the subjects in the experimental group had audiologic evaluations prior to testing which indicated normal hearing.

Other explanations for the significant difficulties in auditory processing come from behavioral research. It has been suggested that the Down Syndrome child's rehearsal mechanism may be defective and that he/she has impairments in storing information as a result of inadequate language skills (Rohr & Burr, 1978). Also, the child's slower encoding at progressively deeper processing levels may account for the reduced auditory processing ability. Schultz (1983) has observed that the depth-of-processing approach has proved to be useful in providing information about processing difficulties in numerous populations. He noted that a retarded individual is in need of more time to construct a richer and more elaborate trace.

Furthermore, it is known that Down Syndrome children have a short-term memory deficit (Marcell & Armstrong, 1982). Because there was an interval of several seconds or longer between asking a question and the appearance of a response, the subjects with Down Syndrome had to retain temporarily information contained in questions or directions in order to respond correctly to a stimulus word.

Some other investigators also reported difficulties in auditory processing in children with Down Syndrome. McDade and Adler (1980) assessed the recall and recognition memories using either auditory or visual input with verbal and nonverbal responses. These authors found that children with Down Syndrome displayed deficits in both auditory and visual storage and retrieval. The auditory and visual sequential memory of children with Down Syndrome were also studied by Marcell and Armstrong (1982). These investigators observed poor auditory sequential memory and significant difficulties recalling auditorily presented material in youngsters with Down Syndrome which they feel might have been due to echoic memory deficits.

Other researchers (Bilovsky & Share, 1965; Snart, O'Grady, & Das, 1982) have found the greatest deficit in children with Down Syndrome to be in the area of auditory sequential memory. Das, Kirby, and Jarman (1979) reported that successive coding underlies much of our language production with simultaneous coding and planning contributing to higher level thought processes. Also, Rohr and Burr (1978) noted that persons with Down Syndrome were the only group with a specific pattern of abilities having visual task performance consistently higher than the auditory task performance. Analogous to results obtained in the present study, these investigators observed significantly lower verbal abilities. These findings were corroborated by Lincoln et al. (1985) who reported that children with Down Syndrome process some types of auditory information significantly slower than do mental age-matched and chronologically age-matched nonretarded children.

It is anticipated that future neurochemical research together with auditory evoked potential studies, investigations of central auditory processing, and specific cognitive and language assessments will provide a greater insight into the underlying pathogenetic mechanisms that lead to auditory processing deficits in children with Down Syndrome. The recent increase in technical and conceptual strength in both psychology and biology makes it possible now to confront the boundary between these two disciplines, and questions posed by both fields are beginning to converge on a common ground.

Another important aspect of this investigation concerns the psychoeducational implications of the study. In order to foster developmental progress of children with Down Syndrome, test scores need to be translated into appropriate programs for effective educational intervention. Although the Mental Processing Scales of the Kaufman test do not predict school success as certain other achievement tests do, they might hold the key to selecting the appropriate strategies for teaching a given child. Since a child's preferred mode of processing information is related closely to his or her learning style, and since research supports the notion that effective learning takes place when the mode of teaching matches an individual's preferred style of processing, investigations employing the Sequential and the Simultaneous Processing Scales of the Kaufman test could provide suggestions for the effective teaching of specific content.

Although our data do not indicate a significant difference between the Sequential and Simultaneous Processing Systems, it was apparent in further analysis of our data that the auditory-vocal and the auditory-motor channels of communication were more affected than other areas of central nervous system processing in children of the experimental group. Thus teaching strategies should capitalize on the children's strengths and should focus on visual-vocal and visual-motor processing modalities in remediation of children with Down Syndrome. An increased emphasis on auditory teaching strategies may lead to frustration in the child, which could impede academic progress.

While it has been shown to be beneficial for children with a decided strength in one type of processing to be taught by methods that feature the child's strong areas, other teaching strategies should not be excluded in the remedial efforts. A built-in flexibility that takes into consideration the individual child's strengths and weaknesses should be the central theme of any intervention program. Other elements such as adaptive functioning, affective behavior, and additional assessment data will need to be integrated into an effective remedial program.

Thus the Kaufman test can be used not only to learn more about the child's approach to solving problems and his/her way of learning but it also will help with the design of intervention programs. This may permit us to do something about the future beyond simply predicting it (Kaufman & Kaufman, 1983b).

Of course, the skillful teacher should realize that no amount of talking or reading or writing is as effective in teaching as it is for the child to feel a tangible object or to participate in real life situations which are more creative learning experiences. Watching snowflakes gently coming down from the sky or seeing rain spattering against the window is infinitely more meaningful to the child than having another adult telling him/her about it. Opportunities for field trips provide the child with Down Syndrome a chance to learn how to live in the community with other people. Expeditions to zoos and parks gives him/her the opportunity to see real life animals, trees and plants, and let him/her view the beauty of nature. Watching the mailman or policeman at work and interacting with them is a much more sustaining experience for the child with Down Syndrome than abstract presentations or even pictures in books. Schools should provide the kind of stimulating enriching experience in which the world appears as an interesting place to explore. Learning situations at school should help a child with Down Syndrome obtain a feeling of personal identity, self-respect, and enjoyment. Schools should give him/her an opportunity to engage in sharing relationships with others and prepare the child so that he/she can later contribute productively and meaningfully to society.

REFERENCES

Belmont, J. M. (1971). Medical-Behavioral Research in Retardation. In N. R. Ellis (Ed.), International Review of Research in Mental Retardation: Vol. 5 New York: Academic Press.

Bilovsky, J. E., & Share, J. (1965). The ITPA and Down's Syndrome: An exploratory study. American Journal of Mental Deficiency, 70, 78-82.

Carr, J. (1970). Mental and motor development in young mongol children. Journal of Mental Deficiency Research, 14, 205-220.

Cornwell, A. C., & Birch, H. G. (1969). Psychological and social development in home reared children with Down's syndrome. American Journal of Mental Deficiency, 74, 341-350.

Corri, J. (1975). Young Children with Down Syndrome. Boston: Buttersworth.

Dameron, L. E. (1963). Development of intelligence of infants with mongolism. Child Development, 34, 733-738.

Das, J. P., Kirby, J., & Jarman, R. F. (1979). Simultaneous and successive cognitive processes. New York: Academic Press.

Dicks-Mireaux, M. J. (1972). Mental development of children with Down's syndrome. American Journal of Mental Deficiency, 77, 26-32.

Down, J. L. H. (1866). Observations on an ethnic classification of idiots. London Hospital, Clinical Lectures

214 Pueschel

and Reports, 3, 259-262.
Dunn, L., & Dunn, L. (1981). Manual for the Peabody Pic-
ture Vocabulary Test-Revised (PPVT-R). Circle Pines,
MN: American Guidance Service.
Fishler, K. (1975). Mental development in mosaic Down's
syndrome as compared with trisomy 21. In R. Koch, &
F. F. de la Cruz (Eds.), Down's syndrome (mongolism):
Research, Prevention and Management. New York: Brunner/
Mazal.
Gesell, A., & Amatruda, C. (1941). Developmental Diag-
nosis. New York: Paul Hoeber, Inc.
Gibson, D. (1978). Down's syndrome. Cambridge: Cambridge
University Press.
Girardeau, F. L. (1959). The formation of discrimination
learning sets in mongoloid and normal children. Journal
of Comparative and Physiological Psychology, 52, 566-
570.
Gramza, A. F., & Witt, P. A. (1969). Choices of colored
blocks in the play of preschool children. Perceptual
and Motor Skills, 29, 783-787.
Kaufman, A. S., & Kaufman, N. L. (1983a). K-ABC Kaufman
Assessment Battery for Children Administration and
Scoring Manual. Circle Pines, MN: American Guidance
Service.
Kaufman, A. S., & Kaufman, N. L. (1965). K-ABC Kaufman
Assessment Battery for Children Interpretive Manual.
Circle Pines, MN: American Guidance Service.
Knights, R. M., Hyman, J. A., & Wozny, M. A, (1965).
Psychomotor abilities of familial brain-damaged and
mongoloid retarded children. American Journal of Mental
Deficiency, 70, 454-457.
Lincoln, A. J., Courchesne, E., Kilman, B. A., &
Galambos, R. (1985). Neuropsychological correlates of
information-processing by children with Down syndrome.
American Journal of Mental Deficiency, 89, 403-414.
Lodge, A. L., & Kleinfield, P. B. (1973). Early behavior-
al development in Down's syndrome. In M. Coleman (Ed.),
Serotonin in Down's syndrome. New York: American
Elsevier Publishing Company.
Marcell, M. M., & Armstrong, V. (1982). Auditory and vis-
ual sequential memory of Down syndrome and nonretarded
children. American Journal of Mental Deficiency, 87,
86-95.

Masland, R. L., Sarson, S. B., & Gladwin, T. (1958). Mental Subnormality. New York: Basic Books, Inc.

McDade, H. L., & Adler, S. (1980). Down syndrome and short-term memory impairment: A storage of retrieval deficit. American Journal of Mental Deficiency, 84, 561-567.

O'Connor, N., & Berkson, G. (1963). Eye movement in normals and defectives. American Journal of Mental Deficiency, 68, 85-90.

O'Connor, N., & Hermelin, B. (1961). Visual and stereognostic shape recognition in normal children and mongol and non-mongol imbeciles. Journal of Mental Deficiency Research, 5, 63-66.

Oster, J. (1953). Mongolism. Copenhagen: Danish Science Press.

Penrose, L. S., & Smith, G. F. (1966). Down's Anomaly. Boston: Little Brown & Company.

Pueschel, S. M., Reed, R. B., Cronk, C. E., & Goldstein, B. I. (1980). The effect of 5-hydroxytryptophan and/or pyridoxin in young children with Down syndrome. American Journal of Diseases of Children, 134, 838-844.

Rohr, A., & Burr, D. B. (1978). Etiological differences in patterns of psycholinguistic development of children of IQ 30 to 60. American Journal of Mental Deficiency, 82, 549-553.

Rosecrans, C. J. (1968). The relationship of normal 21-trisomy mosaicism and intellectual development. American Journal of Mental Deficiency, 72, 562-569.

Rosner, F., Ong, B. H., Paine, R. S. & Mahanand, D. (1965). Blood serotonin activity in trisomic and translocation Down's syndrome. Lancet, 1, 1191-1193.

Sachs, E. S. (1971). Trisomy G/Normal Mosaicism. Leiden: H. E. Stenfert.

Sattler, J. M. (1982). Assessment of children's intelligence and special abilities. (2nd ed.). Boston, London, Sydney, Toronto: Allyn and Bacon, Inc.

Scheffelin, M. (1968). A comparison of four stimulus-response channels in paired-associate learning. American Journal of Mental Deficiency, 73, 303-307.

Schnell, R. R. (1984). Psychomotor development. In S. M. Pueschel (Ed.), The young child with Down syndrome (pp. 207-226). New York: Human Science Press, Inc.

Schultz, E. E. J. (1983). Depth of processing by mentally retarded and MA-matched nonretarded individuals. American Journal of Mental Deficiency, 88, 307-313.

Share, J., Koch, R., Webb, A., & Graliker, B. (1964). The longitudinal development of infants and young children with Down's syndrome (mongolism). American Journal of Mental Deficiency, 68, 685-696.

Sinet, P. M., Lejenue, J. & Jerome, H. (1979). Trisomy-21 (Down's syndrome), glutathione peroxidase, hexose mono-phosphate shunt and I.Q. Life Science, 24, 29-32.

Snart, F., O'Grady, M. & Das, J. P. (1982). Cognitive Processing by subgroups of moderately mentally retarded children. American Journal of Mental Deficiency, 86, 465-472.

Stratford, B. (1980a). Perception and perceptual-motor processes in children with Down's syndrome. Journal of Psychology, 104, 139-145.

Stratford, B. (1980b). Preferences in attention to visual cues in Down syndrome and normal children. Journal of Mental Deficiency Research, 24, 57-64.

Zekulin, X. Y., Gibson, D., Mosley, J. L., & Brown, R. I. (1974). Auditory-motor channelling in Down's syndrome subjects. American Journal of Mental Deficiency, 78, 571-577.

Zellweger, H., & Abbo, G. (1963). Chromosomal mosaicism and mongolism. Lancet, 1, 829-835.

7

DETERMINANTS OR RATE OF LANGUAGE
GROWTH IN CHILDREN WITH DS

Anne E. Fowler
Haskins Laboratories
270 Crown Street
New Haven, CT 06511

The questions addressed in this paper concern the effect of greatly impoverished general intellectual endow-
ment on the acquisition of language structure over time,
focusing upon children with Down Syndrome (DS). In asking
this question, it is necessary to resolve two very well-
documented findings regarding the language structures associated with DS. On the one hand, children with DS often
have great difficulty acquiring language, generally showing delays relative to traditional motor, intellectual or
social indices (Gibson, 1978). Indeed, it appears that
children with DS may have even more difficulty in acquiring language structures than other subgroups of retarded
children; this difficulty is most pronounced in the syn-
tactic-grammatical domain (e.g. Burr and Rohr, 1978; see
Fowler, in press for a review).
On the other hand, despite this marked difficulty in
acquiring language structures, a sizable literature has
consistently maintained that the products of this acquisition are "normal", with no hint of deviant learning
processes. This robust conclusion is generally agreed
upon regardless of the language level (e.g. Stage I versus Stage III); language area (e.g. vocabulary, semantic
relations, syntax, or grammatical morphology) or language
task (production or comprehension) under study. (For
reviews, see Fowler, in press; Miller, in press; Rondal,
1975).
What these two findings suggest is a greatly slowed
down, but normal, learning process. In this paper, the
aim is to better understand the actual course of learn-

ing, paying particular attention to rate of development over time. Is learning slow and steady over time? Or does the child make insights over widely-spaced intervals? What are the relevant factors in accounting for rate of acquisition? In this study, the approach taken is longitudinal, adding to a heretofore extremely limited pool of data. Of special interest is the maturational hypothesis invoked by Lenneberg, Nichols and Rosenberger (1964) to account for the overall pattern of acquisition apparent in 63 children with DS studied over a three-year period. In brief, Lenneberg et al. suggested that language learning followed a timetable much like that assumed to underlie the unfolding of motor development; that IQ played but a minimal role in determining the prognosis of language skill; and that a critical period for language learning shut down with the onset of puberty, preventing further language growth in children whose acquisition was less than complete.

Background

The research presented here and the hypothesis guiding it stem from work first presented in Fowler, Gelman and Gleitman (1980). In that initial study, we addressed the issue of language deviancy in children with DS showing massive delays in language skill. Specifically, 12 year old children with mental age (MA) scores of 5 to 6 years (Stanford-Binet) appeared to be speaking at the level of a normally developing toddler of 2.6 years. To pinpoint areas of differential difficulty in the retarded child, we matched groups on a global language measure -- mean length of utterance in morphemes (MLU) -- rather than on the then more standardly used MA score. We suspected that MA so vastly overestimated language skills as to mask any potential qualitative differences or any interesting discrepancies between skills, such as between closed class and open class vocabulary knowledge.

The results of that study were interesting on two counts. First, as indicated by comparative studies before and since, the language produced by the children with DS contained no hint of deviancy. Despite the advantage of general cognitive level and of impressionistic conversational skill, the children with DS performed remarkably like their MLU controls on a sizable battery of internal measures. They had made the same progress as their MLU peers in regard to the grammatical morphology; produced similar negative and interrogative forms; relied equivalently on open-class and closed-class vocabulary items; encoded similar thematic roles; and used similar sentence structures. In short, the two groups were at the same language stage. This finding is highly consistent with reports since from other labs.

The second conclusion of interest concerned the consistency of the language level observed across the four children with DS. The children with DS were not pre-selected for language level, but fell together as a natural class in our original observations of retarded children generally. Despite this fact, the analyses performed showed them to be operating with highly coherent, internally consistent grammars. Indeed, they were even more consistent than were the normally developing children, who were specifically selected for this language level from among a large number of youngsters between 30 and 36 months of age.

The particular language level observed, characterized as Stage III in Brown's (1973) schema of development, with a mean MLU of 3.0, allows for some primitive concatenation of phrases. It emphatically precedes the development of the verbal auxiliary system and of complex sentence subordination. We were led to ask why this particular stopping point, so consistently evident here and yet, from all reports including observations of our own, so rapidly traversed by the normally developing child.

Input from two other sources shed some potential light on the subject. First, a careful rereading of the available literature on the development of language in children with DS was undertaken, this time looking beyond the claims of normalcy to focus on what language structures the children with DS had acquired in absolute terms (Fowler, in press). The results of this review were startling: children with DS, by and large, do not progress beyond the language level (Stage III) attained by adolescents studied in Fowler et al. (1980). Several studies of language structure in DS have focussed on this stage (Rondal, 1980; Layton and Sharifi, 1979; Ryan, 1975,

1977). An even greater number of studies of language
structure in DS have focused on stage I of language development; here one sees early two-word combinations
characteristic of normally developing children from 18 to
24 months of age (e.g. Beeghly and Cicchetti, 1985;
Coggins and Morrison, 1981; Rondal, 1980; Coggins, 1979;
Dooley, 1977). The low levels characteristic of language
in children with DS were not, of course, restricted to
studies where MLU was the matching criterion. As pointed
out by Rosenberger (1982), even the classic study of
Lenneberg, Nichols and Rosenberger (1964), so often cited
as testimony to the triumph of maturation over general
cognitive disability in determining the course of language development, reported that a total of 3 out of 63
children studied had moved beyond the stage of "primitive
phrases".

The second piece of data available to us was a quick
trip to a younger classroom in the school from which we
had derived our adolescent subjects. There, we found 7 to
9 year old children were using language seemingly indistinguishable from that spoken by our adolescents.

Hypotheses

These data led to the formulation of three hypotheses
regarding the course of language development in children
with DS, and regarding the determinants of when progress
occurs and when it will not. Hypothesis #1 is a stage-
related hypothesis proposed to account for the consistency of language levels across children with DS, and the
lack of movement beyond particular periods of development. According to Hypothesis #1 (a variant of proposals
in the normal literature by Bowerman, 1982 or Karmiloff-
Smith, 1979), language learning might best be characterized as a series of stages in which available information
is reorganized and resystematized by learners -- retarded
and not. Acquisition of a structure, or movement into a
stage should require generalizations of the same scope,
no matter who the learner. A child, who, either because
of age or intellectual constraints, cannot acquire a
structure or system in full, should stall altogether in
the face of it. On the other hand, because a structure

can only be acquired in one form, once within a stage, groups should be indistinguishable. On this account, what should differentiate the retarded child is an extreme difficulty moving from one stage to another together with an early cutoff at a linguistically well-defined ceiling below some next more difficult and unattainable level of development.

Hypothesis #2, the "shallow generalization hypothesis" (Gleitman, 1981), is the implicitly assumed model of slow learning, that learning should be slowed down, uniformly and commensurately, relative to the normal case across the entire learning period. Under this view, language might proceed as a single accretion of facts over time and practice conditions. Rate of growth should be a direct function of IQ with flatter curves and shallower generalizations at all points. Hence, faced with the acquisition of a structure such as the past tense marker, the less well-endowed child might acquire the past tense marker for an individual subclass of verbs, or in the extreme case, verb by verb.

Each of these hypotheses, is, in turn, to be considered in light of yet a third hypothesis, Lenneberg's (1967) critical period hypothesis. Hypothesis #3 suggests that language learning in DS (and in individuals generally), is far more a function of general maturational factors (on a schedule with walking, running, etc.) than it is tied to general intelligence factors. A crucial component of Lenneberg's theory was the notion of a biologically imposed critical period of language development. Lenneberg's data, from work on DS and on aphasia, pointed to a shut-down of the specialized language learning faculty at puberty; such an account has also been invoked to explain effects of age on second language learning.

Two lines of longitudinal research are presented here to bear upon these competing hypotheses. Experiment I (presented in detail in Fowler, 1984) provides indepth data on one child, Rebecca, whose language development from Stage I to Stage V has been studied intensively, both for overall pattern of development and for internal acquisitions. Intensive study of Rebecca occurred between 51 and 89 months of age. Experiment II involves the comparison of Rebecca's overall developmental course with that of 10 other children with DS, varying in IQ and chronological age at the onset of study. This larger data sample was collected over a 7 year period, and collectively spans the chronological age range of 4 to 19 years.

Experiment I

Rebecca (Stanford-Binet 57) was selected for study at the age of 51 months, at which point she was in early Stage I, where Brown began his longitudinal study. She was observed in hour-long play sessions at home on a nearly-monthly basis from 51 to 89 months; since then her progress has been monitored at 6-month intervals (last visit 108 months). Procedures for collection, transcription and analyses of language samples were adapted from the classic normative studies of Bellugi (1967), Brown (1973), and Bloom (1970). The major findings are reviewed here to provide context for Experiment II.

Rebecca's development consisted of two quite distinct phases: Stage I to III; and Stage III and beyond. (See Figure 1). After a slow start in early Stage I, Rebecca proceeded from Stage I up to early Stage III (55 to 66 months) in an absolutely normal fashion. On all measures taken, her growth was unremarkable both in rate and character. This was true not only for the general measure of MLU, which progressed rapidly and consistently upward, but for internal measures as well. During this time, four of Brown's 14 grammatical morphemes (in, on, progressive and plural) were acquired to 90% criterion, the same four were the first acquired by each of Brown's three subjects within comparable language stages. Rebecca's early negative and interrogative constructions also paralleled normal development as set forth by Bellugi (1967), with a heavy reliance on intonation (I play this?, this is yours?); negative modals (I can't shut it), and the unadorned NOT (her not go). Present at this stage was a whole repertoire of unanalyzed wh-questions (e.g. where's NP?, what's this?). Encoding of thematic relations also advanced in an orderly fashion, although slightly in advance of other measures, when compared to normally developing subjects studied by Bloom, Lightbown and Hood (1975). Even the relative distribution of thematic categories relied upon was consistent with norms, with the only difference concerning a consistently greater tendency on Rebecca's part to pad her utterances with such non-developmental categories as stereotyped phrases, adverbs and vocatives. Finally, no unusual or persistent misanalyses were noted during the period from I to III.

Figure 1: Growth in mean utterance length of Rebecca (Down Syndrome) COMPARED TO THREE CHILDREN STUDIED BY BROWN (1973)

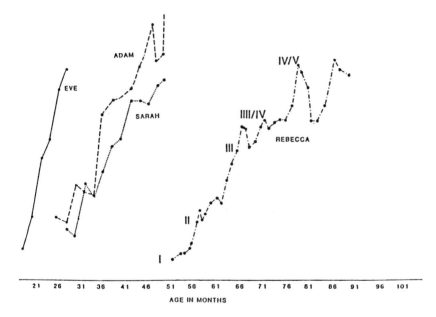

Once having achieved Stage III (MLU 3.5; 67 months), Rebecca's progress slowed sharply and began to deviate from the norm. Growth in MLU ceased altogether for 10 months and further gains were offset by large and erratic shifts downward. By the end of the study almost two years later (89 months), Rebecca had met the criterion for only one additional morpheme, the contractible copula. Even there, despite its consistent appearance in appropriate contexts (e.g. it's gone), the contractible copula also appeared in a wide variety of inappropriate contexts. Note, for example: "she's eat", "what's you want", "mommy's go water". This misanalysis appeared from the onset of Stage III and persisted to the end of the study (67 to 89 months). Other grammatical morphemes previously

acquired were now used inconsistently. Rebecca also plateaued at the Stage III level in terms of her progress in
mastering questions and negation. The auxiliary system
underlying mature constructions involving subject-auxil-
iary inversion and do-support were almost totally lacking
in her grammar, with substantial progress apparent only
at the final session. Between 67 and 89 months, a second
misanalysis appeared, this time involving wh-terms. The
term "what" frequently replaced other wh-terms to yield
constructions like "what's you go" (meaning "where") and
"What's you gonna bring it, Mom? 20 minutes?" (meaning
"when").

The case of Rebecca bears interestingly upon the three
hypotheses proposed. First, despite the fact that Rebecca
has ultimately acquired more language skills than the adolescent children studied in Fowler et al. (1980), and
than other children with DS generally, the changes in her
developmental pattern which occurred at Stage III support
the view that Stage III may indeed constitute a special
blocking point for the child with DS; this is consistent
with Hypothesis #1, the stage-related hypothesis of language acquisition. In contrast, Rebecca's course of development does not appear to be consistent with Hypothesis #2, the shallow generalization hypothesis. Under that
hypothesis, one would have expected a slower progression
across the period studied, rather than the sharp break
between the near normal growth rate and the absolute plateau actually observed.

On the other hand, these data are also not inconsistent
with Hypothesis #3, that age-related factors may account
for Rebecca's change in growth rate as she reached
school-age. Although not discussed in any detail by
Lenneberg (1967), maturational growth curves need not be
a simple case of normal rate of development up to a cutoff at puberty. That language is acquired more quickly --
and more readily -- in the pre-school years than in the
middle childhood years is an idea that is gaining some
currency from work with the deaf, a population which is
of particular interest because of an all-too-frequent
lack of exposure to any language during early childhood.
Newport (1986) reports that deaf first exposed to a formal language model (ASL) during middle childhood show
significant decrements in asymptotic skill in ASL when

compared to their luckier counterparts who learned ASL before five or six years of age.

Experiment II

Subjects - To validate these findings on other subjects, we have now collected extensive longitudinal data on 10 other children with DS, differing widely in terms of IQ_1 starting CA, and language stage. Stanford-Binet IQ scores[1] in this group cluster around 50, but range from 38 to 64. Starting age ranged from 4 to 13 years; the sample includes the four adolescents first studied in Fowler et al. (1980). Although all the children had to be forming at least some two word combinations to be included in the sample, several of the children were well beyond Stage I when they were first interviewed. All children were tested at least once every six months for a minimum of four and a maximum of seven years. As in the case study of Rebecca, procedures for collection, transcrin, and coding of data followed canonical methods of classic normative studies. Taped conversations lasted a minimum of 30 minutes, yielding at least 100 child-initiated non-stock utterances.

Measures - The primary index of grammatical growth and complexity was the Mean length of utterance in morphemes (MLU), an optimal and standardly used measure of early language development, which has proven extremely useful in predicting other aspects of internal development in both normally developing children and in children with DS up to MLU 4.0 or approximately 3;6 years of age (e.g. Fowler, 1984; Brown 1973: Shipley, Smith & Gleitman, 1969). Procedures for calculating MLU were similar to those outlined by Brown (1973) with modifications as outlined and justified in detail in Fowler (1984). These modifications involved basing the analysis upon an entire session rather than just the first 100 utterances; and excluding from the analysis all elicited responses to questions, stock phrases (defined as any single expression occurring in identical form more than 5 times in a transcript), lists without internal structure (counting, naming friends, etc.), and immediate repetitions of self or other. This means differences in language use were systematically removed from our analyses that we might focus on structural competence.

As a second, internal, measure of grammatical complexity, the Index of Productive Syntax (IPSyn - Scarborough, 1985) served to validate the MLU results as well as to aid in those cases where language development had progressed to the point where MLU was no longer reliable or valid (Scarborough, 1985; Chabon, Kent-Udolf, Egolf, 1982). The IPSyn is based on a 100 utterance sample and involves awarding points for the occurrence of 56 kinds of morphological and syntactic forms, for a maximum score of 112. The measure, based on a previous scale devised by Miller (1980), provides a quick quantitative means of detecting growth in internal language structure, for which norms are currently available on a total of 48 sessions collected from 12 children ranging from 24 to 48 months. The syntactic/morphological forms coded for are divided into four categories: Nounphrase, Verbphrase, Question/ Negation and Sentence Structure, each with separate normed scores. Although this measure of optimal performance is not intrinsically tied to MLU, which is a measure of mean performance, Scarborough finds correlations of .72 to .96 between 24 and 36 months of age.

Use of the IPSyn measure with children with DS shows it to be convergent with the MLU measure in this population. This convergence is supported by a correlation of 0.95 between the two measures in Rebecca; this is made graphic in plots of growth for MLU and IPSyn presented together in Figure 2. (See Tager-Flusberg, 1986, for supporting results from other children with DS).

Analysis and Results

As a first look at the data collected from the total sample of 11 children (including Rebecca), all MLU and IPSyn data points were entered into regression analyses calculating growth in these measures as a simple function of chronological age. As seen in Figure 3, the most obvious result of the analysis of growth in MLU is its nonlinearity; using goodness-of-fit statistics, the first acceptable fit is a cubic. Although the overall linear slope is .11 MLU points a year, three distinct periods

Figure 2: Rebecca Total Growth in MLU

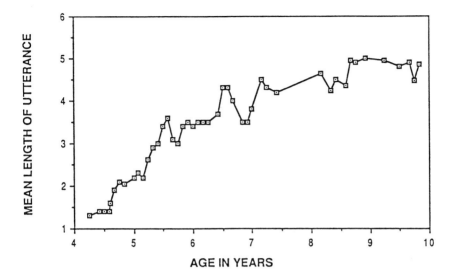

Rebecca Total Growth in IPSyn Measure

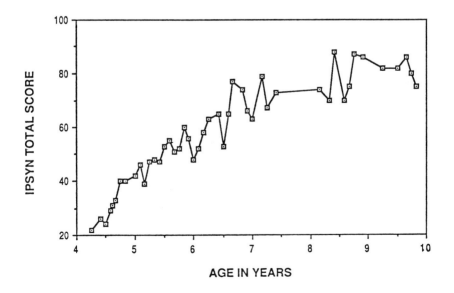

Figure 3: Growth in MLU as a function of age.

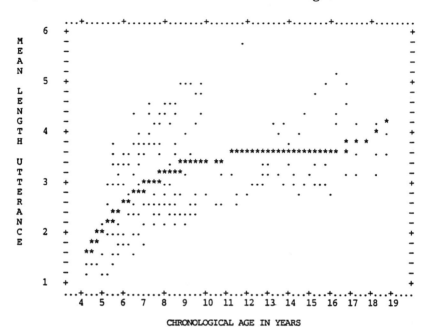

CHRONOLOGICAL AGE IN YEARS

* Data points weighted such that each child represented once in every 6 month interval during the years they were observed. Interpolations were made in those (few) instances in which an observation was not made in a particular 6 month interval.

---

reflecting different growth rates are indicated on this growth curve. Period I (MLU < 3.5; CA 4 to 8 years) is a period of relatively rapid growth with a linear slope of 0.48 MLU points per year. Period II (mean MLU 3.2; CA 8 to 15 years) is characterized by a plateau of no growth with a slope of 0.04. A third period (MLU 3.5 to 4.0; CA 13 to 19 years) reflects modest growth beyond puberty; linear slope is 0.06 MLU points per year.

The data presented in Figure 4 rely upon the same data sessions, but, in this case, reflect growth in IPSyn as a function of age. The pattern is very similar to that found for MLU growth, again suggesting three separate periods of growth. Period I is again characterized by

Figure 4:   Growth in IPSyn as a function of age.

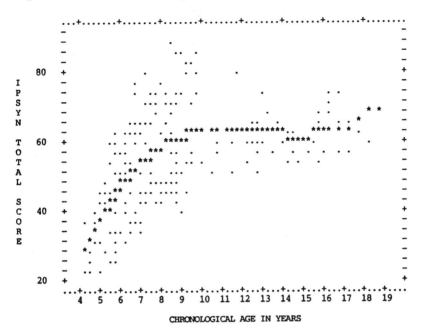

CHRONOLOGICAL AGE IN YEARS

* Data points weighted such that each child represented once in every 6 month interval during the years they were observed. Interpolations were made in those (few) instances in which an observation was not made in a particular 6 month interval.

relatively rapid growth, with a linear slope of 8.0 IPSyn points per year, compared to an overall slope of 1.6 per year. At age 8, just as with the MLU measure, growth in IPSyn virtually ceases, levelling off between 62 and 64. This IPSyn level, like the MLU score of the plateau, is just beyond the 30 month level described by Scarborough (1985). The extended plateau (linear slope = 0.3) lasts throughout middle childhood. The IPSyn measure also reveals a third period of growth beyond puberty; this slight upswing is reflected as an overall linear slope of 2.0 points per year.

Patterns of Development as a Function of IQ - Although the regression analyses presented in Figures 3 and 4 are

Table 1
Mean MLU As a Function of Age and IQ[a]

	Lower IQ 38-48	Higher IQ 55-64
Younger (4 to 7 years)	1.94	3.00
Middle (7 to 12.6 years)	2.56	4.03
Older (12.6 to 19 years)	3.58	3.78

[a] This preliminary analysis is based upon all data points in the sample, with no weighting procedures applied.

Results of 2-way Analysis of Variance on these data
Age: $F(2,207) = 71.06$, $p < .0001$
IQ: $F(1,207) = 125.28$, $p < .0001$
Age x IQ: $F(2,207) = 14.12$, $p. < .0001$

consistent with both stage- and age-related hypotheses, the fit itself is quite bad. The correlation between pre- dicted and observed points (R-squared) is only 0.32 for MLU and 0.44 for IPSyn. A better fit of the data was sought by separating children on the basis of IQ and/or CA. Such a division was justified by a preliminary two- way analysis of variance based upon the entire pool of data presented in Figure 3 (see Table 1). Observed MLU data points were classified according to IQ ("low" vs. "High" with a cutoff of 50) and CA at time of measure ("Young": 4 to 7 years; "Middle": 7 to 12.6 years; and "Older": 12.6 to 19 years). The results of this analysis revealed highly significant effects of CA and IQ as well as a significant CA x IQ interaction.

One seemingly anomalous result of this ANOVA is the finding that the mean MLU for the higher-IQ children is greater in the "middle" than in the "older" years. A more careful examination of individual curves indicated three

distinct groups of children among the 11 subjects analyzed. Whereas the growth patterns of different-aged lower-
IQ children (n = 5) converged to yield a single curve ap-
plicable across all of childhood (4 to 18 years), this
was not the case for higher-IQ children, those scoring
above 50 on the Stanford-Binet IQ test. The higher-IQ
children entering the study before 7 years of age (IQ
56-64; n = 3) were characterized by rapid early growth;
all, for example, had already attained the 3.0 MLU
threshold by 6 years of age; all had moved beyond that
threshold by the close of the study. Other young children
with DS observed by us and others (Tager-Flusberg, 1986;
Beeghly and Cicchetti, 1986) also evidence this rapid
early growth. However, higher IQ adolescents did not obviously fall into this subgroup. When first tested, at 10
to 12 year of age, their MLU scores (approximately 3.0)
were markedly below the level achieved by two of the
three younger higher-IQ children well before that time.
Indeed, the pattern of these two older children with
higher-IQ scores was not markedly dissimilar from the
pattern observed for lower-IQ children overall. Because
of the apparent mismatch between young and older subjects
with IQ's over 50, we treat younger and older subjects
separately, awaiting further data regarding the ultimate
fate of the higher-IQ children followed from an early
age. Although statistical comparison of group patterns is
precluded by the small number of children per cell, the
coherence within groups and differences across groups
regarding developmental course are quite striking.

Effect of Chronological Age - Figures 6 through 8 portray
averaged growth curves for the three chronological age
growth periods emerging from the curve fitting procedures
discussed above. For each of three phases, the two IQ
groups are plotted separately in order to highlight the
effect of IQ. In the earliest phase (4 to 8 years, CA,
Figure 6), note that the six children in our sample began
at the same MLU level. This was a function of subject selection procedures, which required only that the child
show some evidence of two-word combinations. IQ data were
not available at this age, due both to the difficulty of
testing such young children and the policy of the school
in which these children were then enrolled. Thus, they

232   Fowler

Figure 5: Averaged growth in MLU in 11 children with DS.

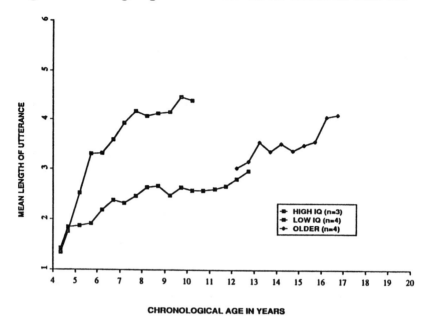

CHRONOLOGICAL AGE IN YEARS

Figure 6: Growth in MLU in lower IQ children.

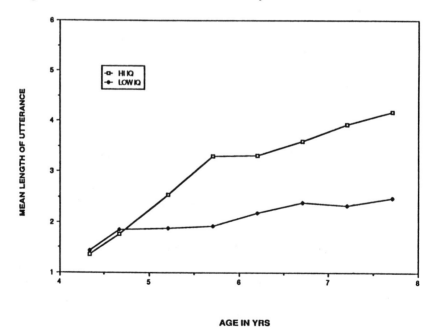

AGE IN YRS

Figure 7: Growth in MLU for Higher IQ children (Younger).

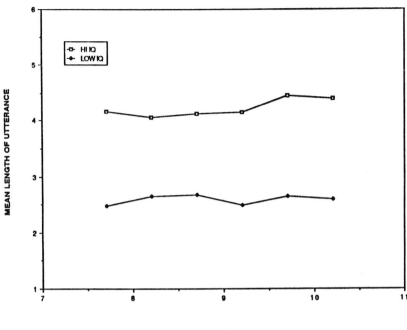

AGE IN YRS

were treated as single group. Differences only emerged after age 5, when the higher-IQ group made and maintained rapid progress upward. Whereas the higher-IQ group continued to progress upward even after 6 years of age, monthly visits to the lower-IQ children (not yet labeled as such) yielded frustratingly small progress. Despite anticipation of a similar spurt in these children, progress remained slow throughout the early childhood period. Linear slope measures for the lower IQ children in this period was 0.28 points per year; the higher-IQ figure was 0.81.

As seen in Figure 7, between the ages of 7;6 and 10;6 years, rate of growth was near a standstill across the two IQ groups (lower-IQ slope in MLU = 0.07; higher-IQ slope = 0.15), despite substantial differences in absolute language level.

Effect of Language Stage on Rate of Growth - The evidence presented thus far, based upon averaged growth curves, points quite compellingly to a maturationally

234   Fowler

Figure 8: Growth in MLU for higher IQ children (Older).

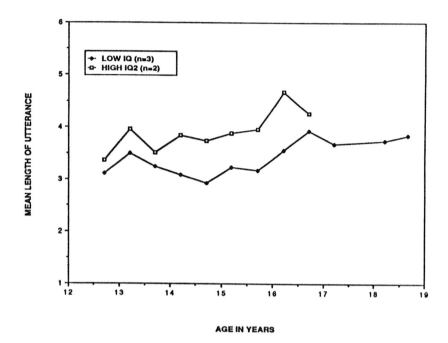

AGE IN YEARS

determined plateau in language growth in middle childhood. The effect of IQ is evident not so much in determining when these plateaus occur, but in how much growth
actually occurs during critical periods of language
growth. In this last section, individual growth curves
are presented based on the raw data collected from each
of the 11 subjects, suggesting that language stage too
may make a significant contribution to language growth
over and above the effects of CA and IQ. Much as was suggested in regard to Rebecca in Experiment I, there appear
within an overall growth curve of an individual to be de-
finable plateaus, with sharp -- if quite brief -- movements to an upper MLU point. These apparent language
"stages" received considerable support on the basis of
internal analyses in the case of Rebecca; similar analyses have been carried out on other children, though not
in as great detail. For the present purpose of highlight-
ing this pattern of development, only the MLU curves are
presented for each of the 11 children studied. Plateaus
apparent on the basis of lack of MLU growth (and fre-

quently supported by internal measures such as IPSyn) are
indicated with straight lines on the growth curves pre-

Table 2
Growth in MLU - Individual Data

ID	S.B.	Age Studied	Mean	Range	Linear Slope
HI#1	IQ57	4;3 to 8;10	3.33	1.30-5.0	0.68(+.048)
HI#2	IQ56	5;7 to 9;2	3.41	2.50-4.35	0.08(+.072)
HI#3	IQ64	6;8 to 9;6	3.93	3.10-4.50	0.30(+.120)
LO#1	IQ47	4;3 to 8;9	2.39	1.28-2.85	0.04(+.048)
LO#2	IQ48	4;11 to 8;8	2.40	1.67-3.06	0.24(+.036)
LO#3	IQ38	5;3 to 9;0	2.21	1.60-2.80	0.21(+.048)
LO#4	IQ48	7;5 to 12;7	2.61	2.26-2.97	0.09(+.030)
AD#1	IQ56	10;8 to 16;8	3.75	2.73-5.15	0.38(+.048)
AD#2	IQ55	12;3 to 18;3	3.47	2.90-4.19	0.07(+.060)
AD#3	IQ48	12;7 to 18;8	3.76	2.86-4.65	0.02(+.036)
AD#4	IQ44	12;8 to 18;8	3.76	2.70-3.55	0.07(+.005)

sented in Figures 9 through 11. The criterion for definition as a plateau is that the slope of the curve defined
within these points is significantly below that of the
overall growth curve for the child.

At the outset of this group study, it was hypothesized
that a plateau between 3.0 and 3.5 would be important in
children with DS generally. Rebecca, studied in Experiment 1, spent 10 months at this level, corroborated by
lack of internal growth measures. A second higher-IQ
child (JH), studied at a similar age period as Rebecca,
has spent four years at this level. Unfortunately, although the third child (KH) was at this level in our
first two sessions with her, it is not known how long she
had been at this stage prior to her participation in the
study (see Figure 9). This plateau is even more evident
in the lower-IQ, group, reaching an extreme in the case
of GW, whose MLU remained virtually constant (3.0) between 12.6 and 19 years of age. The three other adolescent children in the study showed similar plateaus lasting for 3 to 7 years, but two had definitely moved beyond
this level at 14 and 16.6 years, respectively (see Figure

236 Fowler

Figure 9: Individual Growth Curves for Young Higher-IQ
Children

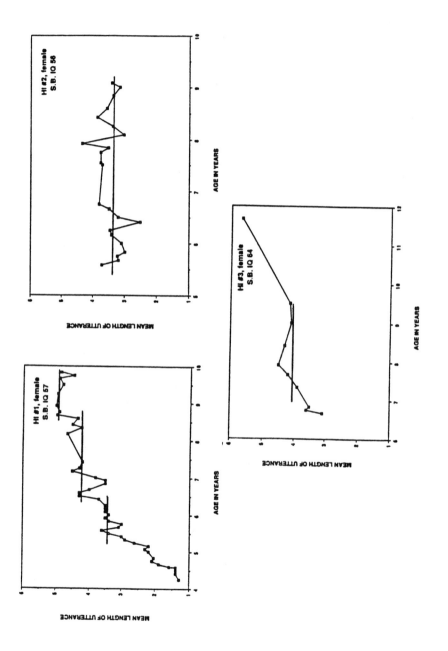

11). The three youngest low-IQ children had not yet attained the 3.0 as they approached 10 years of age. The
one child (KC) who has reached this age, however, does
appear quite recently to have entered Stage III; on the
basis of comparability of IQ, age, and internal measures,
it appears that she, like GW, may remain at this stage
indefinitely. (See Figure 10).

Although there is less relevant data speaking to plateaus at other language stages, extended lack of growth
is apparent at MLU 2.5 in each of the four lower-IQ
children studied between the ages of 4 to 12 (see Figure
10). Similarly, not all that far beyond the 3.0 - 3.5
threshold the growth patterns of Rebecca, KH, and the
older adolescents do seem to indicate a second slow-down
at MLU 4.0. Finally, although our data sampling procedures did not allow us to observe such an early plateau,
there is substantial evidence in the literature, and
emerging from current longitudinal research of Beeghly
and Cicchetti (1986) and Tager-Flusberg (1986) to suggest
a lengthy plateau at early Stage I development in the
pre-school child with DS (see Dooley, 1977, for a
compelling case study).

There are three sources of evidence supporting the view
that these slowdowns constitute real plateaus in development. This thesis has been explored in the greatest depth
in regard to Stage III. First, on the most general measures, e.g. MLU, mean growth rate within a stage is slower than overall growth rate for that child. That is, the
child is not passing through that stage as through any
arbitrary interval. As a rough index of this difference,
mean slope measures for Stage III versus the overall
growth rate are presented in Table 3, averaging the slop-
es of individual children for the relevant periods. Second, there is little evidence for internal growth within
a period isolated on the basis of MLU growth patterns, as
measured by the IPSyn measure, for example. One way of
demonstrating this, which we are currently exploring, involves correlating CA with MLU or IPSyn both within and
across stages. The hypothesis is that such correlations
should be lower within stages than across stages (see
Scarborough, 1985). The third piece of evidence speaking
to stage-determined plateaus in development derives from
data showing that the same MLU stage seems to have great

Figure 10: Individual Growth Curves for Young Low-IQ
Children

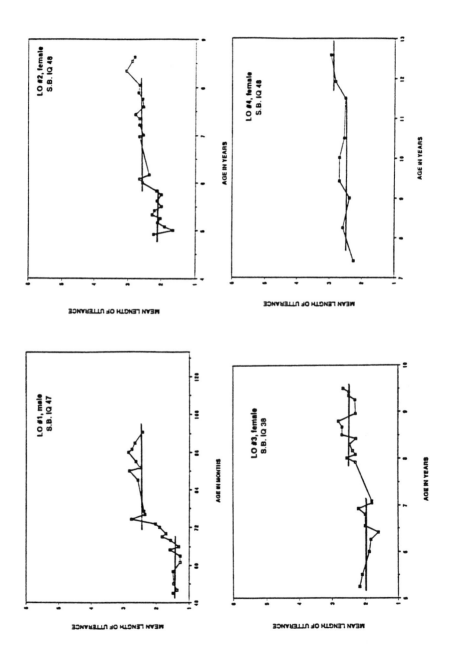

Figure 11: Individual Growth Curves for Adolescent Children

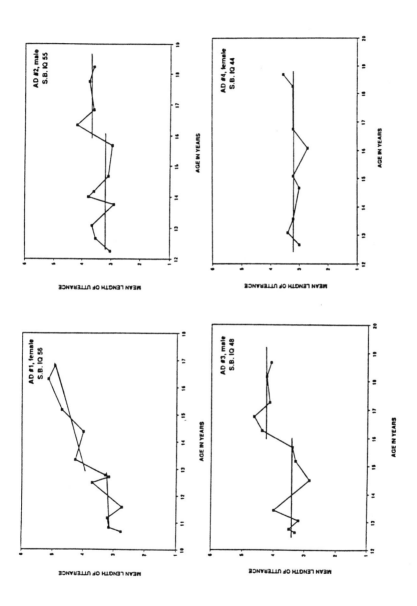

Table 3
Rate Of Growth In MLU as a Function of Language Stage
(Pts. of MLU Per Year)

	Stage III	Overall
Lower IQ	0.004 (+0.001)	0.015 (+0.008)
Higher IQ	0.012 (+0.027)	0.026 (+0.019)

coherence and consistency across children regardless of age or IQ level. As demonstrated in Fowler et al. (1980) and also supported by many other studies (see Fowler, in press; or Miller, in press; for reviews), this stage coherence cuts across both retarded and normal populations alike. On the basis of analyses to date, and based upon Rebecca and the older adolescents, there does appear to be considerable evidence that Stage III, at least, is a verifiable and internally coherent stage which serves as a very real and often extended stumbling block for many children with DS.

Discussion

The purpose of the research presented here was to provide insight into learning processes leading to greatly delayed, but essentially "normal" language output characterizing the productions of children with DS. Although the sample is less than ideal for a definitive test of the hypotheses posed, multiple measures over extended periods of time upon a small, mixed group of children with DS have yielded some rather striking results. First, although the critical period as defined by Lenneberg (1967) would not accurately predict these particular growth curves, chronological age seems to exert considerable influence on the rate of language learning. Whereas Lenneberg suggested a cutoff at puberty, these data, and data from others (Rondal, personal communication) suggest that at least some children with DS make substantial progress in syntactic development during their teen-age

years. On the other hand, these data suggest a virtual
halt in development during the middle childhood years.
Interestingly, such a slowdown in middle childhood is also apparent in the growth curves of general intellectual
development in DS, as presented by Gibson (1966) (see
Figure 12). He reports a marked plateau at eight years of
age, equivalent to mental age of 31 months. This is of
interest not only because of the close correspondence in
regard to CA, but also because a mental age of 31 months

Figure 12: Taken from Gibson, D. (1966), American Journal
of Mental Deficiency.

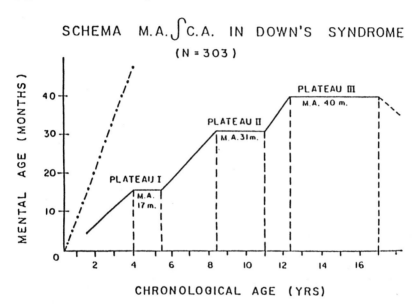

SCHEMA   M.A. ∫ C.A.   IN   DOWN'S   SYNDROME
(N = 303)

corresponds well with the plateaued language level characterizing many of our subjects.

IQ, too, appears to play a substantial role in determining the prognosis of language learning in children
with DS. Although the effects of chronological age remain
apparent across the IQ-levels observed here, an IQ level
greater than fifty seems critical to assuring substantial
growth when maturational factors permit it. Lenneberg
(1967) suggests a similar IQ cutoff to explain differences of language level achieved in his subjects.

242 Fowler

Although more internal analyses on the order of those which are provided for Rebecca in Experiment I are required to support a stage hypothesis in its strongest form, the data presented here support the position that language in DS may best be characterized by discrete periods of development, affected both by chronological age and by language stage. Growth in a child with DS, as in any normally-developing child, is not a steady accumulation of facts. Indeed, the data appear to suggest that the child with DS will provide insight into language stages that the normally developing child passes through at rapid speeds.

Acknowledgments

Draft of a paper delivered at the Boston University Child Language Conference, October, 1986, to be submitted for publication. Much of the impetus and conceptual framework of this work was provided by my collaborators, Lila Gleitman and Rochel Gelman. I am indebted to the parents, teachers and children of St. Katherine's Day School for their active participation and cooperation. The sheer magnitude of collecting transcribing and coding this data was accomplished only with the diligent and dedicated assistance of Elizabeth St. Andre and Martha Loukides. This research was funded by a grant (12-113) from the March of Dimes Birth Defects Foundation to L. Gleitman, R. Gelman and A. Fowler; an NICHHD post-doctoral fellowship (1-F32-HD-06543) funded the author in the writing of this paper. Correspondence should be addressed to A. Fowler, Haskins Laboratories, 270 Crown Street, New Haven CT 06511.

Footnotes

1. To adjust for the known effect of chronological age on IQ scores in children with DS, we report the Stanford Binet assessment made nearest the child's 8th birthday.

REFERENCES

Beeghly, M., & Cicchetti, D. (1985). Development of functional communication during Stage I of syntactic development by children with Down syndrome. Presented at 10th Annual Boston University Conference on Language Development, October, 1985.

Beeghly, M., & Cicchetti, D. (1986). Early language development in children with Down syndrome: A longitudinal study. Presented at 11the Annual Boston University Conference on Language Development, October, 1986.

Bellugi, U. (1967). The acquisition of negation. Unpublished doctoral dissertation, Harvard University.

Bloom, L. (1970). Language development: form and function in emerging grammars. Cambridge, MA: MIT Press.

Bloom, L., Lightbown, P., & Hood, L. (1975). Structure and variation in child language. Monograph of the Society for Research in Child Development, 40(2).

Bowerman, M. (1982). Reorganizational processes in lexical and syntactic development. In E. Wanner and L. R. Gleitman, (Eds.), Language Acquisition: State of the Art. Cambridge MA: Cambridge University Press.

Brown, R. (1973). A first language. Cambridge, MA: Harvard University Press.

Burr, D. B., & Rohr, A. (1978). Patterns of psycholinguistic development in the severely retarded: A hypothesis. Social Biology, 25, 15-22.

Chabon, S., Kent-Udolf, C., & Egolf, D. (1982). The temporal reliability of Brown's Mean Length of Utterance (MLU-M) measure with post-Stage 5 children. Journal of Speech and Hearing Research, 25, 117-124.

Coggins, T. E. (1979). Relational meaning encoded in the two-word utterances of Stage 1 Down's Syndrome children. Journal of Speech and Hearing Research, 22, 166-178.

Coggins, T. E., & Morrison, J. A. (1981). Spontaneous imitations of Down's Syndrome children: A lexical analysis. Journal of Speech and Hearing Research, 46, 303-308.

Dooley, J. (1977). Language acquisition and Down's Syndrome: A Study of Early Semantics and Syntax. Unpublished doctoral dissertation, Harvard University.

Evans, D. (1977). The development of language abilities

in mongols: A correlational study. Journal of Mental Deficiency Research, 21, 103-117.

Fowler, A. (in press). The acquisition of language structure in children with DS. To appear in D. Cicchetti & M. Beeghly, Down Syndrome: The Developmental Perspective, Cambridge MA: Cambridge University Press.

Fowler, A. (1984). Language acquisition in Down's Syndrome children: Production and Comprehension. Ph.D. dissertation, University of Pennsylvania.

Fowler, A., Gelman, R., & Gleitman, L. (1980). A comparison of normal and retardate language equated on MLU. Presented at the 5th Annual Boston University Conference on Child Language Development.

Gibson, D. (1966). Early developmental staging as a prophecy index in Down's Syndrome. American Journal of Mental Deficiency, 70, pp. 825-828.

Gibson, D. (1978). Down's Syndrome: The psychology of Mongolism. London: Cambridge University Press.

Gleitman, L. R. (1981). Maturational determinants of language growth. Cognition, 103-114.

Karmiloff-Smith, A. (1979). Language as a formal problem space for children. Paper presented at Beyond Description in Child Language. Max Planck Gesellschaft, Nijmegen, The Netherlands.

Layton, T. L., & Sharifi, H. (1979). Meaning and structure of Down Syndrome and non-retarded children's spontaneous speech. American Journal of Mental Deficiency, 83, 439-445.

Lenneberg, E. H. (1967). Biological Foundations of Language. New York: Wiley.

Lenneberg, E. H., Nichols, I. A., & Rosenberger, E. F. (1964). Primitive stages of language development in mongolism. Research Publications, Association for Research in Nervous and Mental Disease, 42, 119-147.

Miller, J. F. (1980). Assessing language production in children: Experimental procedures. Baltimore: University Park Press.

Miller, J. F. (in press). Language and communication characteristics of children with Down syndrome. In A. Crocker, S. Pueschel, J. Rynders, & C. Tinghey (Eds.), Down Syndrome: State of the Art. Baltimore: Brooks Publishing.

Newport, E. (1986). Paper presented at the 11th Annual

Boston University Conference on Child Language.

Rondal, J. A. (1975). Developpement du langage et retard mental: Un revue critique de la litterature en langue anglaise. Annee Psychologique, 75, 513-547.

Rondal, J. A. (1980). Verbal imitation by Down Syndrome and nonretarded children. American Journal of Mental Deficiency, 85, 318-321.

Rosenberg, S. (1982). The language of the mentally retarded: Development, processes and intervention. In S. Rosenberg (Ed.), Handbook of Applied Psycholinguistics. Hillsdale, NJ: Erlbaum.

Ryan, J. (1975). Mental subnormality and language development. In E. Lenneberg and E. Lenneberg (Eds.), Foundation of Language Development, Vol. 2, New York: Academic Press.

Ryan, J. (1977). The silence of stupidity. In J. Morton and J. C. Marshall (Eds.), Psycholinguistics: Developmental and Pathological. Ithica, NY: Cornell University Press.

Scarborough, H. S. (1985). Measuring syntactic development: The Index of Productive Syntax, Presented at the Biennial Meetings of the Society for Research in Child Development, Toronto.

Shipley, E., Smith, C., & Gleitman, L. (1969). A study in the acquisition of language: Free responses to commands. Language, 45, 322-342.

Tager-Flusberg, H. (1986). Paper presented at the 11th Annual Boston University Conference on Child Language.

8

USING COMPUTERS TO TEACH CHILDREN WITH DOWN
SYNDROME SPOKEN AND WRITTEN LANGUAGE SKILLS

Laura F. Meyers, Ph.D.
Department of Linguistics
University of California, Los Angeles

Introduction

This paper describes computer-enhanced intervention
strategies designed to facilitate language development in
children with Down Syndrome. First, play and language interventions to facilitate beginning language learning by
young children from 14 months to 44 months old will be
described. Then, interventions using creative writing on
computers with speech output to promote spoken and written language learning by school-aged children will be
discussed.

Background

Effective language intervention strategies for children
with Down Syndrome are critically needed because severe
language delays are consistently reported in the literature beginning with first words and continuing throughout
the school years (Miller, 1988; Miller Streit, Salmon and
LaFollette, 1987; Miller, Budde, Bashir and LaFollette,
1987; Stoel-Gammon, 1980). Miller found that language
skills become increasingly deviant compared to other cognitive skills as the children develop (1987).
Two new studies reported in this volume document the
severity of language disabilities in children with Down
Syndrome (Fowler; Miller). Miller found that young children with Down Syndrome produce new words at a slower rate
than normal children matched for mental age. Looking at

the number of different words produced by children with Down Syndrome 17 to 36 months old in a 20 minute language sample, he found that the children with a mental age of 30 months are delayed 10 months, compared with normal controls. He points out that "This trend is alarming because it suggests a progressive deficit" (Miller, pp. 190).

In addition, while children with Down Syndrome continue to expand their expressive vocabularies, they are limited in the productive use of their early lexicons. In particular, use of the vocabulary in word combinations is considerably delayed. He found no word combinations in the children with Down Syndrome with mental ages of 17 and 20 months, although the normal controls were combining words at these chronological ages. He then studied nonhandicapped children and children with Down Syndrome who had a group mean mental age of 36 months. The average length of utterances of the nonhandicapped children (mean length of utterance - MLU) was 3.6 words. By contrast, the MLU of the children with Down Syndrome at the mental age of 36 months was only 1.6 words. Miller found that delays in productive language grow more severe with age. In his subjects with Down Syndrome who were older than 18 months, 60 - 75% had production skills that were significantly behind their comprehension and cognitive development.

Fowler found that children with Down Syndrome are considerably delayed in their acquisition of first words. Her subjects learned to combine words into two, three and four word combinations between ages four and eight, but failed to acquire most grammatical markers. Their acquisition of the structure of language plateaued after about age eight. Her subjects for the most part failed to gain additional skills in production of language structure, both morphology and syntax. However, a few of her subjects began to gain some expressive language skills in their late teens.

How can Computers Help Children with Down Syndrome Learn Language Structure?

In order for children to learn language they must con-

struct a grammar linking the speech sounds that they hear
around them with meaning, as shown in Figure 1.

Figure 1: The process of beginning language acquisition
(Meyers, L., The Language Machine, College-Hill Press, in
press)

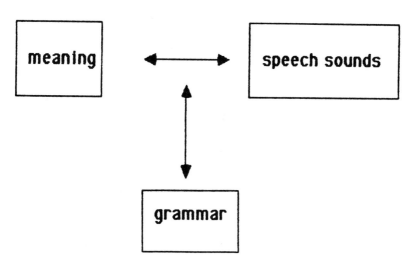

To function as competent users, children must be able
to figure out the meaning of the speech of other people,
and they must be able to express their own communicative
meanings in speech. To participate in the process of language learning, children must be able to hear, remember
and analyze the rapidly occurring constantly changing
acoustic signal of speech, and they must be able to produce the rapidly articulated fine motor movements of
speech. As children figure out how language works, they
develop internalized grammars that let them say utterances that they have never before said, and understand
sentences that they have never before heard.
The speech signal of language presents problems to
children with Down Syndrome. Comprehension of the speech
signal is adversely affected by a high incidence of otitis media and associated hearing loss, and by problems
with rapid auditory processing and memory for auditory
stimuli (Down, 1980; Bivlosky and Share, 1965; Marcell
and Armstrong, 1982; Semmel and Dolley, 1972). Human
speech occurs at a very rapid rate. The syllables of

speech occur at an average rate of 2 to 5 syllables per second. Since a syllable consists of at least two segments, this means that in normal conversation 10 or more segments often occur in a single second, each segment lasting only 1/10th of a second or less (Pickett, 1980). To make matter worse, each time an individual speaker or different speakers say the same word, phrase or sentence the acoustic signal changes slightly or dramatically. These characteristics of the speech signal make it difficult for children with Down Syndrome to develop comprehension skills.

If the children do not process the speech signal correctly, i.e. if they are not able to hear, perceive or remember the "primary linguistic data" in the speech that occurs around them, they do not have an "empirical basis for language learning" (Chomsky, 1965, p. 32) and they will not adequately construct grammars to understand or produce the language that occurs around them. The development of production of speech by Down Syndrome children is further affected by hypotonia and other neurological conditions resulting in poor coordination of respiration and phonation, poor fine motor control of the tongue and lips, and structural abnormalities of the palate (Rosin, Swift and Bless, 1987). Production of language is important for the process of language learning as a whole. It provides a method of testing linguistic hypotheses (Chomsky, 1965). It allows the child to practice moving towards a linguistic target, a well-established part of language learning, as shown by records of monologues of children practicing alone in their cribs (Weir, 1962). It triggers use of simplified input by caretakers (Snow, 1977). It allows the child to experience the powerful function of language, to communicate important personal messages during conversations with peers and adults.

Computers can help the children with Down Syndrome to learn to understand and produce the speech signal of language. Synthesized speech output can give children with Down Syndrome control of a slow, consistent, non-varying speech signal. When computer software and hardware lets them generate unlimited exact repetitions of words and phrases, they can use the speech output to develop an understanding of the sound patterns of words and sentences. They can immediately use the computer-generated speech output as a productive voice to participate in conversations. They can improve their articulation skills by repeatedly generating the speech signal for words and phrases, imitating the signal, gradually improving their approximations of the correct articulation. Since the visual skills of children with Down Syndrome are often at a higher level than the auditory skills, the speech signal should be accompanied by the stable visual cues of keyboard and monitor graphics and text (Bivlosky and Share, 1965; Marcell and Armstrong, 1982).

In the language interventions described here, the computer functions as a powerful cognitive scaffold, helping the children learn language in much the same way that scaffolding helps in the construction of a building (Greenfield, 1983). The computer provides support; it functions as a tool for the children; it extends the range of the children; it allows them to accomplish tasks that are not otherwise possible, and it is used selectively by the children to help them only when they need help (ibid). In order for computer use to be effective, the technology must be incorporated into a meaningful, developmentally appropriate activity (Meyers, 1984a, 1984b, 1986a, 1986b, 1988). Examples well be provided below.

Incorporating Computers with Speech Output into Beginning Language Interventions with Toddlers with Down Syndrome

Computer-enhanced language interventions should always be based on the information that is known about normal development. At the beginning stages of normal language learning, toddlers are learning how to link the speech sounds of the words they hear with the meaningful objects and events in the nonlinguistic context around them. Prior to beginning to learn language, infants and toddlers have developed conceptual structure, organized internalized knowledge of what objects, people and events are like (Jackendoff, 1983). They gain the information they need to develop concepts through exploration of and acting on the environment. The toddlers use their conceptual knowledge of the world to help them understand the speech signal. They use the skills that they have developed during play and exploration to call attention to objects and events as part of their first meaningful productive utterances.

Children's production and comprehension of first words are always augmented by the objects, events, and human interaction in their environments. They use their understanding of the nonlinguistic context to break the language code. Their first utterances are partially encoded in the nonlinguistic context and partially encoded in words. Next, toddlers encode their utterances in two and three words, still depending partially on the context to convey meaning. They build on these skills when they begin to produce their first simple sentences. There is a structural continuity from use of first words combined with nonlinguistic context to use of simple sentences as shown in Table 1 (Greenfield and Smith, 1976).

A second important development in the second year of normal language acquisition is use of words to convey a wide variety of different functions, also shown in Table 1 (ibid). Children first use words as performative and labels, then use the same words to indicate objects, to ask for objects, to describe actions and the agents and objects of actions, to talk about possession, location and modifications of events. First, children convey these different semantic functions by combining single words with the linguistic context. Then, they encode the same message in beginning word combinations and beginning sentences.

We are currently studying the effectiveness of beginning computer-enhanced language intervention for toddlers with Down Syndrome, based on this normal developmental model. The computer is integrated into a typical normal beginning language learning environment, filled with objects, events and human interaction. The toddlers are free to explore and act on this environment. Since toddlers with Down Syndrome are often delayed in fine motor skills and play skills, helping them learn how to effectively participate in play with toys is an important goal of the intervention. The research compares the use of computer-generated speech output, as well as keyboard and monitor graphics, with a standard intervention without a computer present. The goal is to determine the most effective language scaffolding for toddlers with Down Syn-

Table 1
Examples of Functional and Structural Continuity in the
Encoding of Single Words Plus Nonlinguistic Context, Word
Combinations, and Beginning Sentences

FUNCTION	DEFINITION OF FUNCTION	ONE WORD + CONTEXT	WORD COMBINATION	SENTENCE
Performative	words that occur as part of child's action, or as part of a routine	bye-bye (+wave)	bye-bye Mommy	Bye-bye Mommy.
Indicative Object	words that refer to an object that child indicates with gaze or gesture	Mommy (+look or point at mother)	that Mommy	That's Mommy.
Volitional	words that refer to object of demand, or to ask intervener to obtain object while reaching or whining	Mommy (+reach for mother) Mommy (+reach for or orient towards banana)	want Mommy Mommy nana	I want Mommy. Mommy, get the banana.
Agent	words used to name agent of an activity	Mommy (+ watch mother writing)	Mommy write	Mommy is writing
Action or state of object	word describing own or others actions	down (+ watch mother sit down during rosy game)	Mommy down	Mommy is sitting down.
Object	word referring to object of action	Mommy (+ kiss mother)	kiss Mommy	I'm kissing Mommy.
Dative	specifies indirect object	Mommy (+ hand mother object)	give Mommy	I'm giving it Mommy
Object or person associated with an object	names object or person in relation to an object	Mommy (+ points mother's books)	Mommy book	Those are Mommy's books.
Location	names the location of an object	Mommy (+ puts car on mother's lap)	car Mommy	Mommy has the car.
Modification of an event	words that modify an entire event	more (+shows wants mother to wind toy car), fast (+ after swing slows down	more wind car swing fast	Wind the car more, Mommy. Push the swing faster.

(from L. Meyers, The Language Machine, based on Greenfield and Smith, 1976)

drome, to motivate them to develop comprehension and production skills at the developmentally appropriate age.
For example, in one of the computer-enhanced language
activities, the toddlers play with a set of cause and
effect toys, a wind-up helicopter, car and shoes, and a
bottle of soap bubbles. They can touch pictures of the
toys on a membrane keyboard overlay to label the toys, to
ask for one of the toys, saying I want that on the computer. They can use the computer to talk about winding the
toys, opening, blowing or popping the bubbles, to ask for
more of any activity, or to terminate play with a toy by
saying all done. When the children touch a picture on the
membrane keyboard, in addition to the speech output, the
software generates an identical picture on the computer
monitor. The children are introduced to each of the toys,
shown how to label and ask for the toys, how to act on
the toys and describe the action, and how to ask to go on
with or end their play. Then, they can freely explore the
play context and the speech output, both to learn the
sound patterns of the words and to talk about their play.
Instead of taking the children's part by speaking for the
children who cannot produce their own utterances, the researchers can play the role of discourse partners, encouraging the children to communicate through vocalizations, signs, gestures, speech output and through their
own speech.
The toddlers with Down Syndrome using this software immediately begin to imitate the precise articulation of
the speech output. For example, one 30 month boy with
Down Syndrome activated the speech output for the word
more by touching the picture of a child signing the word
in Ameslan on the computer keyboard. An identical graphic
appeared on the computer monitor. He had never said the
word in his own speech, but did know the sign for the
word. He turned to the caregiver and immediately signed
the word, saying "[or]". Then he touched the keyboard two
more times, first mastering the bilabiality of the initial consonant "[bor]", and then mastering the nasality,
saying "[mor]". As soon as he could say the word in his
own speech, he no longer used the computer-generated
speech output.
Annie, a 30 month old girl with Down Syndrome, used the
same activity to move structurally from the use of single
word utterances to word combinations and short simple

sentences. First, she learned to label the wind-up helicopter and car, and to ask for the toys using single
words. Then, she learned to wind up the toys and talk
about winding them, using word combinations (<u>wind</u> <u>heli-</u>
<u>copter</u>, <u>wind</u> <u>car</u>). Next, she was shown that she could ask
for the toys by using the simple sentence, <u>I want that</u>,
available on the keyboard. Finally, she combined that
phrase with her one-word vocabulary to form the sentences
<u>I want that helicopter</u>, <u>I want that car</u>. At first, she
used speech output plus the objects to convey her messages. Then, she combined words on the computers, moving
into saying one word in her speech and the other using
the speech output. Gradually, she became able to combine
the words in her speech, and to say an occasional simple
sentence. The scaffolded computer-enhanced language intervention allowed her to move on to her next level of
complexity, each time she had succeeded at a lower level
(Meyers, 1988).

Data is gathered from vocabulary tests given before and
after each set of intervention sessions, and from videotapes of the language sessions that are coded for motivation measures (time on/off-task, solution behaviors), and
language measures. Preliminary analysis of results for
our first group of ten subjects indicates that use of the
computer with speech output only or with speech output
and monitor graphics is twice as effective in promoting
comprehension and production of language than the intervention without the computer present.

This project will help determine how best to use computer technology in interventions to facilitate beginning
language acquisition and initiate speech in young children at high risk for severe language delay. It is the
first study to determine the link between mastery motivation and language learning in young children. The study
will provide much needed statistical data supporting the
use of augmentative communication with very young children, using computer technology. At present, many speech
and language professionals recommend delaying introduction of augmentation with speech output until children
have a trial of purely oral therapy and fail to initiate
speech. Their assumption is that children may rely on the
speech output, rather than developing their own speech
skills. The pilot study, as well as preliminary results

on this project, show that augmenting language intervention with the speech output helps toddlers enter the di-
alogue of language. Their success as communicators motivates them to make more attempts to perform on their own,
discarding the computer-scaffold as they become autono-
mous.

*Using Writing on Computers with Speech Output to Help
School-aged Children with Down Sydnrome Learn Spoken and
Written Language*

In an ongoing project, severely language delayed
school-aged children with Down Syndrome are writing 30
page "books" using computers with speech output. The project compares the effectiveness of various methods of implementing a language experience approach to creative
writing in developing spoken and written language skills
in the subject population. Written language is being used
in the interventions because prior research has shown
that the visual skills of children with Down Syndrome are
at a higher level that their abilities using the auditory-vocal modalities of spoken language (Bivlosky, D.
and S. Shoare, 1965; Marcell, M. and V. Armstrong, 1982).
    In the research project, the children are given ten
sessions in each of the three interventions: a. writing
with pencils and paper; b. writing on a computer without
speech output; and c. writing on a computer with speech
output. The order of interventions is rotated to rule out
possible order effects. Standardized language and literacy tests are given before and after each set of sessions. Selected sessions are videotaped and the tapes are
coded for spoken and written language measures and measure of motivation, self-confidence, and self-acceptance
    During the intervention with speech output, the soft-
ware the children are using "says" the letters that they
are typing in speech output, "says" the words when the
children type the space bar, and "says" the sentences
when sentence punctuations are added. The children can
use the speech output to read the entire computer monitor
screen, can print their pages on an attached printer,
save and find pages on the disk, and get a new screen.
    The subjects in this project range in age from five to

19 years old, their developmental quotients are between
20 and 65, with the majority of the subjects functioning
in the mid to lower range. Their receptive and expressive
language is more severely delayed than their overall cognitive performance. Most speak in single words or tele-
graphic word combinations. Some use simple grammatical
sentences inconsistently. Data is gathered from standardized language and literacy tests given before and after
each set of interventions. Videotapes of language samples
and of selected language sessions are coded for measures
of utterance complexity, grammaticality, motivation (on/
off task behaviors), memory, self-confidence and self-
praise.

As in the work with toddlers, the design of the computer-enhanced writing intervention is based on a normal
developmental model. In normal beginning literacy development:

> Children learn to read by reading and to spell by
> spelling on the basis of observing models of whole
> language in meaningful contexts, by practicing their
> initial gross skills in a safe environment, and by
> receiving feedback that acknowledges the content of
> their incomplete work, but expands its form.
> (Forester, A. 1980, p. 191)

Nonhandicapped children do not begin the process of acquisition of literacy skills by first learning the mechanics of literacy (letter name, shape and form, sight vocabulary, etc.). In fact, one researcher points out that
"not only are the formal mechanics of reading unnecessary
in the initial stages, they may well be a hindrance. It
is the ability of children to make sense...that will enable them to make use of mechanics" (Smith, F., 1976, p.
298). The research shows that when normal children participate actively in beginning literacy activities, and
experience functioning as readers and writers, they begin
to have a growing control of form (Harste, J.and C.
Burke, 1980). In order to motivate children to participate in the process of becoming literate:

> We need to make it possible for children to see them-
> selves behaving as literate people. They need to make

sense of reading and writing as they use them to represent their own meanings and fulfill their own purposes. They must experience the satisfactions and
pleasure in achievement that make the learning worth-
while. (McKenszie, M., 1977, p. 316)

With the help of the computer scaffolding, the subjects
in this project can immediately function as readers and
writers, experiencing the pleasure in achievement that
motivates them to learn both spoken and written language
structure.

Some of the children with Down Syndrome enter the project with beginning literacy skills, i.e. they know some
letter names and a few words of sight vocabulary. A few
have the ability to write simple sentences when they enter the project. Others have no literacy skills. No project time is spent teaching the formal mechanical skills
of keyboarding, letter recognition, letter names, sound-
symbol correspondence, sight vocabulary, or the software
commands. Instead, the children immediately begin writing meaningful sentences, with the researchers' help. If
they don't know how to spell the words they need, the researcher prints them on a file card or post-it and puts
them on the keyboard for the children to copy. The researchers sound out the letters as the children type
them. Soon, the children begin to sound out parts of
words, and whole words on their own. As was predicted
from the research on normal acquisition of literacy, the
children quickly acquire the formal skills as a result of
writing about meaningful topics.

When they start the project, the children are invited
to write a book. As examples, they are shown books that
other children in the project have written. Each session
begins with the researcher asking the child what (s)he
wants to write about during the session. At first, most
of the children have difficulties choosing a topic and
remembering their topic so that they can develop it with
a set of sentences. As the project progresses they improve in this skill. The children tend to write about
their daily activities (school, Special Olympics, friends, and family), about rock musicians, movie stars and
videos, about vacations, pets, and in one case, God. Some
children bring photographs from home or cut pictures out

of magazines, write about the pictures, and then illustrate the page with them.

Quite often it is very difficult to understand what the
children want to write about, because their articulation
is so poor. To compensate for this, parents are interviewed at the start of the project to obtain information
about each child, including names of family members, how
the children pronounce them, favorite activities, foods,
movies, pets, friends, etc. Parents are asked to write on
the backs of the photographs or pictures that the children bring to the sessions, explaining who is in the picture, and what events are taking place.

Once the topic of the day's writing has been established, the children tell the researchers what they want to
say about the topics. They often use sequences of single
words, or two, three or four word combinations. The researchers translate the children's utterances into grammatical sentences, accepting the contents of the children's messages, but expanding the form. For example, one
15 year old boy, Charlie, who was performing at an overall cognitive level below three years, said, "Cat. Tree.
Jump. Roof." The researcher said, "Oh, you want to say,
"The cat climbed the tree and jumped onto the roof,
right?". Charlie nodded "yes" and the researchers showed
him how to type the grammatical sentence on the computer,
pointing out the necessary grammatical markers and function words.

Another subject, Mark, also 15 years old and performing
at the three year level or below, wanted to talk about
what gifts he would receive on Christmas. He said, "Santa
bring toys!". The researchers showed him that he needed
to include the word will, since he was talking about what
would happen in the future, two weeks from the session.
As he added to his text, he quickly learned that all of
his sentences about Christmas needed to include the word
will, and he wrote:

SANTA CLAUS WILL BRING EVERYBODY TOYS. MARK WILL OPEN
TWO PRESENTS. HE WILL GET A VOTRON AND A WATCH. HE
WILL GET A NEW GAME SHOW GAME IN A BOX. IT WILL BE
FAMILY FEUD. MARK WILL BE HAPPY.

At the next session, which took place after Christmas, he

wanted to report on what had happened at Christmas, and talk about what would happen on his birthday in January. He wrote:

ON CHRISTMAS I GOT A VOTRON. I DID NOT GET A WATCH OR FAMILY FEUD. ON MY BIRTHDAY I WILL GET A WATCH AND FLOWERS. CHRISTY WILL COME TO MY HOUSE.

He knew from the preceding session that he needed to use the word will to talk about the future (his birthday), and he did so spontaneously. He needed to be shown how to describe the events that had happened or did not happen at Christmas using the past tense. Notice that the researcher did not control the topic or sentence content so that specific lessons in grammar could be taught. Rather, she followed the child's choice of topic and content, and demonstrated grammar based on the child's choice. While the clear focus of the session was showing the subject how to get his immediate meaning into grammatical sentences, the session included a nice contrastive lesson on the uses of tense. The new information was enhanced when the speech output on the computer linked the text on the monitor screen with the signal of the speech synthesizer, helping the child link sound and meaning through grammar.

The main hypothesis of the project is that the children can learn to speak in grammatical sentences through a language experience approach to written language using computers with speech output. Mark demonstrated this process during one session, when he wrote:

DEAR CHARLIE,
YOU ARE MY BEST FRIEND. PLEASE EAT AT MACDONALD'S WITH ME NEXT WEEK ON TUESDAY. YOU CAN HAVE A BIG MAC AND FRENCH FRIES.
SINCERELY,
MARK

Although the researcher's help was needed to translate Mark's content into grammatical written sentences, he immediately generalized the new information to his spoken language. First, he had the computer re-read his entire letter in speech output, closely monitoring the screen as the words were read. Then, he planned how he would print what he had written. The researcher pointed out that he needed to print out two copies, one for his book, and one for his friend, Charlie, who he was actually asking out to dinner. Mark immediately responded, "That's right - next week on Tuesday!", pointing to the text on the screen.

In addition to improving both the children's spoken and written language skills, this project clearly changes the children's attitude towards themselves and their own competence. In the initial testing session with each subject, a sample of the children's language is elicited and videotaped. Mark's performance during this session was typical of most of the subjects. He used poorly articulated single, two and three word utterance, and some ungrammatical sentences under four words long. For example, talking about his girlfriend, he said, "Her nice". He looked down, putting his hand in front of his face. The researcher often had difficulties understanding him and asked him to repeat. He soon gave up on communication, saying, "I don't know" or " I can't remember". On the videotape of his fifth session on the computer with speech output, his affect had visibly changed. He acknowledged, smiling, the researchers comment that he was a fast learner, spontaneously applauded his own work, and expressed a new confidence in his abilities, saying to the researcher, several times during this session, "Don't tell me. I know how to do that."

A similar contrast in affect is being found when comparing sessions during which the children write with pencils with those during which they write on the computer with speech output. One subject's behavior was typical. Frances, 13 years old with a developmental level of six to eight years, was cooperative, very enthusiastic, and an eager learner on the computer. When writing with pencils she was often hostile and uncooperative, arguing with the researcher about the spelling of words and the structure of sentences. She resented suggestions and corrections because the struggle to produce accurate written text with a pencil and paper was extremely stressful. In the middle of one session, she started crying because she had made errors in her work. On the computer, on the other hand, where she produced perfect text that was easily edited, she asked for new vocabulary, and enjoyed exploring novel and more sophisticated ways to express her thoughts. The scaffolding provided by the computer frees the learners to take in new information.

The children's books also provide important cognitive scaffolding. In addition to providing tangible evidence of their growing competence, the books serve as references for the sight word vocabulary and language structure that they have already mastered. The children are shown how to refer back to their own prior work to find information they need in a session. They learn to depend on themselves to solve their problems. One research assistant watching a child look up the structure of a sentence in his book, commented, "It's lucky that the children have such good memories." She said this because she had found that her subjects remember everything that they have written. The children's memory for the project material contrasts sharply with prior reports in the literature, documenting the poor memories of children with Down Syndrome (Bivlosky and Share, 1965; Marcell and Armstrong, 1982). The children take their books home with them at the end of the project to use as references in their daily lives.

Preliminary data analysis of the results of the standardized language and literacy tests on the first group of subjects showed a very definite trend indicating that the intervention using synthesized output is more effective in helping the children develop both spoken and written language skills than either writing with pencils and paper or writing on computers without speech output.

School-aged children with Down Syndrome almost universally use sequences of one-word utterances, three to four word utterances, or many ungrammatical sentences in their speech. The grammatical markers are often never acquired, due, at least in part, to problems perceiving the reduced stress, low volume, short duration affixes and grammatical markers (such as plurals, tense markers, and articles). The children have poor auditory memory for the speech signal. Text makes speech visible for them and the speech synthesis links the text to the clear, slow auditory sig- nal of the synthesizer. This project is theoretically interesting because it teaches the spoken language structure through the visual modality of writing augmented with speech output. Most of our subjects are beyond the critical period for language learning, yet, beyond the critical period for language learning, yet, are making impressive progress in learning the structure of language. The children are also making progress in written language skills. If our hypotheses are proven, our results will support the use of writing on computers with synthesized speech output in language intervention with children who have not yet mastered spoken language.

Conclusion

Computer-enhanced language interventions can provide much needed cognitive scaffolding to help toddlers and school-aged children with Down Syndrome learn language. These interventions do not cure the problems presented by the genetic disorder, but they can help the children more actively participate in the process of language learning. The technology is a tool that helps the children play their own roles in the rich human interaction provided during the interventions. How well the interventions work depends on the skill of the caregivers, as well as on the children's individual ability to use the tools that are provided.

REFERENCES

Bivlosky, D., & Share, S. (1965). The ITPA and Down's syndrome: An exploratory study. AJMD, 70, 78-82.

Chomsky, N. (1965). Aspects of the Theory of Syntax, Cambridge, MA, MIT Press.

Downs, M. (1980). The hearing of Down's individuals. In M. Downs (Guest Ed.). Seminars in Speech, Language and Hearing, Vol. 1, No. 1.

Forester, A. (1980). Learning to spell by spelling, Theory Into Practice, Vol. XIX, No. 3, pp. 186-193.

Greenfield, P. (1983). A theory of the teacher in the learning activities of everyday life. In B. Rogoffand and J. Lave (Eds).Everyday Cognition: Its Development in Social Context, Boston, University Press.

Greenfield, P., & Smith, J. The Structure of Communication in Early Language Development. New York, Academic Press.

Harste, J., & Burke, C. (1980). Examining instructional

assumptions: The child as an informant. Theory Into
Practice, Vol. XIX, No. 3, pp. 170-178.
Jackendoff, R. (1983). Semantics and Cognition, Cambridge, MA, M.I.T. Press.
Marcell, M., & Armstrong, V. (1982). Auditory and visual
sequential memory of Down syndrome and nonretarded
children. AJMD, 87, No. 1, 86-95.
Meyers, L. (1984a). Use of microprocessors to initiate
language use in young non-oral children. In W. Perkins
(Ed.). Current Therapy of Communication Disorders: Language Handicaps in Children. New York, Thieme-Stratton.
Meyers, L. (1984b). Unique contributions of microcomputers to language interventions with handicapped children. In L. Meyers (Guest Ed.) Augmenting Language
Skills with Microcomputers. Seminars in Speech and Lan-
guage. Vol. 5, No. 1.
Meyers, L. (1986a). By-passing the prerequisites: The
computer as a language scaffold. Proceedings of the
1986 Closing the Gap Conference. Minneapolis.
Meyers, L. (1986b). Teaching language, The Exceptional
Parent. November.
Meyers, L. (1988). The Language Machine: Using Computers
to Teach Language Skills. College-Hill Press, San
Diego, CA, in press.
McKenzie, M. (1977). The beginnings of literacy. Theory
Into Practice. Vol. XVI, No. 5, pp. 315-323.
Miller, J. (1987). Language and communication character-
istics of children with Down syndrome. In S. Peuschel
et al. (Eds.), New Perspectives on Down Syndrome,
Baltimore, MD: Brookes, pp. 233-262.
Miller, J., Budde, M., Beshir, A., & Lafollette, L.
(1987). Lexical productivity in children with Down syn-
drome. Paper presented at ASHA, New Orleans, LA.
Miller, J., Streit, G., Salmon, D., & Lafayette, L.
(1987). Developmental Synchrony of children with Down
Syndrome. Paper presented at ASHA, New Orleans, LA.
Pickett, J. (1980). The Sounds of Speech Communication,
Baltimore, University Park Press.
Semmel, L.,& Dolley (1972). Comprehension and imitation
of sentences by Down syndrome children as a function of
transformational complexity. AJMD, 75, 739-45.
Smith, F. (1976). Learning to read by reading. Language
Arts, 53, 297-299.

Snow,   C.   (1977). Mothers' speech research: From input to interaction.   In C. Snow and C. Ferguson (Eds.), <u>Talking to Children</u>, Cambridge, MA, Cambridge University Press.

Stoel-Gammon,   C. (1980) Speech development of infants and children with Down's syndrome. In J. Darby (Ed.) <u>Speech Evaluation in Medicine</u>, New York, Grune and Stratton.

Weir,   R. (1962). <u>Language in the Crib</u>, The Hague, Mouton.

PART II

NEUROBIOLOGICAL PERSPECTIVES

9

NEUROPATHOLOGY OF DOWN SYNDROME

Thomas L. Kemper, M.D.

Down Syndrome (DS) is one of the most common identifiable causes of mental retardation. It is invariably associated with triplication (trisomy) of chromosome 21, with
triplication of the distal third of this chromosome, the
21q21 band, being sufficient for the full clinical syndrome. In 95% of patients there is meiotic non-disjunction with triplication of the entire chromosome. In 4-6%
there is translocation of part of chromosome 21 to another chromosome and in 1-4% the cells are a mosaic of normal and trisomic cells as the result of non-disjunction
in early embryonic development. The majority have IQ ratings of 45-55, with a rare case approaching a normal IQ
(Zellweger, 1977; Coyle, Oster-Granite, & Gearhart,
1986). In this review we will focus on cortical architecture, neuroanatomical development, age-related changes
and the relationship of age-related changes to dementia
in older individuals with DS.

Brain weight in DS is reduced as compared to controls
(Benda, 1969; 1971; Friede, 1975; Jacob, 1956; Urich,
1976; Whalley, 1982; Wisniewski, Wisniewksi, & Wen, 1985)
with the average DS brain weight decreased by 24%
(Whalley, 1982). In a series of 34 cerebra, Benda (1969)
found only one that exceeded 1300 grams. In a larger series of 80 cases Benda (1971) noted that the brain weight
of the majority of infants with DS was nearly normal at
birth with a clear decrease in expected brain weight by
two years of age. Measurements of head circumference is
only slightly decreased at birth and then declines in the
first two years to three standard deviations below expectation (Roche, 1966). Using a variety of skull measurements as an index of cranial volume, Schmid, et al.
(1969) came to a similar conclusion. Their calculated

volume was in the low normal range until 6 months of age and then lagged behind controls with the greatest percentile decrease occurring between two and four years of age. The major decrease in linear measurements of the skull was in the fronto-occipital diameter with relative preservation of the biparietal diameter (brachycephaly). The shape of the brain closely mirrors that of the skull with a fore-shortened fronto-occipital diameter and a steeply sloping occipital pole. The exact contribution of the various lobes of the cerebrum to this foreshortening has not been determined. Benda (1971) and Crome and Stern (1972) commented on a hypoplasia of the frontal lobes and Benda (1971) on a "compression" of the occipital lobes. Friede (1975) reports a short occiput. Our own measurement of the position of the central sulcus relative to the maximum fronto-occipital length of the hemisphere in 10 DS brains and 10 controls revealed essentially the same measurements for both (respectively, 0.42, 0.02, and 0.41, 0.06), indicating no disproportionate decrease in size of the frontal lobes in our material (Kemper, personal observation). A consistently reported finding is a narrowed superior temporal gyrus in approximately one half of the brains (Friede, 1975; Urich, 1976; Zellweger, 1977). In some brains it is unilateral and in others bilateral (Fig.1). In our own material it is twice as likely to occur in the left cerebral hemisphere (6/10) than in the right cerebral hemisphere (3/10). In addition Urich (1976) has commented on decreased development of secondary gyri, Zellweger (1977) on hypoplasia of the operculum in some brains and Gullotta and Rehder (1974) on hypoplasia of the corpus callosum in some brains. An increased size of the ventricles has only been noted in the brain of older individuals in association with gyral atrophy (Wisniewski, French, & Rosen, et al., 1982; Zellweger, 1977).

Many observers have noted a disproportionate decrease in the size of the cerebellum and brain stem in the DS brain (Crome, Cowie, & Slater, 1966; Davidoff, 1928; Friede, 1975; Gandolfi, Horoupian, & DeTeresa, 1981; Gullotta, & Rehder, 1974; Jacob, 1956; Urich, 1976; Wolstenholme, 1967). According to Crome et al., (1966) the ratio of the brain stem and cerebellum weight to that of the cerebrum is 1:9 in DS and 1:7 in controls. Benda

Figure 1: Right and left cerebral hemisphere of the same DS brain. Note its globular configuration and steeply sloping occipital pole. In this brain the superior temporal gyrus is small bilaterally. Photographs courtesy of Yakovlev collection, AFIP.

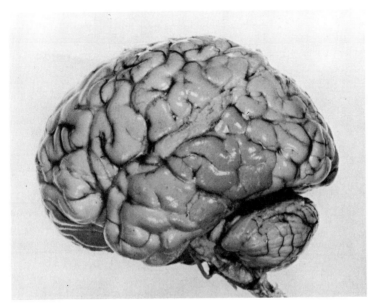

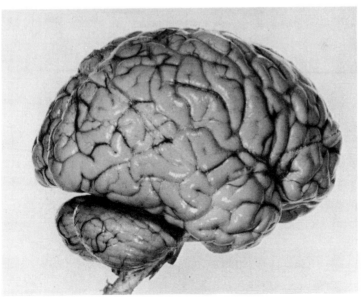

(1971) attributes this decrease to both the brain stem
and cerebellum. He noted that the cerebellum is very
small in DS infants and that it often remains hypoplastic
throughout their life. According to Zellweger (1977) the
decrease in size of the cerebellum predominately affects
the "middle lobes". Both Gans (1925) and Benda (1971)
refer to "cerebellar heterotopias" in a region of the
cerebellum that they call the "tuber flocculi". Their
illustrations locate this malformation to the region of
the flocculus lateral to the medulla oblongata. Benda
(1971) illustrates this malformation as heterotopic
disorganized cortex in the white matter.

The most consistently reported microscopic abnormality
in the cerebral cortex is a decreased neuronal cell packing density (Apert, 1914; Colon, 1971; Crome, Cowie, &
Slater, 1966; Davidoff, 1928; Ross, Galaburda, & Kemper,
1984; Urich, 1976; Wisniewski, Laure-Kamionowska, &
Wisniewski, 1984; Wong, Quaranta, & Glenner, 1985), par-
ticularily in layer III (Davidoff, 1928; Purpura, 1974).
Only one quantitative study has reported an increased
cell packing density (Norman, 1938). Sylvester (1983) has
noted a decreased total number of neurons in the hippocampus, Gandolfi and Horoupian (1981) a decrease in total
number of neurons in the ventral cochlear nucleus and
Casanova et al. (1985) a decreased number of neurons in
the nucleus basalis in DS. Some authors have noted irreg-
ular grouping of neurons in the cerebral cortex, with
areas of apparent decrease in neuronal density inter-
spersed with more densely distributed neurons (Davidoff,
1928; Norman, 1938; Urich, 1976; Zellweger, 1977). In the
quantitative study of Norman (1938) this variation in
cell packing density was found to be significantly
greater than in controls. Difficulty in recognizing cortical layers and cytoarchitectonic areas was noted by
Zellweger (1977). In our own observations of the cerebral
cortex in DS (Galaburda and Kemper, personal observations) we were also impressed with the difficulty in
identifying cytoarchitectonic areas, primarily due to a
paucity of small neurons. These studies were done on
whole brain serial sections of DS brains from the Yakovlev Collection using age- and sex-matched controls. With
a comparison microscope we viewed side-by-side comparable
cytoarchitectonic areas in eight DS brains and controls

Figure   2: Nissl stained section of the auditory cortex in
DS   (A)   with   age- and sex-matched control at B. Note the
paucity   of   small   neurons   in the DS brain. From Ross et
al. (1984).

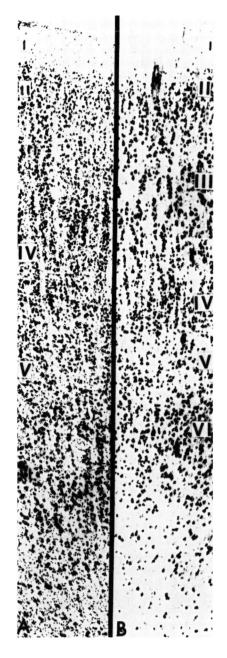

at identical magnification. The observed paucity of small neurons was confirmed by quantitative study of four different cytoarchitectonic areas in two of these brains (Ross, Galaburda, Kemper, 1984). Both DS brains showed a consistent deficit in small neurons while the larger neurons showed a variable pattern without consistent trend (Fig.2). Rapid Golgi impregnated neurons from two of these areas in an additional brain showed the expected pyramidal and non-pyramidal morphology in all cortical layers. Since the decreased density of small neurons occurred in all layers it was suggested that the most likely cells to be decreased in density were the small aspiney or spine-poor non-pyramidal neurons, the only small non-pyramidal neuron to occur in all layers (Feldman, Peters, 1978). This decrease in neuronal cell packing density appears to be congenital. Wisniewski et al. (1984), in a study of the visual cortex of 60 DS brains from birth to 14 years of age, noted 20% to 50% fewer neurons throughout this time. They suggested a prenatal rearrangement of neurons, mainly in Layer IV. Little attention has been paid to myelination in DS. Our own observations indicate that myelination is on schedule at birth and during early childhood (Fig.3).

Rapid Golgi impregnation of individual cortical neurons of children and adults has shown decreased number of synaptic spines and spines with unusually thin, long necks. The latter finding is not unique to DS. Purpura (1974) has noted similar changes in profoundly retarded individuals without chromosomal defect. Suetsugu and Mehraein (1980), in a study of seven DS brains, ages two to 23 years, noted a reduced number of spines on the apical dendrites of pyramidal cells in the subiculum and in layer V in the cingulate cortex. Marin-Padilla (1972; 1974; 1976) noted spines with long, thin necks and small terminal heads in two children ages 18 and 19 months. This latter finding has been confirmed by Takashima et al. (1983), Scott et al. (1983) and in our own material. These abnormal synaptic spines on pyramidal cells appear to develop after birth. Takashima et al. (1981) noted, in a rapid-Golgi study of the visual cortex from 14 fetal weeks to two years of age, that in DS the morphology of the neurons, number of dendrites and number of synaptic

Figure 3: Myelin stained sections of a 4 and 47 year old DS brain (A and B) and normative controls, 53 and 87 years of age (C and D). The density of myelin staining in the 4 year old DS brain is comparable to controls at this age. The 47 year old DS (at B) shows age-related pallor of myelin staining greater than that shown by the 87 year old normative control (at D) Loyez stain. Photographs courtesy Yakovlev Collection, AFIP.

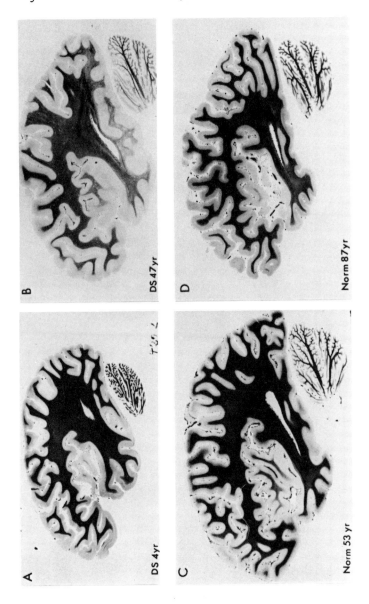

spines was indistinguishable from controls until birth at term. However, by the fourth postnatal month the dendritic spines appear thin and were reduced in number. Similarly Becker et al. (1986) noted, in eight children with DS from four months to five years of age, that the total number of dendritic intersections at predetermined distances from the cell body were normal up to six months and then decreased steadily below expectation for age. Fabreques and Ferrer (1983) have noted perisomatic processes on non-pyramidal neurons and Purkinje cells at birth in DS.

In summary, it appears that the weight of the brain, skull size and linear dimensions, myelination and development of individual cortical neurons are within the normal range up until birth. There is then a progressive curtailment of brain development during the first postnatal years. This curtailment is evident in brain weight, head circumference and development of individual neurons. A decrease in density of cortical neurons is present at birth and is seemingly unaffected during postnatal development. This pattern of development, a curtailment of growth and maturation of the brain in infancy and early childhood, is also noted in other aspects of their postnatal growth and maturation (see Barden, 1983; Zellweger, 1977, for reviews). Of particular interest is data indicating that the major curtailments occur in early childhood. Koch et al. (1963), in a study of 76 infants and children from 2 to 48 months, noted a decline in the score of the Gesell development scale from 71 at two to 13 months of age to 45 in estimated IQ during this time. An example of a similar decline 38 to 48 months. Similarly Melyn and White (1973) noted a 20 point statistically significant decline is provided by Cronk (1978) for body weight and length. In this study ninety DS children were followed from birth to 3 years of age. At birth the body weight and length was decreased to 0.5 standard deviation from controls and by age 7 the respective deviation was 1.5 and 2.0. Measurements of an additional subset of DS children, ages four to six years suggest that growth velocity was then normal. Thus it appears that a progressive curtailment of growth and maturation of both brain and somatic tissue occurs in infancy and early childhood in DS. An explanation for this curtailed maturation during early childhood is not apparent. It closely resembles that seen in metabolic diseases in which the placenta compensates for the deficit during pregnancy, with the deficit becoming progressively more apparent following birth. A well studied example of this is classical phenylketonuria where all parameters of growth and maturation are on schedule at birth and then become progressively more apparent after birth. A comparable metabolic defect in Down Syndrome has not been identified.

Another interesting aspect of the DS brain is the premature appearance of a variety of age-related changes. Following the early reports of Bertrand and Koffas (1946) and Jervis (1948), numerous studies have documented the premature appearance and unusual density of senile plaques (SP) and neurofibrillary tangles (NFT) in DS (Allsup, Kidd, Landon, & Tomlinson, 1986; Burger, & Vogel, 1973; Crapper, Dalton, Skopitz, Scott, & Hachinski, 1975; Ellis, McCulloch, & Corley, 1974; Haberland, 1969; Hooper, & Vogel, 1976; Mann, Yates, & Marcynuik, 1985; Neuman, 1967; Olson, & Shaw, 1969; Roizon, Jervis, Kaufman, Popobitch, & Hashimoto, 1972; Ropper, & Williams, 1980; Schochet, Lampert, & McCormick, 1973; Solitar, & Lamarche, 1966; Wisniewski, Laure-Kamionowska, Wisniewski, 1984; Wisniewski, Wisniewski, & Wen). According to Burger and Vogel (1973) and Wisniewski et al. (1985) they first appear in the second decade in DS. In contrast, in individuals without DS the SP first appear in the fifth decade (Jordan, 1971) and the NFT in the fourth decade (Forno, & Alvord, 1971; Matsuyama, & Nakamura, 1978). In both normative aging (Kemper, 1984) and DS (Ropper, & Williams, 1980; Wisniewski, Wisniewski, & Wen, 1985) there is an age-related increase in the incidence and density of these changes. In normative aging the number of SP and NFT anywhere in the neocortex in individuals less than 50 years of age should not exceed two to five per 200x microscopic field and in those greater than 75 years of age should not exceed an occasional NFT and 15 SP per 200x field (Khachaturian, 1985). This field is approximately 2.6×10^6 microns^2. In a smaller field (1.5×10^6) Wisniewski et al. (1985) noted in fourth decade DS brains numbers of SP comparable to that found in the normative brains greater than 75 years of age. In this comparison the number of NFT in the DS brain in the fourth decade was higher than

Table 1
Number of Neurofibrillary tangles and senile plaques per
mm^2 in Down Syndrome and in senile dementia of the
Alzheimer type (SDAT).

	Downs[1]	SDAT[2]	SDAT[3]
	Neurofibrillary Tangles		
CA1	40.1 ± 68.6	24.7 ± 37.1	34.4 ± 16.1
CA2			14.9 ± 12.1
CA3	8.1 ± 10.5	0	1.1 ± 1.1
CA4	11.1 ± 10.8	0	0.7 ± 0.7
Subiculum	15.4 ± 23.5	20.5 ± 20.6	21.0 ± 7.1
	Senile Plaque		
CA1	25.4 ± 36.7		4.4 ± 3.2
CA2			1.7 ± 3.3
CA3	10.0 ± 17.8		0.0
CA4	26.9 ± 36.1		1.2 ± 1.7
Mol. layer			
fasc. dentata	38.6 ± 82.7		0.6 ± 1.2
Subiculum	10.8 ± 11.2		4.7 ± 2.7

1. Roper and Williams (1980), 12 brains, ages 31-64 yrs.
2. Kemper (1978) 9 brains, SDAT.
3. Wong and Kemper, unpublished data, 10 brains, SDAT.

that found in normative brains greater than 75 years of
age. At older ages the DS brains showed progressively
higher SP and NFT densities in their sample areas, the
prefrontal and hippocampal cortex.

Little information is available on the distribution of
the SP and NFT according to cytoarchitecture in aging,
Alzheimer's disease (AD) or in aged DS brains. Such comparison is possible for the hippocampus. This is shown in
Table 1 taken from Kemper (1983), Roper and Williams
(1980) and unpublished data. It can be seen that the density of NFT in CA1 and subiculum is similar in older DS
brains and in senile dementia of the Alzheimer type

(SDAT). A possible exception, according to Roper and Williams (1980) is inconsistent involvement of the subiculum in DS. However the DS hippocampus shows greater involvement of CA4 and possibly CA 2-3 with the NFT than that found in SDAT. Ball and Nuttal (1981), in a study of the distribution pattern of the NFT in the hippocampus of four DS brains, ages 21 to 65, found a similar emphasis on CA1 and subiculum. The most striking difference between SDAT and DS can be seen in the distribution of the SP. They occur at much greater densities in DS than in SDAT, with major emphasis on the molecular layer of the fascia dentata, CA4 and CA1 in DS. In SDAT the major emphasis is on the subiculum and CA1. Thus the main difference between SDAT and DS is the exaggerated SP density in DS in a different distribution pattern than that found in SDAT.

Data on the density of SP and NFT in comparable cytoarchitectonic areas in the neocortex in DS and AD is not available. However, Jamada and Mehraein (1968) noted in the prefrontal area 9 (of Brodmann) a density of 26.3 SP per mm^2 and 17.1 NFT per mm^2 in presenile AD. Wisniewski et al. (1985) noted in the prefrontal cortex (without specifying the cytoarchitectonic area) a comparable SP densities in the seventh decade in the DS brain and comparable NFT densities in the sixth decade of the DS brains. When compared to SDAT, comparable SP levels were reached in DS in the fourth decade and NFT in the fifth decade.

The other age related changes are less well documented. The presence of the granulovacuolar degeneration in the hippocampal complex has been noted in the 4th decade (Burger, & Vogel, 1973; Olson, & Shaw, 1969). According to Hooper and Vogel (1976) its density in the older DS brains (age 53-55) is similar to that found in AD. Ball and Nuttal (1981), in a single brain of a 54 year old DS patient, found its rank order of density distribution by cytoarchitectonic zones the same in SDAT, rather than the rank order found in aged controls.

The Hirano body appears to be infrequent in elderly DS brains. There is a single case reported by Ellis et al. (1974) and Schochet et al. (1973). Burger and Vogel (1973) noted the Hirano body in only one of 13 patients ages 12 to 65.

Bertrand and Koffas (1946), in their case report, in which they called attention to the occurrence of SP in DS, also noted perivascular mineralization in the globus pallidus. This age-related change has been subsequently noted by others (Haberland, 1969; Schochet, Lampert, & McCormick, 1973; Solitar, & Lamarche, 1966; Wisniewski, French, & Rosen, et al., 1982). Wisniewski et al. (1982) noted it in all brains one year of age to greater than 40 years with a striking age-related increase. They viewed it as premature aging. Although generally described as occurring in the globus pallidus perivascular mineralization also occurs in the striatum and thalamus (Wisniewski, French, & Rosen, et al., 1982). Haberland (1969) also noted it in the cerebellum. In personally observed cases it has been noted in the cerebral white matter (Fig. 4).

Little has been written about congophilic angiopathy. Haberland et al. (1969) noted it in six brains of DS with dementia, ages 34 to 74. According to Glenner and Wong (1984) and Wong et al. (1985) SP and vascular amyloid in both DS and AD stain with the same specific probe for B amyloid.

There is only one report on the nucleus basalis of Meynert. Casanova et al. (1985) noted in 5 DS brains, ages 16 to 56, cogenitally less neurons and neuronal loss in the older brains.

Gyral atrophy and ventricular dilation are frequently commented on in old DS patients (Burger, & Vogel, 1973; Crapper, Dalton, Skopitz, Scott, & Hachinski, 1975; Ellis, McCulloch, & Corley, 1974; Hooper, & Vogel, 1976; Schochet, Lampert, & McCormick, 1973; Solitar, & Lamarche, 1966; Wisniewski, French, & Rosen, et al., 1982). In a small series Haberland (1969) found gyral atrophy mild in the 4th to 5th decade, then moderate to severe. Wisniewski et al. (1982) found it present in the second decade, with many brains showing moderate to severe atrophy by the fourth decade.

Another age-related change is pallor of myelin staining. In normative aging this appears in about the eighth decade and involves primarily the cortical-cortical fiber systems of the corona radiate (Kemper, 1984). In personally observed whole brain serial sections in the Yakovlev Collection at the Armed Forces Institute of decade and involves primarily the cortical-cortical fiber systems of

Figure 4: Age-related mineralization at two different levels in the serial sections of a 56 year old DS individual (A and V). The areas of mineralization are indicated by arrows. Note the pallor of myelin staining in the adjacent myelin stained sectiona at C and D. A and B, Nissl stain; C and D Loyez stain. Photographs courtesy Yakovlev collection, AFIP.

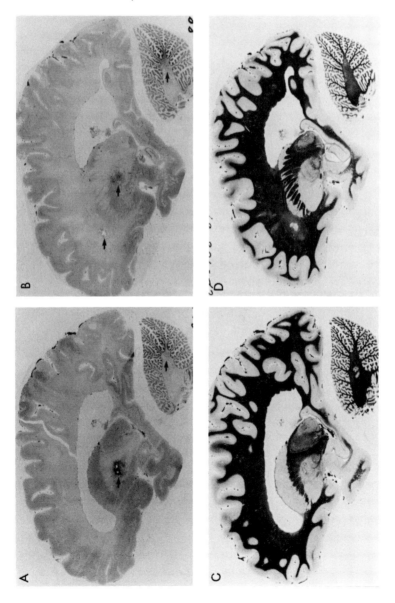

the corona radiate (Kemper, 1984). In personally observed whole brain serial sections in the Yakovlev Collection
at the Armed Forces Institute of Pathology, this change
appears in the second decade in DS (Fig. 3).
Thus there is abundant evidence in DS for premature
onset of many age-related changes and for their exaggerated expression. Perivascular mineral deposits occur early in the first decade, SP, NFT, gyral atrophy, ventricular dilation and age-related changes in myelin stain appear in the second decade. All these progress in severity
with DS brains showing SP and NFT densities comparable to
that found in (presenile) Alzheimer's disease in the 6th
and 7th decade where they occur in association with advanced gyral atrophy and ventricular dilation.
Engrafted on this process is clinical deterioration in
approximately one third of all older DS individuals. This
is usually diagnosed as Alzheimer's disease because of
its association with a striking proliferation of SP and
NFT, (Karlinsky, 1986; Wisniewski, & Rabe, 1986). The
problem with a straightforward diagnosis of Alzheimer's
disease is that most older DS individuals fail to show
evidence of a progressive dementia despite AP and NFT
proliferation that is nearly universal. After age 35
(Karlinsky, 1986) the densities of these changes are
comparable to or above that seen in Alzheimer's disease
(see above; Karlinsky, 1986; Wisniewski, Wisniewski, &
Wen, 1985; Wisniewski, & Rabe, 1986). Wisniewski and Rabe
(1986) suggest a threshold effect, since demented DS patients have higher SP and NFT densities than age matched
non-dementia DS patients. Another possibility is that
lesion topography may be more important for a diagnosis
of Alzheimer's disease than density. What may be unique
to Alzheimer's disease is the distribution pattern of NFT
and SP. The most exact data for the distribution of the
SP and NFT in AD and DS is in the hippocampal complex
(Hyman, Van Hoesen, Kromer, & Damasio, 1986; Kemper,
1978; Ropper, & Williams, 1980; and above). As noted
(above) there are striking differences between their distribution patterns in DS and AD. It may be that only when
specific critical regions become involved with appropriate densities of SP and NFT that clinical dementia will
be evident in DS. In this regard the amygdala has received little attention in DS. It is heavily involved in Alz-

heimer's disease (Kemper, 1983) and in some brains SP and NFT are primarily in the amygdala (Jamada, & Mehraein, 1968). A further point to be considered is the topographic distribution of NFT and SP in aging and dementia. Is it the same in both? Available evidence indicates differences (see Kemper, 1984; for a review). If they are different, does DS fit into one of these patterns? Is it possible that the distribution pattern of the SP and NFT in older DS individuals is an extreme exaggeration of an age-related distribution pattern?. Examples of other exaggerated age-related changes in DS are perivascular mineralization and gross brain atrophy. Another possible explanation for the failure of many older DS individuals to develop dementia is that altered brain circuity due to a decrease in non-pyramidal cells, somehow makes the brain more resistant to the effects of NFT and SP. With all these uncertainties, it might be more accurate to use a less committal term than Alzheimer's disease for the dementia in DS, such as Down-related dementia or Alzheimer-like dementia.

REFERENCES

Allsup, D., Kidd, M., Landon, M., & Tomlinson, A. (1986). Isolated senile plaque cores in Alzheimer's disease and Down's syndrome show different morphology. J. Neurol. Neurosurg. Psychiatr., 49, 886-892.

Apert, E. (1914). Mongolism. Le Monde Medicale, 24, 201.

Ball, M. J. (1978). Histopathology of cellular changes in Alzheimer's disease. In K. Nandy (Ed.), Senile Dementia: A Biomedical Approach, pp. 89-104, Elsevier, New York.

Ball, M. J., & Nuttall, K. (1981). Topography of neurofibrillary tangles and granulovacuoles in hippocampi of patients with Down's syndrome; Quantitative comparison with normal aging and Alzheimer's disease. Neuropath. Appl. Neurobiol., 7, 13-20.

Barden, H. S. (1983). Growth and development of selected hard tissues in Down syndrome: A review. Human Biology, 55, 539-576.

Becker, L. E., Armstrong, D. L., & Chan, F. (1986). Dendritic atrophy in children with Down's syndrome. Ann. Neurol., 20, 520-526.

Benda, C. (1969). Down's Anomaly, 2nd Edition, Grune Stratton, New York.

Benda, C. E., (1971). Mongolism. In J. Mencken (Ed.), Pathology of the Nervous System, Vol. II, pp. 1361-1371, McGram-Hill, Inc.

Bertrand, I., & Koffas, D. (1946). Cas d'idiotie mongolienne adulte avec hombreuses plaques seniles et concretions calcaries pallidales. Rev. Neurol., 78, 338-345.

Burger, P. C., & Vogel, F. S. (1973). The development of the pathologic changes of Alzheimer's disease and senile dementia in patients with Down's syndrome. Am. J. Pathol., 73, 457-476.

Casanova, M. F., Walker, L. C., Whitehouse, P. J. & Price, D. L. (1985). Abnormalities of the nucleus basalis in Down's syndrome. Ann. Neurol., 18, 310-313.

Colon, E. Y. (1972). The structure of the cerebral cortex in Down's syndrome; A quantitative analysis. Neuropadiatrie, 3, 362-376.

Coyle, J. T., Oster-Granite, M. L., & Gearhart, J. D. (1986). The neurobiologic consequences of Down syndrome. Brain. Res. Bul., 16, 773-787.

Crapper, D. R., Dalton, A. J., Skopitz, M., Scott, J. W., & Hachinski, V. C. (1975). Alzheimer degeneration in Down's syndrome: Electrophysiologic alterations and histopathologic findings. Arch. Neurol., 32, 618-623.

Crome, L., Cowie, V., & Slater, E. (1966). A statistical note on cerebellar and brain-stem weight in mongolism. J. Ment. Defic. Res., 10, 69-72.

Crome, L., & Stern, J. (1972). Pathology of Mental Retardation. William and Wilkins, Baltimore.

Cronk, C. E. (1978). Growth of children with Down syndrome: Birth to age 3 years. Pediatrics, 61, 564-568.

Davidoff, L. M. (1928). The brain in mongolian idiocy. Arch. Neurol. Psychiatr., 20, 1229-1257.

Ellis, W. G., McCulloch, J. R., & Corley, C. L. (1974). Presenile dementia in Down's syndrome. Neurology, 24, 101-106.

Fabregues, I., & Ferrer, I. (1983). Abnormal perisomatic structures in non-pyramidal neurons in the cerebral cortex in Down's syndrome. Neuropath. Appl. Neurobiol., 9, 165-170.

Feldman, M. L., & Peters, A. (1978). The forms of non-pyramidal neurons in the visual cortex of the rat. J. Comp. Neurol., 179, 761-793.

Forno, L. S., & Alvord, E. C., Jr. (1971). Recent advances in Parkinson's disease. In F. H. McDowell and C. H. Markham (Eds.), Contemporary neurology series. Some new Observations and Correlations, No. 8, Pt. 1, pp. 120-130, F.A. Davis Co. Philadelphia.

Friede, R. L. (1975). Developmental Neuropathology, Springer-Verlag, New York, Wien.

Gandolfi, A., Horoupian, D. S., & DeTeresa, R. M. (1981). Pathology of the auditory system in autosomal trisomies with morphometric and quantitative study of the vental cochlear nucleus. J. Neurol. Sci., 51, 43-50.

Gans, A. (1925). Anatomische Beobachtungen bei der Mongoloiden Idiotic. Nederl. Tijdschr. Geneesk, 69, 922-925.

Glenner, G. G., & Wong, C. W. (1984). Alzheimer's disease and Down's syndrome: Sharing of a unique cerebrovascular amyloid fibril protein. Biochemical and Biophysical Research Communications, 122, 1131-1135.

Gullotta, F., & Rehder, H. (1974). Chromosomal anomalies and central nervous system. Beitr. Path., 152, 74-80.

Haberland, C. (1969). Alzheimer's disease in Down's syndrome: clinical-neuropathological observations. Acta Neurol. Belg., 69, 369-380.

Hooper, M. W., & Vogel, F. S. (1976). The limbic system in Alzheimer's disease. Am. J. Path., 85, 1-35.

Hyman, B. T., Van Hoesen, G. W., Kromer, L. J., & Damasio, A. R. (1986). Perforant pathway changes and the memory impairment of Alzheimer's disease. Ann. Neurol., 20, 472-481.

Jamada, M., & Mehraein, P. (1968). Verteilungsmuster der senilen Veranderungen in Gehirn. Die Beteiligung des limbischen systems bei hinatrophischen Prozessen des Senium und bei morbus Alzheimer. Arch. Psychiat. Neurol., 211, 308-324.

Jacob H. (1956). Mongolism. Handbuch der Speziellen Pathologischen Anatomie und Histologie. O. Lubarsh, F. Henke and E. Rossle (Eds.) Vierter Teil. Erkrankurgen des zentral Nervensystem IV., pp. 82-98, Springer-Verlag, Berlin.

Jervis, G. A. (1948). Early senile dementia in mongoloid idiocy. Am. J. Psychiatr., 105, 102-106.

Jordan, S. W. (1971). Central nervous system. Human Pathology, 2, 561.

Karlinsky, H. (1986). Alzheimer's disease in Down's syndrome: a review. J. Amer. Geriatr. Soc., 34, 728-734.

Kemper, T. (1978). Senile Dementia: A focal disease in the temporal lobe. In K. Nancy (Ed.), Senile Dementia: A biomedical approach, pp. 105-113, Elsevier, New York.

Kemper, T. L. (1983). Organization of the neuropathology of the amygdala in Alzheimer's disease. In R. Katzman (Ed.), Banbury Report Biological Aspects of Alzheimer's Disease, pp. 31-35, Cold Spring Harbor Laboratory.

Kemper, T. L. (1984). Neuroanatomical and neuropathological changes with aging. In M. L. Albert (Ed.), The Clinical Neurology of Aging, pp. 9-52, Albert, Oxford University Press.

Khachaturian, K. S. (1985). Diagnosis of Alzheimer's disease. Arch. Neurol., 42, 1097-1105.

Koch, R., Share, J., Webb, A., & Graliker, B. V. (1963). The predictability of Gesell development scales in mongolism. J. Pediatr., 62, 93-97.

Malamud, N. (1964). Neuropathology. In H. A. Steves, and R. Heber (Eds.), Mental Retardation, p. 429, University of Chicago Press.

Mann, D. M. A., Yates, P. O., & Marcyniuk, B. (1985). Some morphometric observations on the cerebral cortex and hippocampus in presenile Alzheimer's disease, senile dementia of Alzheimer type and Down's syndrome in middle age. J. Neurol. Sci., 69, 139-159.

Marin-Padilla, M. (1972). Structural abnormalities of the cerebral cortex in human chromosomal aberrations: A Golgi study. Brain Res., 44, 625-629.

Marin-Padilla, M. (1974). Structural organization of the cerebral cortex (motor area) in human chromosomal aberration. A Golgi study. I.D. (13-15) trisomy, Patua syndrome. Brain Res., 66, 375-391.

Marin-Padilla, M. (1976). Pyramidal cell abnormalities in the motor cortex of a child with Down's syndrome: A Golgi study. J. Comp. Neurol., 167, 63-82.

Matsuyama, H., & Nakamura, S. (1978). Senile changes in the brain in the Japanese: Incidence of Alzheimer's neurofibrillary change and senile plaque. In R. Katzman, R. D. Terry, and K. L. Blick (Eds.), Alzheimer's disease: Senile Dementia and Related Disorders.

(Aging Vol. 7), pp. 287-297, Raven Press, New York.

Melyn, M. A., & White, D. T. (1973). Mental and developmental milestones of non-institutionalized Down's syndrome children. Pediatr., 52, 542-545.

Neuman, M. (1967). Langdon Down syndrome and Alzheimer's disease. J. Neuropath. Expr. Neurol., 26, 149-150.

Norman, R. M. (1938). Some observations on the depth and nervercell content of the supragranular cortex in normal and mentally defective persons. J. Neurol. Psychiatr., 1, 198-210.

Norman, R. M. (1971). Malformations of the Nervous System, Birth Injury, and Diseases of Early Life. In W. Blackwood and J. A. N. Corsellis (Eds.), Greenfield's Neuropathology, pp. 324-337, Edward Arnold Publishers, London.

Olson, M. I., & Shaw, C. M. (1969). Presenile dementia & Alzheimer's disease in mongolism. Brain, 92, 147-156.

Petit, T. L., Le Boutillier, J. C., Alfano, D. P., & Becker, L. E. (1984). Synaptic development in the human fetus: A morphometric analysis of normal and Down's syndrome neocortex. Expr. Neurol., 83, 13-23.

Podlisny, M. B., Lee, G., & Selkoe, D.J. (1987). Gene dosage of the amyloid precursor protein in Alzheimer's disease. Science, 238, 669-671.

Purpura, D. P. (1974). Dendritic spine "dysgenesis" and mental retardation. Science, 186, 1126-1128.

Roche, A. F. (1966). The craium in mongolism. Aeta Neurol. Scand., 42, 62-78.

Roizon, L., Jervis, G., Kaufman, M. A., Popobitch, I., & Hashimoto, S. (1972). Senile plaque pathogenesis in Down's, Alzheimer's and senile dementia. J. Neuropath. Expr. Neurol., 31, 188.

Ropper, A. H., & Williams, R. S. (1980). Relationship between plaques, tangles and dementia in Down syndrome, 30, 639-644.

Ross, M. H., Galaburda, A. M. & Kemper, T. L. (1984). Down's syndrome: Is there a decreased population of neurons?. Neurology, 34, 909-916.

Schmid, F., Duren, R., & Ahmadi, K. (1969). Das Mongolismus - Syndrom, Die mongoloid e Dyszephalie. Fortschr. Med., 87, 1252-1256.

Schochet, S. S., Lampert, P. W., & McCormick, W. F. (1973). Neurofibrillary tangles in patients with Down's

syndrome: A   light and electron microscopic study. Acta
Neuropath., 23, 342-346.
Scott,   B.   S.,   Becker,   L.   E.,   &   Petit,   T.   L.   (1983).
Neurobiology   of   Down's syndrome. Prog. Neurobiol., 21,
199-237.
Scott,   B. S., Becker, L. E., & Petit, T. L. (1983). Prog.
Neurobiol., 21, 199-237.
Solitare,   G.   B.,   &   Lamarche, J. B. (1966). Alzheimer's
Disease   and   senile   dementia   as   seen   in mongoloids:
Neuropathological   observations. Am. J. Ment. Diff., 70,
840-848.
Suetsugu,   M.,   &   Mehshein, P. (1980). Spine distribution
along   the   apical dendrites of the pyramidal neurons in
Down's syndrome. Acta. Neuropath., 50, 207-210.
Sylvester,   P.   E.   (1983). The hippocampus in Down's syn-
drome. J. Ment. Defic. Res., 27, 227-236.
Takashima,   S.,   Becker,   L.   E.,   Armstrong,   D.   L.,   & Chan,
F.   (1981).   Abnormal neuronal development in the visual
cortex   of   the   human fetus and infant with Down's syn-
drome: A   quantitative   and   qualitative   Golgi   study.
Brain Res., 225, 1-21.
Urich,   H.   (1976).   Malformations   of the Nervous System,
Perinatal   Damage   and Related Conditions Early in Life.
In   W.   Blackwood   and   J.   A.   N.   Corellis   (Eds.)
Greenfield's   Neuropathology,   pp.   361-496,   Yearbook
Medical Publishers, Chicago.
Whalley,   L.   J.   (1982). The dementia of Down's syndrome
and   its   relevance   to   aetiological   studies   of   Alz-
heimer's disease. Ann. N.Y. Acad. Sci., 396, 39-54.
Wisniewski,   K.   E.,   French, J. H., & Rosen, J. F., et al.
(1982).   Basal   ganglion   calcification   (BGC) in Down's
syndrome   (DS)   -   Another   manifestation   of   premature
aging. Proc. Ann. N.Y. Ada. Sci., 396, 179-189.
Wisniewski,   K.   E.,   Laure-Kamionowska, M., & Wisniewski,
H.   M.   (1984).   Evidence   of arrest of neurogenesis and
synaptogenesis   in   brains   of patients with Down's syndrome. N.E.J. Med., 311, 1187-1188.
Wisniewski,   K.   E.,   Wisniewski,   H.   M.,   &   Wen,   G.   Y.
(1985).   Occurrence   of   neuropathological   changes   and
dementia   of   Alzheimer-type neuropathology and dementia
in   persons   with   Down Syndrome. Ann. Neurol., 17, 278-
282.
Wisniewski,   H. M., & Rabe, A. (1986). Discrepancy between

Alzheimer-type neuropathology and dementia in persons with Down's syndrome. <u>Ann. N.Y. Acad. Sci.</u>, <u>477</u>, 247-259.

Wolstenholme, G. E. W. (1967). <u>Mongolism: CIBA Foundation Series 25</u>, Little Brown and Company, Boston.

Wong, C.W., Quaranta, V., & Glenner, G.G. (1985). Neuritic plaques and cerebrovascular amyloid in Alzheimer's disease are antigenically related. <u>Proc. Nat. Acad. Sci.</u>, <u>82</u>, 8729-8732.

Zellweger, H. (1977). Down Syndrome. In P. J. Vinken and G. W. Bruyn (Eds.), <u>Handbook of Clinical Neurology</u>, Vol. 31, Pt. II., pp. 367-469, North Holland Publ. Co., Amsterdam, New York, Oxford.

10

Physioanatomical Considerations in Down Syndrome

Eric Courchesne 1,2
1. Neuropsychology Research Laboratory
Children's Hospital Research Center
8001 Frost Street, San Diego, CA 92123

2. Neurosciences Department, School of Medicine
University of California, San Diego
La Jolla, California 92093

Normal human neurophysiological and neuroanatomical development involves gradual changes across more than 20
years. These changes consist of numerous processes such
as neurogenesis, myelinogenesis, synaptogenesis, naturally occurring cell death, and functional differentiation
and organization (Cowan, 1979). The process is one of
progressive and selective changes in the configuration of
complex, integrated neural networks. Changes or activity
in any one segment of these networks invariably affect
others; such effects may have short or long time courses,
so that the effects may not be detected until well after
the precipitating change. Sources triggering change or
neural activity are not only internal, but are also external -- sights, sounds, and chemicals absorbed by the
fetus from the mother or, later, ingested by the infant.
In progressive brain development, the very presence and
activity of the neural community alters the physical and
electrochemical environment in such a way as to create
the opportunity for successively more complex and stable
neural configurations to come into existence. Change is
more rapid during the earliest stages of development than
during later ones; the total number of neural elements
increases initially and an overabundance of neurons, axon
connections and synapses occurs; the size and extent of
neurons and their processes initially increases rapidly
and then stabilizes; the relationship between neural net-

works becomes more complex and specialized; and, eventually, a stage is reached that is quite stable compared to preceding ones. In the process of brain development, naturally occurring cell death and synapse elimination is the norm and more than 50% of a neural group and cortical synapses may be eliminated in the course of development. Many more initial axonal connections are apparently made than will survive the process of development (reviews; Cowan, 1979; 1984). Cell death, synapse elimination, and axonal loss may be attributed to complex interactions between the cells and their trophic, physical, electrochemical environment.

Specific Signs of Cellular Abnormalities
during Late Stages of Development

In DS, these progressive development events go seriously awry, and maldevelopment occurs throughout the cerebrum, cerebellum, and portions of the limbic system. In particular, preprogrammed events that normally occur during late stages of development are apparently truncated or "arrested". There is dysgenesis of small granular cell classes throughout neocortex, especially in layer II and IV (Ross et al., 1984; Wisniewski et al., 1984). The cerebellum is especially hypoplastic (Crome et al., 1966) and, in all likelihood, has granule cell dysgenesis. Nadel (1986) has argued that, if DS results in arrest of late stages of development, granular cell dysgenesis may be expected in the dentate gyrus of the hippocampus as well as in the cerebrum and cerebellum. Dendritic and spine development appears to begin normally, but is then arrested early in postnatal development (Takashima et al., 1981). There are a reduced number of spines (Scott et al., 1983; Suetsugu, 1980), and spines that are present, are long and thin rather than short and mushroom shaped; such long and thin spines are only normal in early stages of development (Marin-Padilla, 1976; Purpura, 1979; Takashima et al., 1981). Cerebellar Purkinje cells have perisomatic processes, dendritic-like elements on the soma, and multiple spines; such elements are also only normal in the early stages of development (Purpura, 1979). Electric membrane properties (Scott et al., 1983), synaptic size (Scott et al., 1983), cortical lamination, neuronal grouping patterns, cell morphology, and myelination are also abnormal (Malamud and Hirano, 1974).

*Possible Neural and Functional Consequences
of Cellular Abnormalities*

Theoretical Considerations - In their model of brain development, Changeux and Danchin (1976) proposed that an overabundance of labile synapses is initially produced; then, the functional activity of the nervous system, both spontaneous and evoked, serves to "selectively stabilize" some synapses in preference to those not experiencing adequate functional activity, which regress and disappear. Thus, synaptogenesis provides the necessary condition for neural organization, but it is the experience of spontaneous and evoked functional activity which actually adaptively sculpts it. In this epigenetic model of development, genetically preprogrammed neural elements (e.g., synapses) and configurations are selectively retained, altered or eliminated by experience. The result is a pattern of precisely adaptive microstructural configurations and functional neural activity which did not exist at birth.

   In DS, there is a shattering of this exquisite epigenetic process. The configuration of synapses that would be "selectively stabilized" must be distinctly different from normal. Normally, excitatory type 1 synapses occur on dendritic spines, and inhibitory type 2 occur mainly on cell bodies (Bindman and Lippold, 1981). In DS, one predicts a paucity of type 2 inhibitory synapses due to the reduction in the number of small interneurons mentioned above. Furthermore, excitatory input onto synapses on long and thin dendritic spines should be significantly attenuated (Purpura, 1979; Rall, 1974), and might contribute less than the normal level of functional activity. They might therefore be gradually and selectively eliminated. Purpura (1979) has suggested that long, thin spines that are maintained would be associated with distorted spatiotemporal patterns of excitatory postsynaptic potentials. On the other hand, excitatory synapses on dendritic shafts might be effective in eliciting the functional activity needed to be selectively stabilized, although, again, effectiveness might be somewhat reduced and spatiotemporal patterns of EPSPs might be abnormal because DS have significantly reduced presynaptic and postsynaptic lengths and widths (Scott et al., 1983).

Thus, cortical neurons in DS would be characterized by hypoinnervation, reduced inhibitory control, and a tendency for excitatory spatiotemporal patterns to be either distorted or abnormal in their effectiveness in triggering axonal output. Input/output functions of cortical columns would by simplified and temporally abnormal and would display a reduced capacity for filtering, integrating, selecting, and storing incoming information. The paucity of small, interneuron cell types would open the opportunity for aberrant axonal connections to be established. From the epigenetic point of view, abnormal output from a damaged network could adversely affect the synapses that will be selectively stabilized in networks to which it projects -- whether or not this receiving network was initially unaffected by the developmentally damaging event.

Neurophysiological Evidence: ERP Findings in DS

Background Information - Event-related brain potentials (ERPs) represent the functional neural activity evoked by discrete stimulus experiences. Their complex and subtle changes during development represent the outcome of the epigenetic process. Based on studies of ERPs (Courchesne, in press) and studies of synaptic numbers (Huttenlocher, 1979; Huttenlocher et al., 1982), it would appear that in humans, this selective, development process is continuous from birth to the teenage years. The ERP research on spatial selective attention in congenitally deaf individuals by Neville and Lawson (in press) demonstrates that ERP responses are sensitive indices of the effects of differential experiences during early development on cortical organization.

ERP technology provides the opportunity to record in vivo the functional activity generated by normal and abnormal neural systems involved in sensory, cognitive, and motor systems (Halliday et al., 1987) (Figure 1). The

Figure 1:
Idealized illustration of a single trial ERP response
elicited by a 70 dB nHL sound -- a click. The ERP is a
continuous series of components occurring at various latencies after stimulus onset and having various amplitudes and durations. Shorter latency components -- Waves
I, II, III, IV, and V, and Na and Pa -- are classic examples of "exogenous" (or sensory) components. The longer
latency component P3b is a classic example of an "endogenous" (or cognitive) component (from Courchesne, 1987).

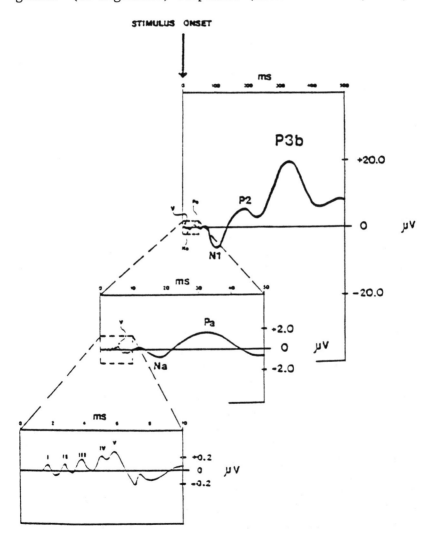

last decade has seen a rapid growth in information about
normal maturation of ERP activity in humans (Courchesne,
1978, 1983, in press; Galambos, 1982; Karrer and Ackles,
in press; Kurtzberg et al., 1985). Simultaneously, there
has been an emergence of information about ERP activity
associated with congenital and childhood developmental
disorders (Courchesne, 1987; Courchesne and Yeung-
Courchesne, 1987; Galambos, 1982; Holcomb et al., 1986;
Neville and Lawson in press; Kurtzberg 1985).

ERP Evidence in DS - Recent neurophysiological evidence
on DS using ERP technology complements the above evidence
of widespread cellular abnormalities and theoretical
microstructural and functional abnormalities in DS. As we
shall see next, this ERP evidence indicates that abnormal
neural activity exists in numerous neural systems ranging
form sensory to cognitive, and including auditory, vis
ual, and somatosensory modalities (e.g., Dustman and
Callner, 1979; Karrer and Ackles, in press; Lincoln et
al., 1985; Squires et al., 1979, 1986). We shall discuss
the ERP evidence that shows that DS patients have reduced
inhibitory control, reduced selectivity and specificity
of responsiveness, increased neural responsiveness, abnormalities in the timing of neural responses, and abnormal mechanisms involved in temporal integration and information storage (e.g., Barnet et al., 1971; Dustman and
Callner, 1979; Karrer and Ackles, in press; Lincoln et
al., 1985; Schafer and Peeke, 1982; Squires et al.,
1979).

Sensory Afferent Information Processing - There are significant abnormalities in the timing of neural responses
in the auditory sensory pathways at the brainstem level
(Squires et al., 1986). The responses measured included
the latencies of Waves I through V which reflect auditory
neural activity in the auditory nerve, pons, inferior
colliculus, medial geniculate body, and auditory thalamo-
cortical radiations (Legatt et al., 1986). Wave II had an
abnormal short response latency; the neural response interval between III and IV was also abnormally short; and
that between Waves IV and V was abnormally long (Squires
et al., 1986) (Figure 2). These abnormalities are independent of high frequency hearing loss, which is often

present in DS (Squires et al., 1986), and appear to
differ from other neurodevelopmental disorders. It will
be important to determine how these abnormalities relate
to the cognitive and language deficits in DS.

Figure 2:
Differences in latency of certain auditory brainstem ERP
peaks between normal and Down Syndrome people (from
Squires et al., 1980).

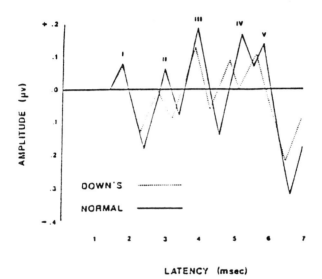

LATENCY (msec)

There are also significant abnormalities in the timing
and amplitude of neural responses associated with cortical sensory-related ERPs in DS (Bigum et al., 1970;
Glidden et al., 1975; Callner et al., 1978; Dustmand and
Callner, 1979; Lincoln et al., 1985). Figure 3 shows that
abnormally increased response amplitudes and response delays exist in numerous cortical sensory-related components of the ERPs elicited by stimuli in auditory, visual, and somatosensory modalities (Dustmand and Callner,
1979).
These cortical sensory-related ERP findings may reflect
the structural and functional abnormalities in granular
cerebral cortex which were discussed earlier. For several
reasons, however, one might also raise the question of

Figure 3:
Averaged evoked responses recorded from normal and Down Syndrome subjects. Each tracing is the average of the responses of 66 individuals. Significant group differences in response amplitudes are given. VER, AER, and SRR are, respectively, average visual, auditory, and somatosensory evoked responses (from Dustman and Callner, 1979).

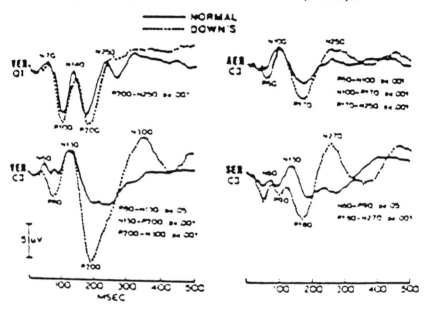

whether cerebellar dysfunction may be involved in these response abnormalities as well as in the abnormal auditory brainstem responses. First, the cerebellum has been shown to modulate cochlear microphonics and auditory nerve action potentials (Velluti and Crispino, 1979). Second, in the normal mammal, cerebellar stimulation (especially in vermal lobules VI, VII, and VIII) modulates brainstem, thalamic and cortical ERP responses to auditory, somatosensory and visual sensory information (Crispino and Bullock, 1984). Third this modulatory function must be defective in DS. As discussed above, cerebellar maldevelopment is one of the primary pathologies in DS. The Purkinje cell abnormalities in DS mentioned earlier are characteristic of granuloprival cerebellar cortex (Rakic, 1984). In mutant mice, granuloprival conditions result in gross distortions of neural circuits in cerebellar cortex (Rakic, 1984). In particular, Purkinje cells receive multiple, perisomatic climbing fiber innervations and mossy fiber innervations (Woodward et al., 1974; Sotelo, 1982). Since DS is thought to be associated with dysgenesis of late forming, small neurons, it remains a possibility that there is a dysgenesis of cerebellar stellate and basket cells as well as the granule cells. In the case of granule cell dysgenesis, Purkinje cells would be functionally hypoinnervated because the excitatory granule cells represent the vast majority of Purkinje cell synaptic input. The granule cell-Purkinje cell synaptic site may be critical in cerebellar plasticity underlying associative learning (Reviews: Gellman and Miles, 1985; Thompson, 1986). Thus, the normal local circuit activity which serves to adaptively integrate incoming information and adaptively modulate Purkinje cell output would be severely compromised; there would be an "information short-circuit" in cerebellar cortex.

Cognition: Memory and Attention - Memory and attention are fundamental to the development of intelligent human thought and action. Habituation to repeated insignificant stimulation is a basic form of memory. Schafer and Peeke (1982) suggested that DS involves deficient inhibitory mechanisms that normally selectively and specifically "suppress response(s) to insignificant or predictable stimuli." To illustrate this, they studied the auditory P2 response (latency ca 150 to 200 msec) which is unusually enlarged in amplitude in DS (Dustman and Callner, 1979; Lincoln et al., 1985). They found that the enlargement of this component and the negative N2 (latency ca 230 msec) that follows it, may be due to deficient modulatory and inhibitory mechanisms.[1] The first of a series of repeated auditory stimuli produces P2 and N2 amplitudes similar to normals. However, with repeated presentations, these responses failed to show the normal pattern of short-term habituation (Figure 4). This failure to find evidence of normal short-term habituation of the cortical sensory ERPs has been reported in DS infants (Barnet et al., 1971) as well as in DS children and adults (e.g., Dustmand and Beck, 1979). Schafer and Peeke (1982) concluded that a deficit in this basic form of learning could help to explain the mental retardation in

Figure 4:

Mean amplitude values for evoked cortical responses to repetitive auditory stimuli from normal and Down Syndrome individuals (Schafer and Peeke, 1982).

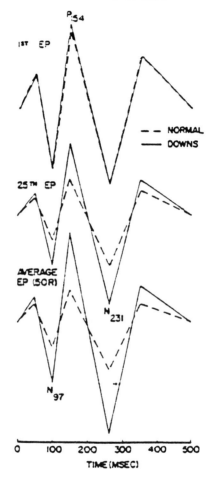

DS.

Memory systems mediated by the hippocampus may provide us with conscious awareness of the memories of specific objects, places, and events that have occurred in the past (Nadel and Zola-Morgan, 1984). Nadel (1986) has suggested that hippocampal maldevelopment may be a key to understanding the mental retardation in DS. Woods et al. (1980) suggested that P3b may depend on controlled, con-

scious processing; it has never been demonstrated in un-
conscious or sleeping people, and it disappears with un-
consciousness under the effects of nitrous oxide (Robert
Sternbach, unpublished data). The visual P3b has not yet
been detected in the ERP responses of infants (Courchesne
et al., 1981; Karrer and Ackles, in press). Interestingly, the P3b has been suggested to be affected by hippocampal damage (Halgren et al, 1980), and the developmental emergence of the visual P3b roughly coincides with
that of memory systems mediated by hippocampus. The study
of the developmental emergence of P3b in DS could add important information regarding this hypothesis; unfortun-
nately, no such information is currently available.

Nonetheless, in older DS children and DS adults, abnormalities in response latency, amplitude, and morphology
of the auditory and visual P3b component of the ERP (particularly over the frontal and central cortical areas) do
occur (Lincoln et al., 1985; Squires et al., 1979). The
abnormalities appeared to be a developmental deviation
rather than lag since the responses were unlike any normal stage of human P3b development (Courchesne, 1983;
Lincoln et al., 1985) (Figure 5), and they were unlike
those present in other developmental disorders (review:
Courchesne and Yeung-Courchesne, 1987).

Lastly, the development of selective attention in normal infants involves an active and selective reaction to
novel and biologically important stimuli, including social cues. The development of the ability to discriminate
new and important information from old and insignificant
information is essential to normal cognitive development.
Since people have a limited capacity to attend to information in their environment, it is equally essential to
develop the complementary capacity for selective and specific responsiveness only to such new, important and
meaningful information. Frontal cortex is important in
the executive control of selective attention (McCallum et
al., 1983; Roland, 1982).

The Nc component, which is recorded from sites over
frontal cortical areas, is a sign of enhanced selective
attention to new, important or meaningful stimuli (Figure
6) (Ciesielski et al., submitted; Courchensne, 1977,
1978, 1983, 1987; Holcomb et al., 1986; Karrer & Ackles,
in press). Nc has been suggested to be generated by cor-

Figure 5:
Evidence that auditory P3b and Nc latencies are longer in 12-year-old Down Syndrome children than in age-matched normal children.   It can also be seen that P3b amplitude is larger at central and frontal sites in Down Syndrome Children than in normal children. (adapted from Lincoln et al., 1985).

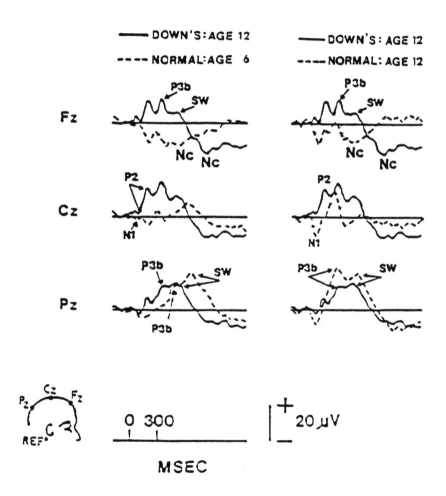

TARGET ERPs

Figure 6:
Nc and visual selective attention. Visual ERP responses recorded over frontal cortex site (Fpz) during three different selective attention tasks. In all three tasks, sequences of stimuli were composed of both visual and auditory stimuli randomly ordered. There were always 2 types of visual stimuli: standards (e.g., a green square) which occurred often, and rares (e.g., a red square) which occurred seldom. Dotted lines are ERPs elicited by ignored visual standard and rare stimuli when subjects selectively attended to auditory stimulation (a "visual ignore" condition). Dashed lines are visual ERPs elicited when subjects were required to selectively respond to the visual rare stimuli, but also were selectively attending to auditory stimulation (a "divided" attention task). Solid line are visual ERPs elicited when subjects were required to selectively respond to visual rare stimuli, but to ignore the auditory stimulation (a "focused" visual attention task). Each ERP trace is the average response of 13 normal adults. Horizontal marks = 100 msec; vertical marks = ± 5 uV. (Adapted from Ciesielski, Courchesne, & Elmasian, submitted).

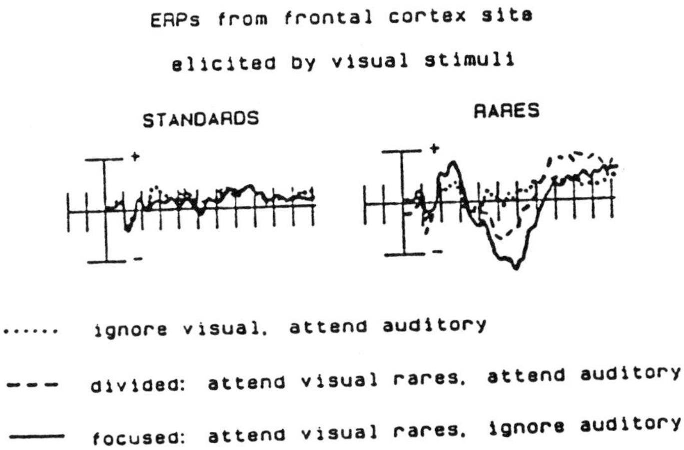

ERPs from frontal cortex site

elicited by visual stimuli

STANDARDS   RARES

...... ignore visual, attend auditory

- - - divided: attend visual rares, attend auditory

——— focused: attend visual rares, ignore auditory

304   Courchesne

Figure 7:
Synapse counts in frontal cortex and Nc amplitude over frontal cortex plotted as a function of age in humans: Curve from Huttenlocher (1979) shows synapse counts (left axis) in layer 3 of middle frontal gryus. Nc amplitude at Fz (right axis) elicited by visual (triangles) and auditory (black circles with star) stimuli which were low in probability and unexpected. Visual Nc amplitude data in 1.5, 6, 12, and 18 month old infants from Karrer and Ackles (1986), and visual data in 7, 11.8, 15.2, and 25 year olds from Courchesne (1977, 1978). Auditory Nc amplitude data in meonates from Kurtzberg (1985; see above Figure 13 anterior electrode site), and auditory data in 4, 7, 11.8, 15.2, and 25 year olds from Courchesne (1983).

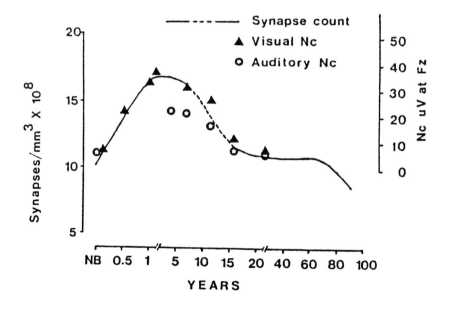

tical postsynaptic potentials that are triggered either by cholinergic-nucleus basalis input or intralaminar thalamic input to cortex. It may index mechanisms designed to increase the temporal resolution of cortex, thereby optimally preparing it to take in and store important information (Courchesne, 1987; Courchesne et al., 1987). Developmental changes in Nc amplitude parallel those in synaptic numbers (Courchesne, in press) (Figure 7). Nc-like responses over frontal cortical areas have been elicited in normal newborns by novel sounds (Kurtzberg, 1985).

Nc responses across early development index a maturing ability to selectively attend to only new, important and meaningful information and to inhibit responses to old and insignificant information (Karrer and Ackles, in press) (Figure 8 and 9). In a study by Karrer and Ackles (in press), novel and surprising visual stimuli were randomly presented amid sequences of visual stimuli to which infants had been previously exposed. By 6 months of age, all stimuli were found to elicit large, distinct Nc responses ("R" or "rares" and "F" or "frequents" in Figures 8 and 9). Between 6 and 18 months of age, normal infants displayed an increased selective enhancement of the Nc response to the novel information relative to the previously seen, non-novel information (Figure 9). Moreover, this selective enhancement displayed a distinct and frontally located pattern of activity.

In 6 to 30 month old DS, measures of Nc indicate an extreme developmental abnormality in frontal attentional selectivity and regional specificity of cortical activation (Karrer and Ackles, in press), and in data from DS 12 year olds, Nc responses are as slow as in DS infants (Lincoln et al., 1985; Figure 5). Across the age range of 6 to 30 months, DS patients showed no evidence of selective enhancement of Nc responses to novel information. Indeed, Nc was as large to the non-novel, insignificant information as to novel information (Figure 10). In addition, patterns of ERP activity elicited by novel information suggested no regional cortical specificity of responsiveness; instead novel stimuli elicited similar activation across wide areas of cortex.

Summary and Concluding Remarks

From an epigenetic point of view, DS brain development, per se, is not "arrested" and does not "cess". Instead,

Figure 8:
Shows normal development of Nc over frontal (Fx) and
central cortex (Cx) across infancy in response to visual
novel stimulation. Nc (stippled areas) elicited by novel
stimuli ("R") that randomly and infrequently occur (p =
20%) in a series of presentations of a frequently presented stimulus ("F"; p = 80%). Novel stimuli (R) elicit
larger amplitude responses than frequent stimuli (F). "n"
refers to the number of infants whose responses are included in the grand average response at each age. Nc is
larger to novel than to the frequent, non-novel stimuli.
Note Nc latency is about 800 msec and amplitudes elicited
by novel stimuli in older infants are about 30 to 40 uV.
(Adapted from Karrer and Ackles, in press.)

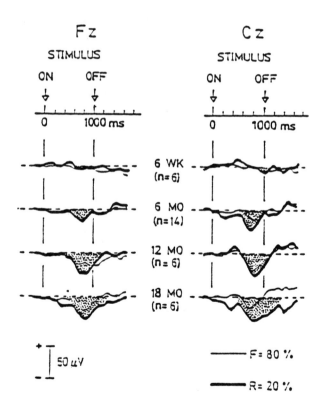

Figure 9:
(Adapted from Karrer & Ackles, in press).

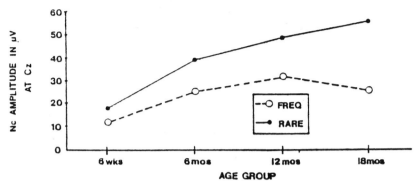

the "arrest" or cessation of <u>specific</u> neural events, such as granule cell migration or spine morphology, only marks the beginning of a sequence of developmental difficulties. The abnormal structural features in DS -- such as dysgenesis of dendritic spines or small cortical cell types -- must necessarily produce abnormal initial neural configurations from which functional neural activity makes cell, axonal, and synaptic selection. These selections from abnormal configurations result in distorted structure and function (e.g., cerebellar local circuitry), and, ultimately, in behavioral expression (e.g., mental retardation).

The initial damage in DS is widespread, including all of the cerebrum, cerebellum, and dentate gyrus. The consequent structural and functional abnormalities are also widespread. At the cellular and local circuit levels, they include reduced inhibitory components, abnormal spatiotemporal patterns of excitation, potential for enhanced excitatory throughput without modulation, general neuronal hypoinnervation with the synapses present being primarily axodendritc excitatory, reduced temporal and spatial filtering and selection, and reduced specificity of responsiveness. These cellular and circuit characteristics are present in the neurophysiological activity that can be recorded in vivo using ERP technology. ERP measures show the presence of widespread abnormal neural functioning in sensory, memory and attention systems in auditory, visual, and somatosensory modalities.

The mental retardation in DS is the product of an epi-

Figure 10:
(Adapted from Karrer & Ackles, in press).

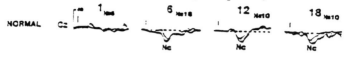

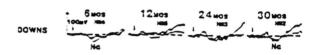

genetic process: Abnormal genetic programming creates abnormal initial structural configurations (too few inhibitory synapses, poorly functioning axospinous excitatory
synapses, functional axodendritic synapses, small synaptic sizes). These abnormal neural configurations produce
abnormal neural activity; and this activity, in turn,
serves as the basis for decisions about what synapses
would be retained (e.g., functional dendritic) and lost
(e.g., axospinous synapses whose excitatory activity
would be too functionally attenuated to be retained and
selectively stabilized). The end result is the sculpting
of maladaptive microstructural configurations and functions throughout vast regions of the brain.

Acknowledgments

Supported by NIMH grant 1-R01-MH36840 and NINICDS grant
5-R01-NS19855 awarded to Eric Courchesne.

Footnotes

1. Primary and secondary auditory cortex are likely to be
involved in the generation of auditory P3 and N2 responses (review: Woods, in press).

REFERENCES

Barnet, A. B., Ohlrich, E. S., & Shanks, B. L. (1971). EEG evoked responses to repetitive auditory stimulation in normal and Down's syndrome infants. Developmental Medicine and Child Neurology, 13, 321-329.

Bigum, H. B., Dustman, R. E., & Beck, E. C. (1970). Visual and somatosensory evoked responses from mongoloid and normal children. Electroencephalography and Clinical Neurophysiology, 28, 576-585.

Bindman, L., & Lippold, O. (1981). The Neurophysiology of the Cerebral Cortex. Austin, TX: University of Texas Press.

Changeux, J. P. & Danchin, A. (1976). Selective stabilization of developing synapses as a mechanism for the specification of neural networks. Nature, 264, 705-712.

Courchesne, E. (1977). Event-related brain potentials: A comparison between children and adults. Science, 197, 589-592.

Courchesne, E. (1978). Neurophysiological correlates of cognitive development: Changes in long-latency event-related potentials from childhood to adulthood. Electroenceph. Clin. Neurophysiol., 45, 468-482.

Courchesne, E. (1983). Cognitive components of the event-related brain potential: Changes associated with development. In A. W. K. Gaillard and W. Ritter (Eds.), Tutorials in ERP research: endogenous components. Amsterdam: North-Holland Publishing Company.

Courchesne, E. (1987). A neurophysiological view of autism. In E. Schopler and G. B. Mesibov (Eds.), Neurobiological issues in autism (pp. 285-324). Plenum Press, New York.

Courchesne, E. (in press). Comparison of neurophysiological and neuroanatomical indices of human postnatal brain development. In K. Gibson, M. Konner, and A. C. Petersen (Eds.), Brain and Behavioral Development: Biosocial Dimensions. Hawthorne, NY: Aldine Press.

Courchesne, E., Elmasian, R. O., & Yeung-Courchesne, R. (1987). P3b and Nc: Basic clinical and developmental research. In A. M. Halliday, S. R. Butler, and R. Paul (Eds.), A textbook of clinical neurophysiology. Sussex, England: John Wiley & Sons Ltd.

Courchesne, E., Ganz, L., & Norcia, A. (1981). Event-related brain potentials to human faces in infants. Child Development, 52, 804-811.

Courchesne, E., Ganz, L., & Norcia, A. M. (in revision). The P3b/SW complex in young children in a face discrimination task. Electroenceph. Clin. Neurophysiol.: Evoked Potentials.

Cowan, W. M. (1979). The development of the brain. Scientific American, 241, 113-133.

Cowan, W. M., Fawcett, J. W., O'Leary, D. D. M., & Stanfield, B. B. (1984). Regressive events in neurogenesis. Science, 225, 1265-1285.

Crispino, L. (1983). Modification of responses from specific sensory systems in midbrain by cerebellar stimulation: experiments on a teleost fish. Journal of Neurophysiology, 49, 3-15.

Crispino, L., & Bullock, T. H. (1984). Cerebellum mediates modality-specific modulation of sensory responses of midbrain and forebrain in rat. Proc. Natl. Acad. Sci. USA, 81, 2917-2920.

Crome, L., Cowie, V., & Slater, E. (1966). A statistical note on cerebellar and brain-stem weight in mongolism, pp. 69-72.

Dustman, R. E., & Callner, D. A. (1979). Cortical evoked responses and response decrement in nonretarded and Down's syndrome individuals. American Journal of Mental Deficiency, 83, 391-397.

Galambos, R. (1982). Maturation of auditory evoked potentials. In G. A. Chiarenza and D. Papakostopoulos (Eds.), Clinical application of cerebral evoked potentials in pediatric medicine. Amsterdam: Excerpta Medica.

Gellman, R. S., & Miles, F. A. (1985). A new role for the cerebellum in conditioning? Trends in Neurosciences, 8, 181-182.

Glidden, J. B., Busk, J., & Galbraith, G. C. (1975). Visual evoked responses as a function of light intensity in Down's syndrome and nonretarded subjects. Psychophysiology, 12, 416-422.

Holcomb, P. J., Ackerman, P. T., & Dykman, R. A. (1986). Auditory event-related potentials in attention and reading disabled boys. International J. of Psychophysiology, 3, 263-273.

Huttenlocher, P. R. (1979). Synaptic density in human frontal cortex developmental changes and effects of aging. Brain Res., 163, 195-205.

Huttenlocher, P. R., de Courten, C., Garey, L. J., & Van Der Loos, H. (1982). Synaptogenesis in human visual cortex -- evidence for synapse elimination during normal development. Neuroscience Letters, 33, 247-252.

Karrer, R., & Ackles, P. K. (in press). Visual event-related potentials of infants during a modified oddball procedure. Electroenceph. Clin. Neurophysiology.

Karrer, R., & Ackles, P. K. (in press). Brain organization and perceptual/cognitive development in normal and Down syndrome infants: A research program. In P. Vietze & H. G. Vaughan, Jr. (Eds.), The Early Identification of Infants at Risk for Mental Retardation. Orlando, FL: Grune & Staton.

Kurtzberg, D. (1985). Late auditory evoked potentials and speech sound discrimination in newborns. Presented at the meetings of the Society for Research in Child Development, Toronto.

Legett, A. D., Arezzo, J. C., & Vaughan, H. G. (1986). Short-latency auditory evoked potentials in the monkey. II. Intracranial generators. Electroencephalography and Clinical Neurophysiology, 64, 53-73.

Lincoln, A. J., Courchesne, E., Kilman, B. A., & Galambos, R. (1985). Neuropsychological correlates of information-processing by children with Down syndrome. Journal of Mental Deficiency, 89(4), 403-414.

Malamud, N., & Hirano, A. (1974). Atlas of Neuropathology (2nd revised ed.). Berkeley: University of California Press.

Marin-Padilla, M. (1976). Pyramidal cell abnormalities in the motor cortex of a child with Down's syndrome. A Golgi study. J. Comp. Neur., 167, 63-82.

McCallum, W. C., Curry, S. H., Cooper, P. V., & Papakostopoulos, D. (1983). Brain event-related potentials as indicators of early selective processes in auditory target localization. Psychophysiology, 20, 1-17.

Nadel, L. (1986). Down syndrome in neurobiological perspective. In C. J. Epstein (Ed.), The Neurobiology of Down Syndrome (pp. 239-251). New York: Raven Press.

Nadel, L., & Zola-Morgan, S. (1984). Infantile amnesia: A neurobiological perspective. In M. Moscovitch (Ed.), Infant memory. New York: Plenum Press.

Neville, H. J., & Lawson, D. (in press). Attention to central and peripheral visual space in a movement detection task: An event-related potential and behavioral study. II. Congenitally deaf adults. Brain Research.

Purpura, D. P. (1979). Pathobiology of cortical neurons in metabolic and unclassified amentias. Congenital and Acquired Cognitive Disorders, 43-68.

Rakic, P. (1984). Defective cell-to-cell interactions as causes of brain malformations. In E. S. Gollin (Ed.), Malformations of Development (pp. 239-285). New York: Academic Press.

Rakic, P. Bourgeois, J. P., Eckenhoff, M. F., Zecevic, N., & Goldman-Rakic, P. S. (1986). Concurrent overproduction of synapses in diverse regions of the primate cerebral cortex. Science, 232, 232-235.

Rall, W. (1974). Dendritic spines, synaptic potency, and neuronal plasticity. In C. D. Woody, K. A. Brown, T. J. Crow, and J. D. Knipsel (Eds.), Cellular Mechanisms Subserving Changes in Neuronal Activity (pp. 13-21)., UCLA: Brain Information Service.

Roland, P. E. (1982). Cortical regulation of selective attention in man: A regional cerebral blood flow study. J. Neurophysiol., 48, 1059-1078.

Ross, M. H., Galaburda, A. M., & Kemper, T. L. (1984). Down's syndrome: Is there a decreased population of neurons? Neurology, 34, 909-915.

Schafer, E. W. P., & Peeke H. V. S. (1982). Down syndrome individuals fail to habituate cortical evoked potentials. American Journal of Mental Deficiency, 87(3), 332-337.

Scott, B. S., Becker, L. E., & Petit, T. L. (1983). Neurobiology of Down's syndrome. Progress in Neurobiology, 21, 199-237.

Soleto, C. (1982). Synaptic remodeling in agranular cerebella. In S. L. Paley and V. Chan-Palay (Eds.), The Cerebellum -- New Vistas (pp. 50-68). Berlin: Springer-Verlag.

Squires, N., Galbraith, G., & Aine, C. (1979). Event-related potential assessment of sensory and cognitive deficits in the mentally retarded. In D. Lehman & E. Callaway (Eds.), Human Evoked Potentials. New York: Plenum Press.

Squires, N., Ollo, C., & Jordan, R. (1986). Auditory brain stem responses in the mentally retarded: Audiometric correlates. Ear and Hearing, 7(2), 83-92.

Suetsugu, M., & Mehraein, P. (1980). Spine distribution along the apical dendrites of the pyramidal neurons in Down's sydnrome. A quantitative Golgi study. Acta Neuropath., 50, 207-210.

Takashima, S., & Becker, L. E. (1985). Basal ganglia calcification in Down's syndrome. Journal of Neurology, Neurosurgery, and Psychiatry, 48, 61-64.

Thompson, R. F. (1986). The neurobiology of learning and memory. Science, 233, 941-947.

Velluti, R., & Crispino, L. (1979). Cerebellar actions on cochlear microphonics and on auditory nerve action potential. Brain Res. Bull., 4, 621-624.

Wisniewski, K. E., Laure-Kamionowska, M., & Wisniewski, H. M. (1984). Evidence of arrest of neurogenesis and synaptogenesis in brains of patient with Down's syndrome. The New England Journal of Medicine, 311, 1187-1188.

Wood, C. C., McCarthy, G., Squires, N. K., Vaughan, Jr., H. G., Woods, D. L., & McCallum, W. C. (1984). Anatomical and physiological substrates of event-related potentials. In R. Karrer, J. Cohen, and P. Tueting (eds.), Brain and Information: Event-Related Potentials. Annals of the New York Academy of Sciences, 425, 681-721.

Woods, D. L., Courchesne, E., Hillyard, S. A., & Galambos, R. (1980a). Recovery cycles of event-related potentials in multiple detection tasks. Electroenceph. Clin. Neurophysiol., 50, 335-347.

Woodward, D. J., Hofer, B. J. & Altman, J. (1974). Physiological and pharmacological properties of Purkinje cells in rat cerebellum degranulated by postnatal X-irradiation. Journal of Neurobiology, 5, 283-304.

11

NEUROLOGICAL AND PSYCHOLOGICAL STATUS
OF INDIVIDUALS WITH DOWN SYNDROME

K.E. Wisniewski, C.M. Miezejeski,
and A.L. Hill
NYS Office of Mental Retardation and
Developmental Disabilities
Institute for Basic Research in
Developmental Disabilities
1050 Forest Hill Road,
Staten Island, New York 10314

Considerable variability of intellectual function has been reported among individuals with Down Syndrome (DS) (Clements et al., 1976; Rynders et al., 1978; Bennett et al., 1979). For institutionalized people with DS severe mental retardation (MR) is the most frequent diagnosis (Johnson & Abelson, 1969; Connally, 1978; Demaine & Silverstein, 1978; Silverstein, et al., 1982)., while mild and moderate MR is more frequently seen among individuals raised at home (Centerwal and Centerwal, 1960; Melyn & White, 1973; Clements, et al., 1976; Cunningham, 1982). This observation, along with recent results of research investigating the effects of early initiation of infant stimulation and educational mainstreaming, has suggested that children with DS may possess previously unrealized abilities and that the abilities of a proportion of the mentally retarded population with DS may have been underestimated (Rynders et al., 1978; Libb et al., 1983; Pieterse & Center, 1984; Rynders, 1986; Pueschel 1987).

Recently, the usefulness of broad measures of function, such as IQ, has been de-emphasized (Silverstein, et al., 1982), and most current research has been concerned with more specific questions (Hartley, 1985; 1986). Many attempts have been made to examine performance profiles of persons with DS to see how their abilities differ from

those of both nondisabled persons and persons with MR due
to other etiologies. For persons with DS relative weakness in language as compared to nonverbal functions has
been frequently reported in the literature (Bilovsky &
Share, 1965; McCarthy, 1965; Share, 1975; Rohr & Buhr,
1978; Greenwald & Leonard, 1979; Silverstein et al.,
1982; Piper, et al., 1986). Some examples of possible
reasons for this relative language deficit include: atypical social environments, hearing loss frequently associated with recurrent otitis media; specific central nervous system (CNS) abnormalities that may be the expression of genetic determinants such as a triple dose of the
gene products of chromosome 21.

A considerable body of literature has been developed
around the issue of environmental factors that influence
the cognitive development of infants and children with
DS. Initially gross differences in environment, i.e., institutionalization versus home-rearing, were the independent variables under consideration. As early as 1945,
through the study of intellectually nondisabled children
who had experienced prolonged hospitalization, it had
been demonstrated that institutionalization has adverse
consequences (Spitz, 1945, 1946). This pioneering work
focussed on maternal deprivation. Of course, infants and
children reared in institutions have been deprived of
much more than contact with their mothers. Often they
have resided in facilities that were not equipped to provide adequate stimulation of positive emotions, sensory
stimulation, and visual-motor development. Institutions
for children with MR were certainly as, if not more, inadequate than those for the nondisabled. As a consequence, there has been both a move away from institutionalization and a proliferation of programs of early stimulation and educational intervention that are frequently
introduced within weeks, if not days, following birth.
Voluminous research has supported the efficacy of these
programs, as well as the importance of early initiation
(for a review, see Hanson, 1981, 1987). Currently, this
area of research appears to be focussed on the quality of
the child's home environment and factors that enhance the
effectiveness of early intervention.

Since the child's parents are most likely the major
critical environmental influence on a child's develop-

ment, differences in parenting behaviors and possible correlates, such as parents' level of education, (Fraser & Sadovnick, 1976; Golden & Pashayan, 1976; Clements, Hafer, & Pollock, 1978; Libb et al., 1983) have been the primary components of home environment that have been investigated. According to Veitze (1987), the longitudinal studies of parent stimulation of their infants in naturalistic settings have revealed quantitative and qualitative differences in the stimulation provided by mothers of children with DS versus mothers of nondisabled children. Mothers of children with DS engaged in much higher levels of activity with their infant but vocalized less frequently than did mothers of nondisabled children. It was suggested that this resulted in the mothers of children with DS less frequently taking turns with their infant when vocalizing. When these mothers were instructed to imitate their child, thereby fostering turn-taking, the infants with DS nearly trebled their vocal output (McQuiston, 1982). These observations suggest that attention should be given not only to the quantity but also the quality of the stimulation provided during early infancy. Research confirming the belief that environmental factors are correlated with the cognitive development of children with DS has provided support for programs of early stimulation and educational intervention, as well as behavior training for parents.

Notwithstanding the proven efficacy of these interventions, Balkany et al. (1979) have questioned their relative importance as compared to the need for medical interventions directed toward early detection, prevention, and treatment of hearing impairment, which occurs with a high incidence in persons with DS. Studies of hearing loss in persons with DS have included samples of children (e.g., Dahle & McCollister, 1986; van Gorp & Baker, 1984), and adults (e.g., Keiser et al., 1981), and both age groups (e.g., Balkany et al., 1979; Brooks, Wooley, & Kanjilal, 1972). The high incidence of abnormal tympanograms reported by these investigators has led to the conclusion that this hearing loss is usually conductive rather than sensorineural, and can be attributed to a high incidence of recurrent otitis media in the population of persons with DS. This relatively higher incidence of conductive hearing loss has been observed even when the investigators have conducted their study during a time of the year (April to June) chosen intentionally to reduce the risk of transient upper respiratory and middle ear infections (Keiser et al., 1981). The latter report cautioned that sensorineural and mixed losses (sensori-neural and conductive) should not be overlooked in that twice as many individuals showed losses of the sensori-neural and mixed types as showed conductive losses alone. Note, however, that this study did not include children with DS, but only adults. In their study of both adults and children, Brooks et al. (1972) observed a significant association of age with type of hearing loss. Most inves-tigators have concluded that persons with DS experience a much higher incidence of conductive and sensorineural hearing loss than do persons with MR of other etiologies and that this loss is due to the equally high incidence of recurrent otitis media in this population. Brooks et al. (1972) also conjectured that the high incidence of sensorineural hearing loss in the adults in their DS sam-ple was the consequence of long-standing middle ear dis-ease. Early diagnosis and treatment could prevent these abnormalities. It has been shown with standardized IQ tests that the general intelligence of both children and adults is diminished by hearing losses, as indicated by abnormal tympanograms (Libb, et al., 1985). This rela-tionship between IQ and hearing loss may reflect the fact that performance on the IQ tests used by Libb et al. (1985) was hindered disproportionately by deficient re-ceptive language. Consequently, these results may reflect a relationship between hearing loss and receptive lan-guage rather than hearing loss and general intelligence.

Observations of motor deficits that include dimin-ished muscle tone, impaired balance (Butterworth & Cicchetti, 1978), early developmental decline in locomo-tor function (Piper et al., 1986), and lower scores on measures of gross motor function as compared to the men-tally retarded peers without DS (Henderson, et al., 1981) have been noted frequently. Despite these general motor deficits, from early in life, children with DS appear to exhibit a selective profile of relative weakness in the development of speech and relative strength in motor functions (Bilovsky & Share, 1965; McCarthy, 1965; Share, 1975; Rohr & Buhr, 1978; Greenwald & Leonard, 1979;

Silverstein et al., 1982; Piper, et al.,1986). While the
latter may sound contradictory, it merely serves to emphasize the need to examine the complex pattern of behaviors and skills of this heterogeneous population. One
frequent observation of persons with DS is their strength
in the use of manual gestures. This may explain their
greater reliance on gestures alone, rather than gestures
and words (Share, 1975; Greenwald & Leonard, 1979). The
more capable is the child with DS, the more he will use
good quality gestures in an apparent effort to circumvent
speech difficulties (Share, 1975). This observation has
repeatedly withstood scrutiny of objective testing. Several investigators have shown that persons with DS perform better on the manual expression subtest of the Illinois Test of Psycholinguistic Abilities (ITPA) than they
do on any of the other nine subtests (McCarthy, 1965;
Bilovsky & Share, 1965; Rohr & Buhr, 1978). These observations suggest that the children with DS may be better
able to demonstrate their comprehension of a verbal instruction via manual expression. This may be the beginning of a nonverbal compensation for a more extensive
language deficit than observed for the mentally retarded
children of other etiologies.

Perhaps due to the greater complexity of the required
skills, the relative performance in academic subjects has
been less frequently examined in persons with DS. Nonetheless, relative deficiency in arithmetic has been observed for persons with DS, who were either mentally retarded (Kostrewski, 1965; Rynders, 1986), of borderline
intelligence (Miezejeski, Wisniewski, & Hill, 1987), or
only learning disabled (Rosecrans, 1971; Miezejeski et.
al., 1987). Observations of children with DS who have
been integrated into regular classrooms suggest that in
some areas of academic achievement, especially reading,
they perform as well as some of their nondisabled peers.
In other areas, especially arithmetic, children with Down
Syndrome consistently perform poorly (Pieterse and Center
1984; Rynders, 1986).

Perhaps the most informative investigations of cognitive and functional profiles of persons with DS have
studied people with moderate and mild MR, as well as
borderline to average intelligence. While it may be argued that such samples are not representative of the en-

tire population of persons with DS, it is also possible
that more severe cognitive impairments are due to the ex-
acerbating effects of undiagnosed sensory impairments or
environmental deprivation (Golden & Pashayan, 1976). Recent reports have indicated that improved health care
(Pueschel, 1982; 1985; 1987) and early educational intervention can boost the level of cognitive functioning of
many children with DS (Smith and Hagen, 1984; Hanson,
1981, 1987). Consequently, the proportion of the population with DS functioning in the lower ranges of MR appears to be diminishing (Cunningham, 1982).

In this chapter we compare the status of persons with
DS below and above 30 years of age. We have also analyzed
the role of nongenetic, environmental factors discussed
above in determination of the degree of MR in DS. Another
goal of our research presented in this chapter is to examine the aging phenomenon in persons with DS. Over the
past several decades the population of older mentally retarded individuals has increased greatly. Future projec-
tions strongly suggest a continuation of this trend
(Lubin and Kiely, 1985). Older mentally retarded individuals with DS are at particularly high risk for developing
dementia of the Alzheimer's type (Wisniewski et al.,
1978; 1983; 1985; Wisniewski and Hill, 1985). However,
detailed descriptions of how dementia is manifested in
this population are scarce, and risk factors defining
specific individuals who will deteriorate are unknown.
Studies specifically designed to look for early indications of dementia among older mentally retarded individuals, i.e., over 30 years, are scarce and confined, almost completely, to subjects drawn from low functioning
and institutionalized populations (Dalton et al., 1974;
Thase et al., 1984; Wisniewski et al., 1978; 1982; 1983;
1985; Hewitt et al., 1985). We could find no prospective
studies which examined cognitive functioning of older
mentally retarded individuals who both resided in the
community and functioned at or above the level of moderate MR. We have initiated such a study.

Method

Patient Groups - Data has been collected from interdis-

ciplinary evaluations of 194 persons with DS (186 triso-
mics, 4 mosaics, and 4 translocations) seen at the IBR
George Jervis Diagnostic Clinic between 1978 and 1987.
Many of our subjects were obtained through interactions
with parents, service providers, and advocates for the
developmentally disabled. Additional referrals were received from local pediatricians and psychologists. This
may have resulted in a bias toward inclusion of high
functioning individuals. Consequently, these data were
viewed as descriptive of our sample and not necessarily
of the DS population. Those DS persons less than 30 years
old were designated Group I, and those more than 30 years
old were Group II.

As indicated above we have also initiated a prospective study of aging, for which we have selected a third
sample of persons with DS (Group III). For inclusion in
Group III, the DS individual had to be above 27 years
old, function at a level greater than severe mental retardation and reside in the community. Also, 29 non-DS

Table 1
Population statistics by group

No.	Age Range in years	Mean (sd) in years
	Group I (N = 133)	
67	2-10	6.4 (1.9)
32	11-20	17.2 (1.9)
34	21-30	25.9 (3.2)
	Group II (N = 61)	
28	31-40	34.6 (3.0)
22	41-50	43.8 (2.5)
8	51-60	52.2 (1.8)
3	61-67	64.7 (2.5)
	Group III (N = 45)	
33	27-40	34.7 (3.2)
8	41-50	43.9 (1.8)
4	51-60	55.7 (4.0)

age-matched controls were available for study. They were required also to have had no prior history of trauma, CNS infections, congestive heart failure, or seizures and no evidence of focal neurological findings or severe sensory or motor impairment. A summary of the three groups is presented in Table 1.

Evaluation Procedures

Medical histories were taken for all individuals in Groups I, II, and III. The members of all three groups received psychological evaluations in which their levels of cognitive function were measured via the Bayley Scales of Infant Development, the Stanford-Binet Intelligence Scale (Form L-M), the Leiter International Performance Scale, or the Wechsler Intelligence Scales (WISC-R and WAIS-R). Group III received additional testing to assess for early signs of accelerated aging. This additional testing consisted of a three choice visually presented Matching to Sample Task employing a simultaneous as well as 0, 5, and 10 second delays similar to that used by Ellis and Meador (1985). In addition, the Buschke Test of Sequential Reminding was used to provide an assessment of verbal memory processes. The Buschke (1973) Test of Sequential Reminding is easy to present and understand and takes about 15 minutes to administer. In this test, the subject is asked to learn a list of words (animals, clothing, etc.) and to recall the list verbally in any order. After each trial, the subjects is selectively reminded of only those items not recalled on the previous trial. Subjects are given ten trials. This procedure permits retrieval from long term memory to be demonstrated simultaneously with retrieval from short term memory. It has been used to study memory and learning in children (Buschke, 1974; 1974; Morgan, 1982) and during aging (Rabinowitz, 1984; Macht & Buschke, 1984), impairment in learning and memory in neurological diseases including primary dementia (Weingartner et al., 1979; Branconnier et al., 1982; Laursen and Netterstrom, 1982; Cherry et al., 1984), and as a measure of the effect of drugs on neurological conditions (Brinkman et al., 1982; Kaye et al., 1982; Ross et al., 1984; Smith et al., 1984)

Five basic scores are obtained.

1. Total Recall is the number of items recalled correctly (possible range: 0-72).

2. Long-Term Storage (LTS) is defined as the number of items which have been retrieved without reminding at least once (possible range 0-72).

3. Long-Term Retrieval (LTR) is defined as the number of items recalled from those items in LTS (possible range: 0-72).

4. Short-Term Recall is defined as the number of items recalled after being presented and prior to storage in Long-Term Storage (possible range: 0-36).

5. Consistent List Learning is defined as the number of items recalled consistently from LTS without further reminders (possible range: 0-72).

Thirty-one subjects with DS (mean age = 38.2; s.d. = 7.2 years) and 29 controls (mean age = 37.8; s.d. = 8.1 years) have been tested so far. With the exception of one subject with DS who was employed as a dishwasher at a hospital, all of the subjects were employed at workshops run by voluntary agencies. The controls were obtained from the same workshops as were the subjects with DS. The mean IQ for the subjects with DS was 49.2 (s.d. = 11.4) and for the controls was 54.9 (s.d. = 8.8).

Results

For all of our clients with DS, our clinical observations suggested a range of cognitive disabilities, speech problems, impairment of fine, gross motor function and relative strength in the use of manual expression. In Groups I and II, we identified eleven children and four adults who were not mentally retarded, as well as two adults whose verbal IQs were within the normal range. The distribution of cognitive function observed within Group I is summarized in Table 2.

Degree of functioning at or above mild MR was most common for persons in their first decade of life. All of the youngest children and some who were in their second decade of life had begun attending infant stimulation pro-

Table 2
Levels of Cognitive Function in Group I

Level of Cognitive Function	Age Range		
	2-10	11-20	21-30
	N	N	N
Nonretarded	10	2	3
Mild MR	47	10	4
Moderate MR	7	17	11
Severe MR	3	3	10
Profound MR	0	0	6
Total No. of Cases	67	32	34

grams as early as one to two weeks of age and had been raised at home by parents who were actively involved in their child's education. Fifteen of the 133 persons in Group I were found to be of borderline to low normal intelligence. All but one of these 15 individuals had received early intervention and academic mainstreaming. The severe MR observed in three of the youngest group of cases may be attributable to other factors (one had meningitis in infancy, a second had cerebral emboli due to complications during cardiac catherization, and a third had head trauma). Whereas 85% of the children in their first decade functioned at a cognitive level ranging from mild MR to low average intelligence, only 37.5% of those in their second decade were found to function within this higher range of ability. Again, the severe MR observed for three of these 32 children could be attributable to nongenetic risk factors causing brain damage (one had uncontrolled seizures secondary to perinatal birth trauma, a second had cerebral emboli as a complication of catherization, and a third had perinatal anoxic encephalopathy). Among the 34 in their third decade of life, 16 (47%) exhibited severe to profound MR and again nongenetic factors were contributory. Among these 16 with severe to profound MR, six had academic deprivation and or undiagnosed severe deafness. Also two out of 16 DS cases

had a past history of status-post brain trauma, two had
CNS infections, and six had perinatal complications. Only
20% of these 34 people also in the 3rd decade of life exhibited cognitive function within the range of mild MR to
low average intelligence. None of these 34 individuals
had attended an early infant stimulation program. A review of past clinical records revealed that a history of
transient hearing impairment associated with recurrent
otitis media was noted in 50 % in Group I.

Group II - The distribution of measured levels of cognitive function for persons in Group II are summarized in
Table 3.

Table 3
Levels of Cognitive Function in Group II

Level of Cognitive Function	Age Range			
	31-40	41-50	51-60	61-70
	N	N	N	N
Nonretarded	2	-	-	-
Mild MR	3	6	-	-
Moderate MR	7	2	1	-
Severe MR	5	5	4	-
Profound MR	11	9	3	3
Total	28	22	8	3

Most of those people in Group II (50/61 cases), were in
their fourth or fifth decade of life. Whereas 5 of those
in their fourth decade (17.8%) and 6 in their fifth decade (27.3%) functioned within the range of mild MR to low
average intelligence, none of the cases from the sixth or
seventh decade functioned above the range of moderate MR.
Forty of the 61 persons in Group II functioned within the
range from severe to profound MR. Of these 40 patients,
30 had been institutionalized for most of their early
lives. Deafness (secondary to recurrent ear infection),
status-post perinatal encephalopathy, CNS infections, and
academic deprivation were noted frequently in the histor-

ies, as well as recurrent otitis media with possible transient deafness especially in those functioning within the ranges of severe and profound MR. Five individuals had histories of seizures and autistic features. In 13 of the 26 persons in Group II who had profound mental retardation, hearing impairment was identified, while among those 19 persons in Group II with mild or moderate mental retardation only four were hearing impaired. In two of these 61 cases, there were focal neurological findings that were secondary to structural CNS lesions associated with perinatal birth trauma. Dementia of the Alzheimer's type was suspected in 5 of the 61 cases all of whom were more than 50 years of age.

Nonretarded Adults with DS: Arithmetic Deficits

Among the adults with DS who had received clinical evaluations in our clinic, there were six (four in Group I and two in Group II) whose WAIS-R full scale or verbal IQ scores were over 70. These scores are presented in Table

Table 4
WAIS-R IQs of Nonretarded Adults in Group I and II

Cases No.	Full Scale IQ	Verbal IQ	Performance IQ
1	73	75	73
2	72	69	77
3	86	88	86
4	62	74	53
5	68	73	65
6	87	86	90

4. Karotyping indicated that four were trisomic (cases no. 2, 3, 4, 5,) and two were mosaic (cases no. 1, 6). Two of these six, one trisomic (case no. 3) and one mosaic (case no. 6) had IQs that placed them in the low average range of intelligence. The latter individual, who was mosaic, not only exhibited average intelligence, but also had none of the specific deficits usually associated

with learning disabilities. Case no. 3, who had trisomy, however, had obtained a profile of subtest scores on both the WAIS-R and Wide Range Achievement Test-Revised (WRAT-R) that indicated a learning disability, characterized by a specific deficit in arithmetic. Her WAIS-R arithmetic scaled score of 5 was her lowest verbal scaled score and her WRAT-R standard score on Arithmetic (79) was lower than that for either reading (120) or spelling (114). In terms of conventional terminology that restricts the designation of "learning disabled" to persons with IQs above 85, cases 4 and 5, who both had trisomy, may not be considered learning disabled per se. However, for both of these individuals, a WAIS-R scaled score of 3 on Arithmetic was their lowest verbal scaled score and WRAT-R standard scores of 46 (case no.4) and 65 (case no. 5) on Arithematic were lower than they had obtained on either Reading or Spelling.

Group III - Preliminary Neurological Findings - We have studied 45 persons with DS and 29 non DS. Forty-four patients with DS were confirmed to have trisomy 21 (one individual refused to have blood drawn for karyotype studies), and none of these cases had evidence of mosaicism or translocation. As noted earlier in our sample, no indications of focal neurological signs (e.g., pyramidal, extrapyramidal and cerebellar signs) were found prior to the study. There were 27 mild and 18 moderate MR DS and 14 mild and 15 moderate non DS persons.

As indicated in Table 5, the occurrence of frontal release signs were in our research sample increased with age in DS but not in non DS persons, e.g., among those individuals with DS who were in their fifth or sixth decade of life (palmo-mental reflexes were seen in 8 of 33 people in the 4th decade, 5 of 8 people in the 5th decade and 3 of 4 people in the 6th decade of life). The presence of soft neurological findings and impairment of fine and gross motor function was a common feature of this syndrome. None of the patients previously examined had new neurological findings except one DS person, 60 years of age, who had developed dementia of the Alzheimer type and was excluded from this study.

Matching to Sample - The preliminary results of the matching-to-sample and delayed matching-to-sample test

Table 5
Number of DS and non DS clients with frontal release signs

| Item | Age Ranges | | | | | |
| | 27-40 | | 41-50 | | 51-60 | |
	DS	Non DS	DS	Non DS	DS	Non DS
Snout reflex	6	0	4	0	2	0
Sucking reflex	0	0	1	0	1	0
Palmo-mental reflex	8	0	5	1	3	0
Myerson's Signs	3	0	2	0	2	0
Total Number Examined	33	21	8	5	4	5

(presented in Table 6) confirmed that as a group the clients were capable of performing the task. However, by one month subsequent to testing the one individual who had to undergo secondary training and who could not perform the zero delay matching-to-sample task above the chance level was no longer able to perform adequately at the workshop and was transferred to a day treatment center. Multidisciplinary evaluation showed that she had developed Alzheimer type of dementia. This is the same 60 year old DS patient that was mentioned above during description of our preliminary neurological findings.

Table 6 presents the preliminary results from one matching to sample test obtained for 30 people with DS and 29 control clients. These data were analyzed using a

Table 6
Percent Correct Responses on Matching-to-Sample Tasks

	Simultaneous	Zero Delay	5 Sec Delay	10 Sec Delay
DS (N = 31)	91.2(17.1)	75.2(19.2)	61.2(16.7)	57.1(20.9)
Control (N = 29)	95.7(9.3)	75.0(23.9)	65.2(23.4)	60.3(22.5)

Group (DS, non DS) by Task (simultaneous, 0, 5, 10 second delay) analysis of variance. Group was a between subjects factor and Task was a within subjects factor. While there was no group main effect or interaction, Fs < 1.0 the Task effect was highly significant, F(3,178) = 72.8, p < .001. Follow up analyses indicated that all Tasks differed from each other with only one exception; performance was equivalent at the 5 and 10 second delays.

In agreement with the results of Ellis and Meador (1985), the greatest decline in correct responses occurred between the simultaneous match-to-sample and the zero delay match-to-sample condition for both groups, and no significant forgetting was found beyond the 5 second delay condition. These results suggest that differences or the lack of differences between conditions cannot be attributed to the discriminability of the stimuli. The stimuli employed here are highly discriminable while those employed by Ellis and Meador were discriminable on a single dimension.

To date, 25 individuals with DS and 16 control subjects have been tested in the follow-up study. Overall, these individuals did as well on the second test as they did on the first. However, the results are not always consistent. For instance, one individual did better on the zero delay condition and on the ten second delay but not as well on the 5 second delay as she had during the original evaluation. This type of variability is to be expected with the limited number of trials (16) within each condition and the loss at 5 seconds does not appear indicative

Table 7
Preliminary Results of the Test of Sequential Reminding

| | For 30 DS and 29 control clients | | | |
| | DS | | Control | |
Totals	Mean	SD	Mean	SD
Recall	44.8	(13.9)	43.9	(17.1)
Short Term Memory	45.5	(16.1)	43.1	(20.3)
Long Term Storage	38.1	(17.2)	36.9	(21.4)
Consistent Recall	24.7	(19.9)	26.3	(23.5)
Short Term Memory	6.9	(4.4)	6.8	(5.1)

of a dementing process.

Buschke Test of Sequential Reminding - The preliminary results are presented in Table 7. The variables were very highly correlated. However, since none of the clients tested to date show any indications of dementia, we believe it is premature to collapse the measures into a single measure of verbal memory until longitudinal testing has been completed. Therefore, for the purposes of the present study, we are continuing to score and analyze all the variables.

Most of the individuals did as well or better on the second test as they did on the first. The exceptions are not considered clinically significant. For instance, one individual (a 40 year old man) had somewhat lower scores on the retest. However, he is doing well at the group home, and is maintaining his level of production at the workshop. He will be reevaluated next year (sooner if any other indications of a loss of function occur). If, at that time, the third test demonstrates continued decreases in functioning, it may be that this slight performance decrement is an early indication of a dementing process. This selective group of DS patients is to be tested on a yearly basis. Future results will determine the neurological and psychological consequences of accelerated aging processes in persons with DS.

Discussion

Among our clinic sample of 194 persons with DS (Groups I and II), we have observed a range of cognitive disabilities. All except one (mosaic DS, age 22 with IQ 87) had cognitive and functional deficits, speech problems, borderline intelligence, or learning disabilities. As previously stated, the degree of some of these cognitive deficits seen in our sample may have been partially ameliorated by early intervention during critical stages of development when brain plasticity is high (Wisniewski, et al., 1984, 1986, 1987; Hanson, 1981, 1987). All persons with DS that were examined in our clinic exhibited relative strength in the use of manual expression, which may have been compensatory for their decreased verbal expressive capacity. The distribution of levels of cognitive function in Group I (age < 30 years) differed from that in Group II (age > 30 years). Fifteen of the 133 persons (11%) in Group I (Table 2), but only two of the 61 persons (3.2%) in Group II (Table 3) were not mentally retarded. Across all the age ranges of Groups I and II, the largest proportion of nonretarded persons were the ten (14.9%) nonretarded children of the 67 children in their first decade of life. All these children had received early intervention that had been initiated before they were six months old. An additional seven nonretarded persons were found to be distributed evenly across ages 11 to 33 years. Among those in our sample of persons with DS who were older than 33 years, all were mentally retarded. In Group I, as compared to Group II, there was a much higher proportion of persons with mild MR, especially among those in their first decade of life, 47 of 67 (70.2%) of whom exhibited only mild MR. These observations, along with recent results of research investigating the effects of early initiation of infant stimulation and educational mainstreaming suggest that the majority of persons with DS are functioning higher and that their abilities have been underestimated previously (Rynders et al., 1978, Libb et al., 1983; Pieterse and Center, 1984, Rynders, 1986; Pueschel 1987). Also, in our sample persons with DS who were lower functioning were often institutionalized, academically deprived, or brain damaged due to nongenetic factors as suggested previously by others, e.g. Clements, et al. (1976, 1978), Cunningham (1982), and Silverstein, et al. (1982).

All but one of the persons with DS in Groups I, II, and III had some degree of speech defect and speech delay. Particular among those in their first decade of life, it appeared to be not merely secondary to mental retardation, but a relatively more specific deficit. Across all levels of cognitive function, we observed language deficits disproportionate to those observed for nonverbal abilities. As discussed above, one of the more frequently suggested potential causes of language deficiency in persons with DS is the existence of transient or permanent hearing impairment due to recurrent otitis media during the critical stage of speech maturation. Based on their past medical histories, 50% of our sample had had recurrent otitis media and transient hearing impairment. DS persons with severe and profound MR showed sensorineural or conductive hearing impairment in 6 out of 16 cases below age 30 years. (Group I), 13 of 36 cases, (Group II) above age 30. Brooks et al. (1972) reported that among 38 persons with DS who were under 20 years of age only 21% had sensorineural hearing loss, whereas among 40 persons with DS who were above age 21, 55% had this type of sensory impairment. They conjectured that the high incidence of sensorineural hearing loss in adults in their DS sample was the consequence of long standing middle ear disease. Early diagnosis of hearing impairment and treatment could prevent these abnormalities. We propose also that, although hearing loss may contribute to the language deficiency exhibited by people with DS, there exists a more specific deficit of auditory processing associated with possible CNS abnormalities that are genetically controlled. Zinkus, Gottlieb, and Schapiro (1978) have reported interesting data regarding the impact of otitis media on profiles of ability and academic achievement. They compared two groups of children both experiencing educational difficulties, but differing in early childhood histories of otitis media. They studied children of average intelligence, however, and consequently their results may have only limited application when viewed relative to persons with DS, who are typically mentally retarded. Nonetheless, relative to the abilities profile that has been observed for the nonretarded adults with DS (Miezejeski, et al., 1987), the findings of Zinkus et al. may contribute to our understanding of this syndrome. They reported that children who had had a history of severe otitis media obtained lower IQs on the Wechsler Intelligence Scale for Children-Revised (WISC-R) than did those children with a history of mild otitis media. Zinkus et al. pointed out that these lower IQs, however, could be attributed entirely to a profile of relatively lower scores on subtests that rely heavily on receptive language, i.e., Arithmetic, Digit Span, Similarities, Picture Arrangement, and Coding. Further, on the Wide Range Achievement Test (WRAT), these same children had obtained relatively lower scores on the subtests of Reading and Spelling, but not Arithmetic. They interpreted these results as indicating that one consequence of severe otitis media during early childhood, a critical period for language development, was a diminished ability in academic and intellectual areas that rely heavily on language ability and auditory processing skills.

In our evaluations of the nonretarded adults with DS (Miezejeski, et al., 1987), we observed an abilities profile that was quite different. With the WRAT-R, we observed higher scores on Reading and Spelling but not Arithmetic. Further, while Zinkus et al. found that subjects with a history of severe otitis media had obtained relatively lower scores on a constellation of three verbal and two performance subtests on the WISC-R, we found that nonretarded adults with DS had obtained a relatively lower score consistently on only one WAIS-R subtest, Arithmetic. Consequently, although there is no doubt that impaired language ability may contribute to the specific deficits observed in persons with DS, we suspect that the language deficits of persons with DS differ from those experienced by persons with early histories of severe otitis media. Be that as it may, other findings suggest that the more specific academic deficit in arithmetic may be less responsive to intervention. The children with DS who have been integrated into regular classrooms may perform in some academic areas, especially reading, as well as some of their nondisabled peers, but in other areas; especially arithmetic, they consistently perform below the range of the nondisabled (Pieterse & Center, 1984). Further participation in a program of early intervention has resulted in improved reading, but not arithmetic, (Rynders, 1986).

Thus, although we accept that hearing loss frequently contributes to the relative language and cognitive deficits observed in persons with DS, we suspect that the abilities profile observed for these individuals is also a function of more specific cognitive deficits associated with CNS abnormalities that are genetically controlled. We have observed characteristic abnormalities in the brains of persons with DS. We have studied during the time of maturation 112 DS brains and those of 80 controls (Wisneiwski et al., 1984, 1986, 1987). We have found that persons with DS have shown prenatal retardation of neurogenesis and pre and postnatal synaptogenesis. The number of neurons in the cortical mantle, especially within the granular layers, is diminished by 20 to 50 percent at the

time of birth (Wisneiwski et al., 1987). In the brains of
33 of 100 persons with DS between newborn to 12 years of
age, the superior temporal gyrus was prominently narrowed. Also, when head circumference and brain weight were
measured after 6 mos. of age, the retardation of brain
growth, especially of the frontal and temporal lobes, was
noted in all cases. Our previous morphometric studies of
the temporal, occipital, and frontal lobes (areas 28, 17,
10) showed significantly decreased neuronal density. In
addition, studies on myelination in persons with DS have
indicated a delay in myelination, especially the association fibers (Wisniewski et al., 1986,). We have suggested that the neurological, psychological and brain abnormalities found in persons with DS are genetically controlled and might be dependent on a gene dose effect
(Jenkins et al., 1983; Wisniewski et al., 1986, 1987).

The most current psychological research on the deficits
exhibited by persons with DS has focussed on the significance of relative cognitive deficits. Most of the results
of these studies of cognitive function appear to lead in
the same general direction. That is, persons with DS exhibit relative deficits in language and possess, perhaps,
relatively more specific deficits in receptive language
processes (Varnhagen, Das, and Varnhagen, 1987) that may
be a function of deficient auditory processing (Marcell &
Armstrong, 1982). As a result of their receptive language
deficits they exhibit secondary deficits in expressive
language and academic skills, such as arithmetic, that
rely heavily on auditory processing and the comprehension
of syntax. We suggest that the neurological and psychological status of persons with DS may be better understood through research that focuses on the higher functioning persons with DS for whom, as we have shown, it is
possible to decipher an abilities profile. Perhaps an increased knowledge of this abilities profile might also
contribute to the more effective study of other concerns
crucial to the entire population of persons with DS, such
as the early onset of dementia.

From our clinical sample of 45 persons with DS (Group
III), we have reported some findings from our study of
aging adults with mild and moderate MR.The development of
methods to detect the early stages of dementia in persons with DS has been hindered previously by the choice

of samples of persons with DS who exhibited much lower degrees of functioning (Dalton et al., 1974; Thase et al., 1984; Wisniewski et al., 1978, 1982, 1983, 1985). Working with such lower functioning samples, researchers are more likely to encounter floor effects in their attempts to measure diminished function. As noted above, our data have not yet revealed any differences between our groups of aging persons with and without DS. On the matching-to-sample task a lack of performance by one person with DS was followed subsequently by an apparent decline in his level of adaptive functioning. Poor performance on the Buschke Test of Sequential Reminding by another person with DS appeared to be unrelated to current level of adaptive function. Should the latter person subsequently dement, however, then it may be that this diminished performance on the Buschke could be predictive of dementia. This individual is continuing to be followed by us.

In conclusion, our observations have indicated that the perception of DS as solely a form of MR, which by definition has been viewed as a disorder in which all functions of adaptation and cognition are equally deficient, may be too limited. That is, there are individuals with DS who function within the borderline to normal range of intelligence, some of whom also exhibit a learning disability in the form of dyscalculia. This learning disability appears to consist of a specific performance deficit in arithmetic that may be secondary to deficient receptive language. Although conventional psychometric assessment procedures are insufficient to demonstrate clearly a relative deficiency in arithmetic among those persons with DS who are also mentally retarded, it appears that such a relative deficiency may exist in this population. At present, much research supports the presence of a relative deficiency of expressive language in mentally retarded persons with DS. Other research reported in this volume suggests that with the aid of computer assisted instruction using speech synthesizers mentally retarded persons with DS who are capable of writing may demonstrate greater expressive language skill than was previously thought possible (Meyers, this volume). Thus, given the means to express themselves, the language deficit exhibited by persons with DS may be seen to be less expressive than receptive in nature. As has been noted, the cause of this language deficit may be multi-factorial, and can be attributed to hearing deficits, impaired social interaction, especially with parents during development, and specific cognitive deficits associated with a characteristic pattern of CNS neuropathology that may be genetically controlled. Consequently, we need to devote attention to the early diagnosis of hearing deficits to enable the initiation of medical, speech, and hearing interventions as early during development as pos- sible. More research on the role of social interactions is needed so that health professionals can be trained to provide instruction in the most optimal approaches to parenting. Additional research, especially with higher functioning persons with DS, should be devoted to determining more clearly their abilities profile and the associated neuropathology and genetic determinants. With a better understanding of the cognitive strengths and weaknesses of higher functioning persons with DS, as well as how aging may affect the skills of such higher functioning individuals, future research will provide us with more effective prevention and intervention for all persons with DS.

Acknowledgments

The authors gratefully acknowledge the editorial comments of Dr. Wayne Silverman, the bibliographical editing by Mr. Lawrence Black, and the secretarial assistance of Ms. Madeline Tinney.

This study is supported partially by NIH Grants 1P01HD22634.

REFERENCES

Balkany, T. J., Downs, M. P., Jafek, B. W., & Krajicek, M. J. (1979). Hearing loss in Down's syndrome. A treatable handicap more common than generally recognized. Clin. Pediatr., 18, 116-118.

Bennett, F. C., Sells, C. J. & Brand, C. (1979). Influence on measured intelligence in Down's syndrome.

Am. J. Dis. Child., 133, 700-703.

Bilovsky, D., & Share, J. (1965). The ITPA and Down's syndrome: An exploratory study. Am. J. Ment. Defic., 70, 78-82.

Branconnier, R. J., Cole, J. O., Spera, K. F., & DeVitt, D. R., (1982). Recall and recognition as diagnostic indices of malignant memory loss in senile dementia: A Bayesian analysis. Exp. Aging Res., 8, 189-193.

Brinkman, S. D., Pomara, N., Goodnick, P. J., Barnett, N., & Domine, E. F. (1982). A dose-ranging study of lecithin in the treatment of primary degenerative dementia (Alzheimer disease). J. Clin. Psychopharmcol., 2, 281-285.

Brooks, D. N., Wooley, H., & Kanjilal, G. C. (1972). Hearing loss and middle ear disorders in patients with Down's syndrome (mongolism). J. Ment. Defic. Res., 16, 21-29.

Buschke, H. (1973). Selective reminding for analysis of memory and learning. J. Verbal Learn. Verbal Behav., 12, 543-550.

Buschke, H. (1974). Components of verbal learning in children: Analysis by selective reminding. J. Exp. Child Psychol., 18, 488-496.

Buschke, H. (1974). Two stages of learning by children and adults. Bull. Psychon. Soc., 4, 392-394.

Butterworth, G., & Cicchetti, D. (1978). Visual calibration of posture in normal and motor retarded Down's syndrome infants. Perception, 7, 513-525.

Centerwall, S. A., & Centerwal, W. R. (1960). A study of children with mongolism reared in the home compared to those reared away from home. Pediatrics, 25, 678-685.

Cherry, N., Venables, H., & Waldron, H. A. (1984). Description of the tests in the London School of Hygiene test battery. Scand. J. Work Environ. Health, 10, 18-19 (Supple. 1).

Clements, P. R., Bates, M. V., & Hafer, M. (1976). Variability within Down's syndrome (Trisomy-21): Empirically observed sex differences in IQs. Ment. Retard., 14, 30-31.

Clements, P. R., Hafer, M., & Pollock, J. L. (1978). Parental education and rate of intellectual development of Down's syndrome (Trisomy-21) individuals. Res. Retarded, 5, 15-19.

Connolly, J. A. (1978). Intelligence levels in Down's syndrome children. Am. J. Ment. Defic., 83, 193-196.

Cunningham, C. (1982). Down's syndrome: A guide for parents, Souvenir Press, London. p. 176.

Dahle, A. J., & McCollister, F. P. (1986). Hearing and otologic disorders in children with Down syndrome. Am. J. Ment. Defic., 90, 636-642.

Dalton, A. J., Crapper, D. R., & Schlotterer, G. R. (1974). Alzheimer's disease in Down's syndrome: Visual retention deficits. Cortex, 10, 366-367.

Demaine, G. C., & Silverstein, A. B. (1978). MA changes in institutionalized Down's syndrome persons: A semi-longitudinal approach. Am. J. Ment. Defic., 82, 429-432.

Ellis, N. R., & Meador, D. M. (1985). Forgetting in retarded and nonretarded persons under conditions of minimal strategy use. Intelligence, 9, 87-96.

Fraser, F. C., & Sadovnick, A. D. (1976). Correlation of IQ subjects with Down's syndrome and their parents and sibs. J. Ment. Defic. Res., 20, 179-182.

Golden, W., & Pashayan, H. M. (1976). The effect of parental education on the eventual mental development of noninstitutionalized children with Down syndrome. J. Pediatr., 89, 603-605.

Greenwald, C. A., & Leonard, L. B. (1979). Communicative and sensorimotor development of Down's syndrome children. Am. J. Ment. Defic., 84, 296-303.

Hanson, M. J. (1981). Down's syndrome children - characteristics and intervention. In M. Lewis and L.A. Rosenblum (eds.), The uncommon child. pp. 83-114, New York: Plenum Press.

Hanson, M. J., edited by Pueschel, S. M., Tingey, C., Rynders, J. E., Crocker, A. C., & Crutcher, D. M., (1987). New perspectives on Down syndrome, Chapter 6, Baltimore/London: Brookes Publishing Co., pp. 149-170.

Hartley, X. Y. (1985). Receptive language processing and ear advantage of Down's syndrome children. J. Ment. Defic. Res., 29, 197-205.

Hartley, X. Y. (1986). A summary of recent research into the development of children with Down's syndrome. J. Ment. Defic. Res., 30, 1-14.

Henderson, S. E., Morris, J., & Frith, U., (1981). The motor deficit in Down's syndrome children: A problem of timing? J. Child Psychol. Psychiatry, 22, 233-245.

Hewitt, K. E., Carter, G., & Jancar, J. (1985). Aging in Down's syndrome. Br. J. Psychiat., 147, 58-62.

Jenkins, E. C., Duncan, C. J., Wright, C. E., Giordano, F. M., Wilbur, L., Wisniewski, K., Sklower, S. L., French, J. H., Jones, C., & Brown, W. T. (1983). Atypical Down syndrome and partial trisomy 21. Clin. Genet., 24, 97-102.

Johnson, R. C., & Abelson, R. B. (1969). The behavioral competence of mongoloid and non-mongoloid retardates. Am. J. Ment. Defic., 73, 856-857.

Kaye, W. H., Sitaram, N., Weingartner, H., Ebert, M. H., Smallberg, S., Gillin, J. C. (1982). Modest facilitation on memory in dementia with combined lecithin and anti-cholinerestase treatment. Biol. Psychiatry, 17, 275-280.

Keiser, H., Montague, J., Wold, D. Maune, S., & Pattison, D. (1981). Hearing loss of Down syndrome adults. Am. J. Ment. Defic., 85, 467-472.

Kostrzewski, J. (1965). The dynamics of intellectual and social development in Down's syndrome: Results of experimental investigation. Rocznicki: Filozoficzne, 13, 5-32.

Laursen, P., & Netterstrm, B. (1982). Psychological function of urban bus drivers exposed to exhaust gases. A cross-sectional study of urban bus drivers in Denmark. Scand. J. Psychol., 23, 282-290.

Libb, J. W., Myers, G. J., Graham, E., & Bell, B. (1983). Correlates of intelligence and adaptive behavior in Down's syndrome. J. Ment. Defic. Res., 27, 205-210.

Libb, J. W., Dahle, A., Smith, K., McCollister, F. P., & McLain, C. (1985). Hearing disorder and cognitive function of individuals with Down syndrome. Am. J. Ment. Defic., 90, 353-356.

Lubin, R., & Kiely, M. (1985). Epidemiology of aging in developmental disabilities. M. Janicki & H. M. Wisniewski (eds.), Aging and Developmental Disabilities: Issues and Approaches, pp. 95-113, Baltimore: Brooks Publishing Co..

Macht, M. L., & Buschke, H. (1984). Speed of recall in aging. J. Gerontol., 39, 439-443.

Marcell, M. M., & Armstrong, V. (1982). Auditory and visual sequential memory of Down syndrome and nonretarded children. Am. J. Ment. Defic., 87, 86-95.

Meyers, L. F., & Beckwith, L. (1987). Using Computers to teach children with Down Syndrome spoken and written language skills. Motivation and Language Learning. Neurobiology of Down Syndrome Session 4, language functions, 12/4/87.

McCarthy, Y. M. (1965). Patterns of psychiatry in the development of mongoloid severely retarded children. Dissertation, University of Illinois.

McQuiston, S. (1982). Mother-infant interaction in infants with Down syndrome: Dissertation Abstracts International, 42, 4534A-4535A (University Microfilms No. 82-38).

Melyn, M. A., & White, D. T. (1973). Mental and developmental milestones of noninstitutionalized Down's syndrome children. Pediatrics, 52, 542-545.

Miezejeski, C., Wisniewski, K. E., & Hill, A. (1987). Non-retarded learning impaired Down's syndrome adults. Neurology, 37, (Supple. 1): 203 (Abstr.).

Miezejeski, C., Wisniewski, K. E., & Hill, A. (1988). Non-retarded and Learning Disabled Adults with Down syndrome. Ann. Neurol., submitted 1988.

Morgan, S. F. (1982). Measuring long-term memory storage and retrieval in children. J. Clin. Neuropsychol., 4, 77-85.

Peiterse, M., & Center, Y. (1984). The integration of eight Down's syndrome children into regular schools. Australian New Zealand J. Develop. Disabil., 10, 11-20.

Piper, M. C., Gosselin, C., Gendron, M., & Mazer, B. (1986). Developmental profile of Down's syndrome infants receiving early intervention. Care, Health Dev., 12, 183-194.

Pueschel, S. M., & Rynders, J. E., (eds. 1982). Down syndrome: Advances in biomedicine and the behavioral sciences. pp. 524, Cambridge, MA: The Ware Press.

Pueschel, S. M. (1985). Changes of counseling practices at the birth of a child with Down syndrome. Appl. Res., Ment. Retard. 6, 99-108.

Pueschel, S. M., Tingey, C., Rynders, J. E., Crocker, A. C., & Crutcher, D. M., (eds. 1987). New perspectives on Down syndrome. pp. 416, Baltimore/London: Brookes Publishing Co.

Rabinowitz, J. C. (1984). Aging and recognition failure.

J. Gerontol. 39, 65-71.

Rohr, A., & Burr, D. B., (1978). Etiological differences in patterns of psycholinguistic development of children of IQ 30 to 60. Am. J. Ment. Defic., 82, 549-553.

Rosecrans, C. J. (1971). A longitudinal study of exceptional cognitive development in a partial translocation Down's syndrome child. Am. J. Ment. Defic., 76, 291-294.

Ross, R. J., Smallberg, S., & Weingartner, H. (1984). The effects of desmethylimipramine on cognitive function in healthy subjects. Psychiatry Res., 12, 89-97.

Rynders, J. E., Spiker, D., & Horrobin, J. M. (1978). Underestimating the educability of Down's syndrome children: Examination of methodological problems in recent literature. Am. J. Ment. Defic., 82, 440-448.

Rynders, J. E. (1986). Always trainable? The need to re-examine educational expectations for school children with Down syndrome. Presented at the National Convention of the American Psychological Association, Washington, D.C.

Share, J. B. (1975). Developmental progress in Down's syndrome. In R. Koch and F. F. DeLa Cruz (eds.), Down's syndrome (mongolism): research, prevention and management, pp. 78-86, New York: Brunner/Mazel.

Silverstein, A. B., Legutki, G., Friedman, S. L., & Takayama, D. L. (1982). Performance of Down syndrome individuals on the Stanford-Binet Intelligence Scale. Am. J. Ment., 86, 548-551.

Smith, R. C., Vroulis, G., Johnson, R., Morgan, R. (1984). Comparison of therapeutic response to long-term treatment with lecithin versus piracetam plus lecithin in patients with Alzheimer's disease. Psychopharmacol. Bull., 20, 542-545.

Smith, L. & Hagen, V. (1984). Relationship between the home environment and sensorimotor development of Down syndrome and nonretarded infants. Am. J. Ment. Defic., 89, 124-132.

Spitz, R. A. (1945). Hospitalism: An inquiry into the genesis of psychiatric conditions in early childhood. Psychonal. Study Child, 1, 53-74.

Spitz, R. A. (1946). Hospitalism: A follow-up report. Psychoanal. Study Child, 2, 113-117.

Thase, M. E., Liss, L., Smeltzer, D., & Maloon, J.

(1982). Clinical evaluation of dementia in Down's syndrome: A preliminary report. J. Ment. Defic. Res., 26, 239-244.

Van Gorp, E. & Baker, R. (1984). The incidence of hearing impairment in a sample of Down's syndrome schoolchildren. Int. J. Rehab. Res., 7, 198-200.

Varnhagen, C. K., Das, J. P., & Varnhagen, S. (1987). Auditory and visual memory span: Cognitive processing of TMR individuals with Down syndrome or other etiologies. Am. J. Ment. Defic., 91, 398-405.

Vietze, P. M. (1987). Parental stimulation of high-risk infants in naturalistic settings. Pediatric Round Table 13. In N. Gunzenhauser (ed.), Infant Stimulation: For Whom, What Kind, When, and How Much?, pp. 136-143, Johnson & Johnson Baby Products Co.

Weingartner, H., Caine, E. D., & Ebert, M. H. (1979). Imagery, encoding, and retrieval of information from memory: Some specific encoding-retrieval changes in Huntington's Disease. J. Abnorm. Psychol., 88, 52-58.

Wisniewski, K., Howe, J., Williams, D. G., & Wisniewski, H. M. (1978). Precocious aging and dementia in patients with Down's syndrome. Biol. Psychiatry, 13, 619-627.

Wisniewski, K. E., & Wisniewski, H. M. (1983). Age-associated changes and dementia in Down's syndrome. In B. Reisberg (ed.), Alzheimer's disease, pp. 319-326. New York: The Free Press.

Wisniewski, K. E., Laure-Kamionowska, M., & Wisniewski, H. M. (1984). Evidence of arrest of neurogenesis and synaptogenesis in brains of patients with Down's syndrome. N. Engl. J. Med., 311, 1187-1188.

Wisniewski, K. E., Dalton, A. J., Crapper McLachlan, D. R., Wen, G. Y., & Wisniewski, H. M. (1985). Alzheimer's disease in Down's syndrome: Clincopathological studies. Neurology, 35, 957-961.

Wisniewski, K. E., Wisniewski, H. M., & Wen, G. Y. (1985). Occurrence of neuropathological changes and dementia of Alzheimer's disease in Down's syndrome. Ann. Neurol., 17, 278-282.

Wisniewski, K., & Hill, A. L. (1985). Clinical aspects of dementia in mental retardation and developmental disabilities. In M. Janicki and H. M. Wisniewski (eds.), Aging and developmental disabilities - Issues and approaches., pp. 195-210. Baltimore/Brooks Publishing Co.

Wisniewski, K. E., Laure-Kamionowska, M., Connell, F., & Wisniewski, H. M. (1985). Quantitative determination of synaptic density and their morphology during the post-natal brain development in visual cortex of Down syndrome brain. J. Neuropathol. Exp. Neurol., 44, 342.

Wisniewski, K. E., Laure-Kamionowska, M. Connell, F., & Wen G. Y. (1986). Neuronal density and synaptogenesis in the postnatal stage of brain maturation in Down syndrome. In C. J. Epstein (ed.), The neurobiology of Down syndrome, pp. 29-44, New York: Raven Press.

Wisniewski, K., & Schmidt-Sidor, B. (1986). Myelination in Down's syndrome brains (pre- and postnatal maturation) and some clinical-pathological correlations. Ann. Neurol., 20, 429-430.

Wisniewski, K. E., Schmidt-Sidor, B., & Sersen, E. A. (1987). Reduction of head circumference and brain weight of DS cases: Birth to 5 years. Neurology, 37 (Suppl. 1), 203.

Zinkus, P. W., Gottlieb, M. I., & Schapiro, M. (1978). Developmental and psycho-educational sequelae of chronic otitis media. Am. J. Dis. Child., 132, 1100-1104.

12

The Relationship Between
Down Syndrome and Alzheimer's Disease

Michael E. Thase, M.D.
Associate Professor of Psychiatry
University of Pittsburgh, School of Medicine
and Western Psychiatric Institute and Clinic
3811 O'Hara Street, Pittsburgh, PA 15213

Introduction

While a possible association between the condition now known as Down Syndrome (DS) and Alzheimer's disease has been described in the literature for over 100 years, interest in the association of these conditions has peaked over the last several years (e.g., Dalton & Crapper-McLachlan, 1986; Karlinsky, 1986; Oliver & Holland, 1986). Such increased interest is likely the result of recognition that Alzheimer's disease is the most common cause of dementia in the general population and because of mounting evidence that the nature of the age-related cognitive decline experienced by persons with Down Syndrome may be similar, if not identical, to dementia of the Alzheimer type (DAT). This paper will begin with a brief review of DAT, and then will proceed to summarize the evidence of its association with Down Syndrome.

Overview of Dementia, Alzheimer's Type

Alzheimer's disease is now known to be the leading cause of dementia in the elderly (Katzman, 1986). It is estimated that at least 10 to 15 per cent of the population will develop this condition if they live past age 65 (Katzman, 1976). As the risk of developing DAT increases with age, it is clear that DAT represents a major, if not the major, public health concern for the coming decades.

Although the clinical and neuropathological syndrome of DAT was first described over 80 years ago (Alzheimer's, 1907), it has only been within the past two decades that DAT has been identified as the cause of a majority of cases of what used to be referred to as senility. Further, it is now well recognized that this is a pathologic condition, not a normal and invariant consequence of aging (Katzman, 1986).

The key clinical features of dementia include impairment of short term and long term memory, impairment of abstract thinking and judgment, disturbances of higher cortical function (such as aphasia, apraxia, or agnosia), personality change and significant change in work, leisure and/or relationships (see Table 2; American Psychiatric Association, 1980). However, dementia may have many causes and it is the characteristic neuropathologic changes of DAT that distinguish it from other forms of dementia. As summarized in Table 1, these changes include diffuse cortical atrophy and, at the microscopic level, neuronal loss (especially cholinergic, e.g. Coyle, Price, & DeLong, 1983), neuritic plaques in the gray matter, perivascular amyloid deposits, and neurofibrillary tangles (Katzman, 1986).

Table 1
Neuropathological Features of Alzheimer's Disease

1. Diffuse cortical atrophy and neuronal loss
2. Neuritic plaques in gray matter
3. Extracellular and perivascular amyloid deposits
4. Neurofibrillary tangles

The structure of the amyloid protein found in senile plaques is identical to that found in perivascular deposits (Katzman, 1986). Interest in the possible etiopathological significance of brain amyloid in DAT has been heightened in recent years, following the identification of the molecular structure of this polypeptide (Glenner & Wong, 1984). Increased levels of amyloid protein also are found in the brains of other aging mammals (Selkoe et al., 1987), suggesting that deposition of this polypeptide may serve as a marker of both pathologic and normal age-related processes.

Because the pathological changes of Alzheimer's disease can only be confirmed at necropsy, clinical criteria for the diagnosis of DAT have been formulated. For example, the criteria for primary degenerative dementia in the third edition of the American Psychiatric Association's Diagnostic and Statistical Manual (DSM-III) are summarized in Tables 2 and 3. The DSM-III system allows for two forms of DAT, a presenile dementia (onset before age 65) and a senile dementia (after age 65), although neuropathological evidence suggests that these conditions may be identical (Katzman, 1986).

Table 2
Key Clinical Features of Dementia *

1. Impairment in short- and long-term memory
2. Impairment in abstract thinking
3. Impairment in judgement
4. Other disturbances of higher cortical function
   (aphasia, apraxia, or agnosia)
5. Personality change
6. Significant impairment in work, leisure, and/or
   relationships

* Adapted from the Diagnostic and Statistical Manual of Mental Disorders, Third Edition (1980).

Table 3   Clinical Diagnostic Criteria for Alzheimer's Disease *

1. Meets criteria for Dementia
2. Insidious onset
3. Generally progressive deteriorating course
4. Exclusion of all other specific causes of Dementia
5. Age of onset: presenile ($\leq$ age 65)
                  senile (> age 65)

* Adapted from the Diagnostic and Statistical Manual of Mental Disorders, Third Edition (1987).

Longitudinal clinical studies indicate that the course of DAT may be subdivided into three phases of progressive deterioration. These phases include: 1) an early phase, marked by subjective memory changes, depression, vague somatic complaints and/or irritability; 2) a middle phase in which definite impairment in memory is apparent, in addition to the development of periods of disorientation, changes in abstraction, in judgment, mood lability, and major personality changes; and 3) a late phase marked by definite and severe dementia, culminating in impaired gait, incontinence, and impaired vegetative functions to the point of bed-ridden existence (Katzman, 1986).

Dementia often goes undetected during the first phase of development of DAT, as affected individuals and their families may minimize the changes and/or develop alternate means for coping with the slowly worsening impairment. The dementia of DAT is irreversible and, ultimately, fatal, although the exact cause of death often is pneumonia or some other complication of severe debilitation (Katzman, 1976). There currently are no effective forms of treatment available for DAT, although this remains an ongoing topic of research of the highest priority. The normal progression of DAT from onset to death may range from 5 to 15 years (Katzman, 1976).

Relationship Between Down Syndrome and DAT

An initial reference to the occurrence of dementia in Down Syndrome may be found in the literature as far back as 1876, when Fraser and Mitchell (1876) noted that death due to a form of "precipitated senility" was observed in a number of instances. Little attention subsequently was given to the possible association for the next 100 years, perhaps because so few persons with Down Syndrome lived into adulthood. Nevertheless, an initial reference to post-mortem detection of Alzheimer-like neuropathological changes in the brains of persons with Down Syndrome is found as early as 1929 (Struwe, 1929). Subsequent reports in the late 1940's and the early 1950's noted cases of clinical dementia accompanied by the neuropathologic changes of DAT in Down Syndrome (Jervis, 1948; Verhaart & Jelgersma, 1952). A number of investigations appeared in the late 1960's and early 1970's which provided further confirmation of the high frequency of neuropathological changes consistent with DAT in Down Syndrome individuals who died past the age of 35 (Burger & Vogel, 1973; Crapper et al., 1975; Ellis, McCulloch, & Corley, 1974; Liss et al., 1980; O'Hara, 1972; Olson & Shaw, 1972; Owens, Dawson, & Losin, 1971; Reid, Maloney, & Aungle, 1978; Schochet, 1973; Solitaire & Lamarche, 1966).

The current evidence of an association between Down Syndrome and DAT is derived from five types of research: 1) neuropathological studies; 2) genetic risk studies; 3) epidemiological trends; 4) clinical findings; and 5) recent molecular genetic research. Pertinent evidence from each of these lines of research supporting the association of DAT and DS is reviewed below.

Neuropathological Studies - There is compelling evidence that post-mortem brain specimens of older persons with Down Syndrome show Alzheimer-like neuropathological changes (see, for example, a review by Oliver & Holland, 1986). As nicely summarized in the recent work of K.E. and H.M. Wisniewski and their associates (1985a, 1985b, 1986), neuropathological examination of brains of persons with Down Syndrome dying past the age of 30 show cortical atrophy, neuronal loss, senile plaques, perivascular amyloid deposits, and neurofibrillary tangles. In fact, it is a virtual certainty that these changes will be found in the brains of all persons with Down Syndrome who die after the age of 35 (e.g., Wisniewski et al, 1985a, 1985b). Although several investigators have described minor morphological differences between the Alzheimer-like changes in the brains of older persons with Down Syndrome individuals and nonretarded adults with confirmed DAT (Allsop et al., 1986; Ball & Nuttall, 1980; Masters et al, 1985), the similarities are far more consistent than the differences.

Two groups of investigators also have reported abnormal deposits of calcium found around the basal ganglia in older Down Syndrome individuals (Wisniewski et al., 1982; Takashima & Becker, 1985). However, this latter finding suggests a more generalized breakdown in the blood-brain barrier in Down Syndrome, which is not a typical feature of DAT.

As discussed by Kemper (this volume), another interesting difference between DS and DAT concerns the marked degree of neuropathological changes observed in Down Syndrome in brain regions which are normally spared in Alzheimer's disease. Thus, the neuropathology of the aging brain in Down Syndrome may not be exactly identical to the normal progression of pathological changes in DAT. As discussed below, evidence from clinical studies of neuropsychological changes in Down Syndrome also show differences when compared with the natural history of DAT.

Such profound neuropathologic findings in Down Syndrome normally <u>should</u> dictate that the clinical evidence of Alzheimer's disease can be found in all older persons with DS. However, this simply is not the case. Cross sectional studies suggest that only 10% to 45% of older persons with Down Syndrome meet clinical criteria for dementia (Dalton & Crapper, 1977; Reid & Aungle, 1974; Ropper & Williams, 1980; Thase et al., 1982; Wisniewski et al., 1985a; 1985b). This observation suggests that in Down Syndrome, unlike DAT in the general population, profound neuropathologic changes may be greatly preceded, or even be unaccompanied, by clinical evidence of cognitive decline (see Figure 1).

Figure 1. Discrepancy between neuropathological (white bars) and clinical (dark bars) evidence of DAT in Down Syndrome (adapted from Wisniewski et al., 1985a).

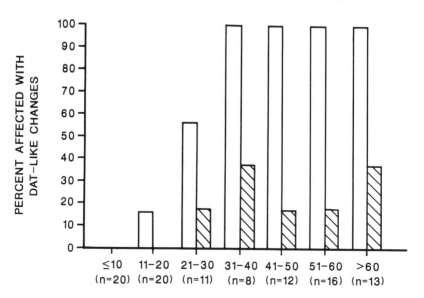

An interesting clarification of the paradox between clinical and neuropathological findings has been provided in a recent paper by H. Wisniewski and Rabe (1986). In this report, the authors documented that clinical evidence of dementia in Down Syndrome is associated with a significantly increased number of plaques and tangles compared to the brains of Down Syndrome individuals who showed no evidence of dementia. While the nondemented persons with Down Syndrome in this series had plaque and tangle counts in the range normally associated with DAT, those with clear-cut dementia had even higher levels of neuropathology. Thus, the lesion count of dementia in Down Syndrome appears to be higher than in DAT as it occurs in the general population (see Table 4). Alternatively, it could be concluded that persons with DS have a higher neuropathological "threshold" for development of dementia as measured by plaque and tangle counts.

Table 4
Relationship Between Plaque and Tangle Density and Clinical Dementia in General Population and Down Syndrome

Group	Plaques **	Tangles **
General Population		
Nondemented	1.4	2.2.
Demented	6.4	15.4
Down Syndrome		
Nondemented	11.4	12.6
Demented	27.2	20.6

* Adapted from Wisniewski and Rabe (1986).
** Mean Number per mm(2).

Genetic Risk Studies - One investigation has studied the possible clinical genetic association between DAT in the general population and Down Syndrome (Heston & Mastri, 1977; Heston, 1982). Results of this project indicate that the risk of Down Syndrome is increased approximately 2-2 1/2 times in the relatives of probands with DAT. Such increased observed risk suggests that a related aberrant

mechanism (or mechanisms) may account for the nondisjunction of chromosome 21 in trisomic Down Syndrome and the
(as yet) unrecognized genetic abnormality in DAT. However, it is alternatively conceivable that a common epi-
phenomenal factor such as maternal age, could account for
such a relationship. The replication of these interesting
findings certainly is needed.

Figure 2. Decline in survivorship with advancing age in
Down Syndrome (reprinted with permission from Thase,
1982a).

Figure 2

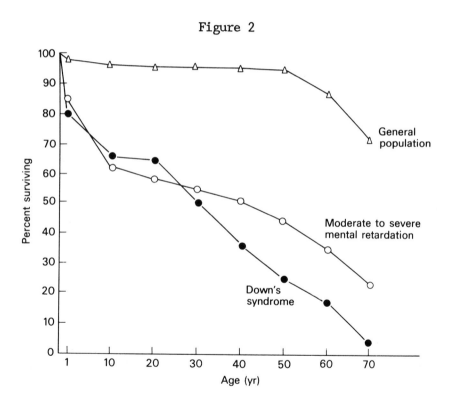

Epidemiologic Trends - In prior generations, an association between age-related cognitive decline and Down Syndrome was little more than a curiosity, since only a
small number of persons with DS lived past age 30 (Thase,
1982a). However, the life expectancy of persons with Down

Syndrome has increased significantly over the past several decades, such that over half of the Down Syndrome population now survives past the age of 30, i.e., into the age range that Alzheimer-like neuropathological changes are observed (Thase, 1982a). Indeed, average life expectancy in Down Syndrome is now approaching 50 years. Such increased longevity is pertinent to study of the potential relationship between Down Syndrome and DAT because there is a marked drop in survival in DS past the age of 30, when compared either to the general population or to the mentally retarded population (see Figure 2). Thus, an unexplained source of mortality is apparent in Down Syndrome past age 30, which very well could be the development of DAT. Moreover, a terminal acceleration of mortality rates is observed in Down Syndrome past age 50 that is comparable to mortality rates in the general population at age 80 (see Figure 3; Thase, 1982a).

Figure 3. Precipitous rise in mortality rates past age 40 in Down Syndrome (reprinted with permission from Thase, 1982a).

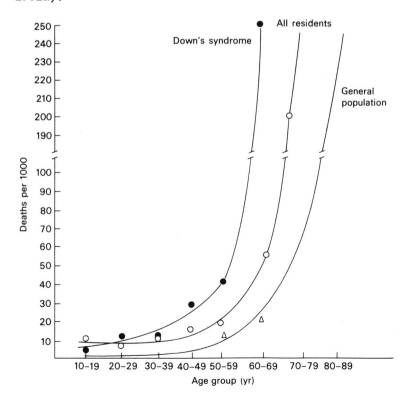

Clinical Findings - With the compelling post-mortem evidence of neuropathologic changes of DAT in persons with Down Syndrome, research addressing the prevalence and significance of cognitive changes in the living DS population remains a logical priority. Unfortunately, most initial studies of this phenomenon are, by and large, of a cross-sectional nature, i.e., a sample of older persons with Down Syndrome is identified and then tested against either samples of other mentally retarded individuals or younger persons with DS. As summarized in Table 5, these studies have documented evidence of impaired orientation, decreased attention span, poor object identification, and impaired short-term visual memory in older persons with Down Syndrome (see Cutler et al., 1985; Dalton, Crapper, & Schlotterer, 1974; Owens, Dawson, & Losin, 1971; Thase et al., 1982, 1984; Wisniewski et al., 1978).

Table 5
Cross-Sectional Evidence of Cognitive Impairment in Older DS Individuals

Abnormality	Strength of Finding
Decreased attention span	+
Impaired orintation	++
Poor object identification	++
Impaired short term visual memory	+++

Our group (Thase, et al., 1982; Thase et al., 1984) has conducted the largest of this type of investigation, with the study of the entire population of persons with Down Syndrome residing at a mental institution -- 165 persons with Down Syndrome -- and an age- and IQ-equated group of 163 mentally retarded controls. As summarized in the final report of the initial assessment (Thase et al., 1984), we demonstrated impairment on a number of cognitive and behavioral measures in Down Syndrome compared to the control group. In particular, we observed a significant age-by-group interaction indicating age-related impairment in performance in older persons with Down Syndrome. For example, attention span, digit span, and visual memory declined with age in DS (but not controls), and test performance was most impaired in persons with DS over age 50 (see, for example, Figure 4). There also were comparable age-associated changes in cooperation and affect. In summary, our cross-sectional data support the notion that there is an age-related cognitive impairment in Down Syndrome that is not likely to be explained by a simple cohort effect. Longitudinal follow-up evaluation of this sample unavoidably has been delayed, but now is underway.

Figure 4. Decline in visual memory performance in older Down Syndrome subjects compared to matched controls (reprinted with permission from Thase et al., 1984).

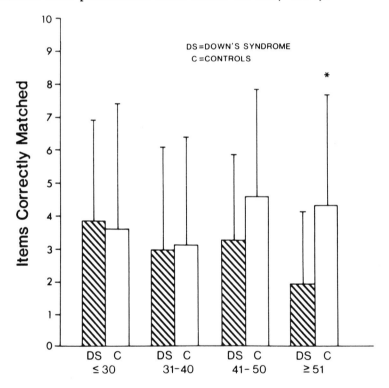

Several investigators have studied behavioral and neurologic parameters in older persons with Down Syndrome. Findings from these studies are consistent with the pro-

files observed in dementia, including deterioration of
self-care skills (Francis, 1970; Miniszek, 1983), the
presence of pathological "released" reflexes (Loesch-
Mdzewska, 1968; Owens et al., 1971; Wisniewski et al.,
1978; Thase et al., 1982, 1984; Sand et al., 1983), and
abnormal electroencephalographic rhythms (Veall, 1974;
Crapper et al., 1975; Tangye, 1979). More recently, preliminary evidence of diminished brain glucose utilization
as detected by the positron emission tomography technique
has been reported in two dementing persons with Down Syndrome (Cutler et al., 1985).

Although studies employing cross-sectional design methodology have provided significant information about cognitive, behavioral, and neurological changes in older
persons with Down Syndrome, these studies are subject to
a variety of criticisms. For example, utilization of institutional samples certainly biases subject selection
towards a more impaired sample. Moreover, neuropathological studies are cross-sectional and, by their very nature, are biased to study a greater proportion of the
most impaired individuals. Cross-sectional studies also
are flawed by possible cohort effects, such as differences in early educational experiences or length of con-
finement in an institution, and group effects, such as
the well-described difficulties in auditory/verbal processing in Down Syndrome reviewed in a number of the
other chapters in this volume. It also is virtually impossible to conduct any form of sophisticated clinical
study in which the examiner is "blind" to the knowledge
of whether a subject has Down Syndrome or is a control.

A further area of difficulty observed in cross-sectional research concerns application of the cognitive and behavioral criteria for dementia in the mentally retarded
population. Such a process usually requires a very well
documented "baseline," which often is not available in
the case of an institutionalized sample. Nevertheless, it
should be recognized that, without such a detailed baseline and rigorous systematic follow-up, a clinical dementia may go undetected in a person with Down Syndrome for
a number of years until the level of deterioration begins
to affect workshop performance or self-care skills. Dementia may thus go undetected for a number of years until
the degree of disability becomes patently obvious. This

observation may account for at least a portion of the disparity between neuropathological findings and clinical diagnosis of dementia, particularly when the history of dementia is based on chart review or a single cross-sectional assessment.

Finally, perhaps the most clinically relevant shortcoming of many cross-sectional studies is the failure to exclude other specific etiologies of dementia. From this vast point, it would be impossible to ascertain if the cognitive impairment detected is actually specifically caused by DAT. I have reported a pertinent case example of this problem in an older person with Down Syndrome who was presumed to have DAT but actually had reversible cognitive impairment due to hypothyroidism (Thase, 1982b). In summary, cross-sectional studies provide only a piece of evidence in the overall puzzle, and their significance pales in comparison to the value of the carefully designed and executed longitudinal studies in which an initial baseline is well established.

To date, such a definitive and comprehensive longitudinal study has not been conducted in a large sample of persons with Down Syndrome. However, several fragments of evidence are available from studies employing prospective methodology. In the first such report, Dalton and Crapper (1977) described a three-year longitudinal follow-up of 11 persons with Down Syndrome aged 35 and over. During the follow-up period, 4 (36%) of the subjects developed clinical evidence of dementia. This finding is striking in two ways: first because a 3-year incidence rate of dementia in 36% of DS subjects is substantially higher than the general population risk, even for persons older than age 80; and second, it is equally striking that the majority of subjects showed no evidence of cognitive decline despite the presumed 100% risk of Alzheimer-like neuropathologic changes.

Comparable findings have been described in longitudinal studies of self-care skills described by Miniszek (1983) and Holland (cited in Oliver & Holland, 1986), as well as in a recent study of the stability of IQ in Down Syndrome (Fenner et al., 1987). These investigations indicate that there also is prospective evidence of cognitive and functional decline in Down Syndrome. However, such deterioration generally is documented in less than half of the

persons studied and, given the strength of the neuropathological evidence, virtually all should show changes of
dementia within a 3 to 5 year follow-up if the deterioration in Down Syndrome was strictly analagous to DAT.
Returning to the issue of diagnosis of dementia in Down
Syndrome, it should be recalled that DAT is a diagnosis
which requires both clinical evidence of cognitive and
functional deterioration and the accompanying neuropathologic findings. It therefore would prove informative to
review cases of DS in which both a clinical history of
dementia has been documented and the subsequent post-mortem examination is available. Pooling the results summarized by Oliver and Holland (1986) and Wisniewski et al.
(1985b), there have been at least 21 such cases described
with sufficient detail in the literature (see Table 6).

Table 6
Clinical Course of Confirmed DAT in Down Syndrome

Number of cases:	n = 21
Mean age of onset:	44 years (range: 18-56)
Mean age at death:	49.6 years (range: 23-65)
Mean length of illness:	5.6 years (range: 2.5-36)

* From Oliver & Holland (1986)
  and Wisniewski et al. (1985a)

It can be gleaned from these case summaries that the average age of onset of dementia in persons with Down Syndrome (44 years) is nearly ten years past the age of apparent 100% neuropathologic risk. However, the mean
length of illness prior to death (5.6 years) is entirely
consistent with the natural history of DAT in the general
population (Katzman, 1976). These observations nicely
parallel the earlier neuropathological-clinical correlation reported by H. Wisniewski and Rabe (1986), as there
is an apparent lag between development of neuropathologic
changes and the onset of a clinical syndrome of dementia.
As we have noted elsewhere (Thase et al., 1982), we examined a number of Down Syndrome persons in our series
over the age of 50 who did not show any of the clinical
signs of dementia. Dr. K. Wisniewski and her associates

(1985a) have noted similar observations in nondemented DS patients who died past age 60 and who were found to have marked Alzheimer-like neuropathological changes. Therefore it seems likely that some persons with Down Syndrome may be able to live for 10, 20 or even 30 years after the presumed onset of neuropathological changes without experiencing cognitive decline. However, as described earlier, when a clinical syndrome of dementia is apparent, the period between the onset of cognitive and behavioral changes and death appears to be essentially the same as observed in the general population.

Recent Molecular Genetic Studies - Perhaps the strongest rationale for the considerable interest in the association between Down Syndrome and DAT is the overall public health significance of Alzheimer's disease. The association of Alzheimer-like neuropathology and Down Syndrome has made molecular genetic study of the chromosome 21 an obvious priority for scientific study. Now that this technology is available, molecular genetic research has proceeded at an amazingly rapid pace over the past several years, such that during 1987 alone a number of key contributions have been published. For example, it is now known that gene coding for the precursor of the amyloid polypeptide (beta amyloid protein) is localized on the q21 region of the long arm of chromosome 21 (Goldgaber et al., 1987; Rabokis et al., 1987; Tanzi et al., 1987a). It should be recalled that this polypeptide forms the basis of the senile plaques and perivascular deposits seen in DAT. Thus, the substrate of one of the key neuropathological features of DAT is controlled by a gene that is duplicated in trisomic Down Syndrome. Further, recent genetic linkage studies suggest a defect in a chromosomal region adjacent to 21q21 in individuals with the familial type of DAT (St. George-Hyslop et al., 1987a; Tanzi et al., 1987a).

The following logic has been proposed to test the association between DAT and Down Syndrome through recent molecular genetic studies: (1) trisomic DS individuals have three copies of chromosome 21 and may have increased levels of all products of this chromosome, including amyloid polypeptide (AP); (2) Alzheimer-like changes in DS thus could be caused by an increased AP gene dosage effect;

(3) genetic linkage studies place the abnormality in familial DAT close to the AP locus; and (4) therefore both sporadic and familial forms of DAT in the general population could be caused by a microduplication of the q21 region of chromosome 21. This explanation has received limited empirical support: duplication of the AP gene recently has been reported in normal karyotypic persons with Down Syndrome, as well as in three apparently sporadic cases of DAT (Delabar et al., 1987).

Several other observations mitigate against the relatively simplistic AP gene duplication theory of DAT. First, the concordance rates of Alzheimer's disease in identical twins is far less than expected 100% rate that would be seen in the case of gene duplication. Second, there are several clinical and neuropathological disparities noted between the dementia of Down Syndrome (a condition with certain AP gene duplication) and DAT in general population. Indeed, three recent studies employing more stringent molecular genetic techniques have failed to find evidence of AP gene duplication in both sporadic (Podlisny et al., 1987; St. George-Hyslop et al., 1987b) forms of DAT. Given the negative findings noted above, it would be of interest to restudy the subjects reported by Delabar et al. (1987) using alternate methods to ascertain if the earlier positive results were artifactual or if a minority of DAT cases indeed manifest AP gene duplication.

It therefore appears that a simple gene dosage effect cannot be invoked to explain the abnormal deposition of amyloid in most cases of DAT. It remains to be seen what role the AP gene actually plays in development of DAT, particularly with respect to adjacent loci which may modulate or regulate its activity. However, it appears quite likely that the actual genetic mechanism of dementia in Down Syndrome may differ from most cases of DAT. This inference amplifies the significance of the otherwise debatable differences in neuropathology (the topography and density of plaque and tangle count) and clinical course (the apparent lag between development of cortical changes and the onset of clinical dementia) observed in Down Syndrome.

Summary and Future Directions

It is now well known that virtually all individuals
with Down Syndrome who die past the age of 35 show the
characteristic neuropathologic changes of Alzheimer's disease. There is sufficient clinical and neurological evidence to indicate that cognitive decline and, less frequently, a clear-cut dementia also occur in a significant
minority of older persons with Down Syndrome. Such observations are remarkable when compared to the risk of development of dementia in the general population, and form
the basis of a conclusion that there is a definite association between Down Syndrome and Alzheimer's disease.
However, this conclusion is tempered by the observation
that dementia in Down Syndrome is observed much less frequently after the age of 35 than would be predicted from
the neuropathological findings. As suggested by several
lines of evidence, there is a higher pathophysiological
threshold (i.e., with respect to the plaque and tangle
counts) for development of dementia in Down Syndrome than
is observed in the general population. It is conceivable
that all individuals with Down Syndrome might develop dementia if they lived long enough and if no other causes
of mortality would circumvent the natural history of progression of DAT. Nevertheless, this speculation is moot
since clearly a substantial number of persons with Down
Syndrome now live into their fifth, sixth, or even seventh decade without manifesting clinical signs of dementia.

A key clinical implication of these findings is that it
should never be assumed Alzheimer's disease is the invariant consequence of longevity in Down Syndrome. It thus
is crucial that the families of, and health care providers for, persons with Down Syndrome know that the association of DS and the full clinical-neurological condition
of DAT is far from absolute. There are a number of age-
related conditions which may either cause, or masquerade
as, dementia in Down Syndrome and it would be harmful to
persons with DS to assume that all cognitive deterioration in older persons with Down Syndrome is the result of
DAT. For example, sensory deprivation associated with
either visual impairments (such as cataracts) or hearing
deficits may produce cognitive and behavioral changes

(Hewitt et al., 1985), as well as thyroid disease and other systemic illnesses. Indeed, the older DS population may be at high risk for such conditions (Hewitt et al., 1985; Thase, 1982a, 1982b). Further, the well described pseudo-dementia syndrome of depression should not be overlooked, nor should the behavioral toxicity of numerous medications. Careful clinical attention to these factors is a necessary part of a standard evaluation of any person experiencing cognitive deterioration and should not be overlooked in persons with Down Syndrome.

Unfortunately, no breakthroughs have yet been established for treatment of DAT. However, there are grounds for at least some degree of optimism that a palliative treatment will be forthcoming. Within the past year, important and still controversial evidence has emerged suggesting that the increased risk of DAT in Down Syndrome is associated with the gene coding for the precursor of the amyloid polypeptide, which is located on the 21st chromosome. However, much needs to be learned about the regulation of the AP gene's activity and it seems clear that increased gene dosage is not the mechanism causing most, if not all, cases of DAT in the general public. Further work in this area may enlighten us regarding the threshold effect for neuropathological changes in Down Syndrome, as well as the parallel clinical observation of significant variability in development of dementia. Such knowledge also might shed light on potential treatment mechanisms to alter the pathophysiology of DAT, with the hope that control or even prevention of dementia in Down Syndrome may be a reality in the future.

Acknowledgement

The author wishes to thank Ms. Nancy Karwowski and Ms. Kelly McGinn for their assistance in preparation of this manuscript.

REFERENCES

Allsop, D., Kidd, M., Landon, M., & Tomlinson, A. (1986). Isolated senile plaque cores in Alzheimer's disease and Down's syndrome show differences in morphology. Journal of Neurology, Neurosurgery, and Psychiatry, 49, 886-892

Alzheimer, A. (1907). Uber eine eigenartige Erkrankung der Hirnrinde. Allgemeine Zeitschrift fur Psychiatrie und Psychisch Gerichtliche Medizine, 64, 146-148.

American Psychiatric Association (1980). Diagnostic and Statistical Manual of Mental Disorders (third ed.). APA: Washington D.C.

Ball, M. J., & Nuttall, K. (1980). Neurofibrillary tangles, granulovacuolar degeneration and neurone loss in Down's syndrome: quantitative comparison with Alzheimer's dementia. Annals of Neurology, 7, 462-465.

Burger, P. C., & Vogel, F. S. (1973). The development of the pathological changes of Alzheimer's disease and senile dementia inpatients with Down's syndrome. American Journal of Pathology, 73, 457-468.

Coyle, J. T., Price, D. L., & Delong, M. R. (1983). Alzheimer's disease: a disorder of cortical cholinergic innervation. Science, 219, 1184-1189.

Crapper, D. R., Dalton, A. L., Skopitz, M., Eng, P., Scott, J. H., & Hachinski, V. (1975). Alzheimer's degeneration in Down's syndrome. Archives of Neurology, 32, 618.

Cutler, N. R., Heston, L. L., Davies, P., Haxby, J. V., & Schapiro, M. B. (1985). Alzheimer's disease and Down's Syndrome: new insights. Annals of Internal Medicine, 103, 566-578.

Dalton, A. J., & Crapper-McLachlan, D. R. (1986). Clinical expression of Alzheimer's Disease in Down's Syndrome. Psychiatric Clinics of North America, 9, 659-670.

Dalton, A. L., & Crapper, D. R. (1977). Down's Syndrome and aging of the brain. In P. Mittler (ed.), Research to Practice in Mental Retardation, Vol. 3, Biomedical Aspects, pp. 391-400. University Press: Baltimore.

Dalton, A. L., Crapper, D. R., & Schlotterer, G. R. (1974). Alzheimer's disease in Down's syndrome: visual retention deficits. Cortex, 10, 366-377.

Delabar, J. M., Goldgaber, D., Lamour, Y., Nicole, A., Huret, J. L., deGrouchy, J., Brown, P., Gajduser, D. C., Sinet, P. M. (1987). Beta-amyloid gene duplication in Alzheimer's disease and karyotypically normal Down Syndrome. Science, 235, 1390-1392.

Ellis, W. G., McCulloch, J. R., & Corley, C. L. (1974). Presenile dementia in Down's syndrome: ultrastructural identity with Alzheimer's disease. Neurology, (Minneapolis) <u>24</u>, 101-106.

Fenner, M. E., Hewitt, K. E., & Torpy, D. M. (1987).
Down's Syndrome: intellectual and behavioral functioning during adulthood. <u>Journal of Mental Deficiency Re-
search</u>, <u>31</u>, 241-249.

Francis, S. H. (1970). Behavior of low grade institutionalized mongoloids: changes with age. <u>American Journal
of Mental Deficiency</u>, <u>75</u>, 92-101.

Fraser, J., & Mitchell, A (1876). Kalmuc idiocy: report
of a case with autopsy with notes on 62 cases. <u>Journal
of Mental Science</u>, <u>22</u>, 161.

Glenner, G. G., & Wong, C. W. (1984). Alzheimer's disease
and Down's syndrome: sharing of a unique cerebrovascular amyloid protein. <u>Biochemistry and Biophysics Research Communications</u>, <u>122</u>, 1131-1135.

Goldgaber, D., Lerman, M. I., McBride, O. W., Saffiotti,
V., & Gajdusek, D. C. (1987). Characterization and
chromosomal localization of a cDNA encoding brain amyloid of Alzheimer's disease. <u>Science</u>, <u>235</u>, 877-880.

Heston, L. L. (1982). Alzheimer's dementia and Down's
Syndrome: genetic evidence suggesting an association.
<u>Annals of the New York Academy of Sciences</u>, <u>396</u>, 29-37.

Heston, L. L., & Mastri, A. R. (1977). Genetics of Alzheimer's disease: associations with hematological mal-
ignancies and Down's Syndrome. <u>Archives of General Psy-
chiatry</u>, <u>34</u>, 976-981.

Hewitt, K. E., Carter, G., & Jancar, J. (1985). Aging in
Down's Syndrome. <u>British Journal of Psychiatry</u>, <u>147</u>,
58-62.

Jervis, G. A. (1948). Early senile dementia mongoloid
idiocy. <u>American Journal of Psychiatry</u>, <u>105</u>, 102-106.

Karlinsky, H. (1986). Alzheimer's disease in Down's Syndrome: a review. <u>Journal of the American Geriatric So-
ciety</u>, <u>34</u>, 728-734.

Katzman, R. (1986). Alzheimer's disease. <u>New England
Journal of Medicine</u>, <u>314</u>, 964-973.

Katzman, R. (1976). The prevalence and malignancy of
Alzheimer's disease. <u>Archives of Neurology</u>, <u>33</u>,
217-218.

Liss, L., Shim, C., Thase, M., Smeltzer, D., Maloone, J.,
& Couri, D. (1980). The relationship between Down's
Syndrome and dementia Alzheimer's type. <u>Journal of
Neuropathological and Experimental Neurology</u>, <u>39</u>, 371.

Loesch-Mdzewska, D. (1968). Some aspects of the neurology of Down's Syndrome. Journal of Mental Deficiency Research, 12, 237-246.

Masters, C. L., Simms, G., Weinman, N. A., Multhaup, G., McDonald, B. L., & Beyreuther, K. (1985). Amyloid plaque core protein in Alzheimer disease and Down Syndrome. Proceedings of the National Academy of Sciences USA, 82, 4245-4249.

Melamed, N. (1964). Neuropathology. In H. A. Stevens and R. Heber (ed.), Mental Retardation: A Review of Research, pp. 429-452. University of Chicago Press, Chicago.

Miniszek, N. A. (1983). Development of Alzheimer's disease in Down's Syndrome individuals. American Journal of Mental Deficiency, 87, 377-385.

O'Hara, P. T. (1972). Electron microscopical study of the brain in Down's Syndrome. Brain, 95, 681-684.

Oliver, C., & Holland, A. J. (1986). Down's Syndrome and Alzheimer's disease: a review. Psychological Medicine, 16, 307-322.

Olson, M. I., & Shaw, C. M. (1969). Presenile dementia and Alzheimer's disease in mongolism. Brain, 92, 147-156.

Owens, D., Dawson, J. C., & Losin, S. (1971). Alzeimer's disease in Down's Syndrome. American Journal of Mental Deficiency, 75, 606-612.

Paulson, G. W. (1977). The neurological examination in dementia. In C. E. Wells (ed.), Dementia, pp. 169-188. F. A. Davies: Philadelphia.

Podlisny, M. B., Lee, G., & Selkoe, D. J. (1987). Gene dosage of the amyloid beta protein precursor in Alzheimer's disease. Science, 238, 669-671.

Reid, A. H., & Aungle, P. G. (1974). Dementia in aging mentally defectives: a clinical psychiatric study. Journal of Mental Deficiency Research, 18, 15-23.

Reid, A. H., Maloney, A. F. J., & Aungle, T. G. (1978). Dementia in aging mental defectives: a clinical and neuropathological study. Journal of Mental Deficiency Research, 22, 233-241.

Robakis, N. K., Wisniewski, H. M., Jenkins, E. C., Devine-Gage, E. A., Houck, G. E., Yao, X. L., Ramakrishna, N., Wolfe, G., Silverman, W. P., & Brown, W. T. (1987). Chromosome 21q21 sublocalization of gene encoding beta-amyloid peptide in cerebral vessels and neuritic (senile) plaques of people with Alzheimer disease and Down Syndrome. Lancet, 1(8529), 384-385.

Ropper, A. H., & Williams, R. S. (1980). Relationship between plaques, tangles and dementia in Down's Syndrome. Neurology, 30, 639-644.

Saint George-Hyslop, P. H., Tanzi, R. E., Polinsky, R. J., Haines, J. L., Nee, L., Watkins, P. C., Myers, R. H., Feldman, R. G., Pollen, D., Drachman, D., Growden, J., Bruni, A., Foncin, J. F., Salmon, D., Frommelt, P., Amaducci, L., Sorbin, S., Piacentini, S., Stewart, G. D., Hobbs, W. J., Conneally, P. M., & Gusella, J. F. (1987). The genetic defect causing familial Alzheimer's disease maps on chromosome 21. Science, 235, 885-888.

Sand, T., Mellgren, S. I., & Hestnes, A. (1983). Primitive reflexes in Down's Syndrome. Journal of Mental Deficiency Research, 27, 39-44.

Schochet, S. S. (1973). Neurofibrillary tangles in patients with Down's Syndrome: A light and electron microscopic study. Acta Neuropathological, 23, 342-356.

Selkoe, D. J., Bell, D. S., Podlisny, M. B., Price, D. L., & Cork, L. C. (1987). Conservation of brain amyloid proteins in aged mammals and humans with Alzheimer's disease. Science, 235, 873-877.

Solitaire, G. B., & Lamarche, J. B. (1966). Alzheimer's disease and senile dementia as seen in mongoloids: neuropathological observations. American Journal of Mental Deficiency, 70, 840-848.

Struwe, F. (1929). Histopathologische Untersuchungen uber Entstehung und Wesen der Senilen Plaques. Zeitschrift fur die gesamte Neurologie und Psychiatrie, 122, 291.

Takashima, S., & Becker, L. E. (1985). Basal ganglia calcification in Down's Syndrome. Journal of Neurology, Neurosurgery and Psychiatry, 48, 61-64.

Tangye, S. R. (1979). The EEG and incidence of epilepsy in Down's Syndrome. Journal of Mental Deficiency Research, 23, 17-24.

Tanzi, R. E., Bird, E. D., Latt, S. A., & Neve R. G. (1987b). The amyloid beta protein gene is not duplicated in brains from patients with Alzheimer's disease. Science, 238, 666-669.

Tanzi, R. E., Gusella, J. F., Watkins, P. C., Bruns, G. A. P., Saint George-Hyslop, P., Van Keuren, M. L.,

Patterson, D., Pagan, S. Kurnit, D. M., & Neve, R. L. (1987). Amyloid beta protein gene: cDNA, MRNA distribution, and genetic linkage near the Alzheimer locus Science, 235, 880-884.

Thase, M. E. (1982a). Longevity and mortality in Down's Syndrome. Journal of Mental Deficiency Research, 26, 177-192.

Thase, M. E. (1982b). Reversible dementia in Down's Syndrome. Journal of Mental Deficiency Research, 26, 111-113.

Thase, M. E., Liss, L., Smeltzer, D., & Maloon, J. (1982). Clinical evaluation of dementia in Down's Syndrome: a preliminary report. Journal of Mental Deficiency Research, 26, 239-244.

Thase, M. E., Tigner, R., Smeltzer, D., & Liss, L. (1984). Age-related neuropsychological deficits in Down's Syndrome. Biological Psychiatry, 19, 571-585.

Tomlinson, B. E., Blessed, G., & Roth, M. (1970). Observations on the brains of demented old people. Journal of Neurological Sciences, 11, 205-242.

Veall, R. M. (1974). The prevalence of epilepsy among mongolia related to age. Journal of Mental Deficiency Research, 19, 99-106.

Verhart, W. J. C., & Jelgersma, H. C. (1952). Early senile dementia in mongolian idiocy. Description of a case. Folia Psychiatrica Neerlandica, 55, 453-459.

Wisniewski, H. M., & Rabe, A. (1986). Discrepancy between Alzheimer-type neuropathology and dementia in persons with Down's Syndrome. Annals of the New York Academy of Sciences, 477, 247-260.

Wisnieswki, K. E., Dalton, A. J., Crapper-McLachlan, D. R., Wen, G. V., & Wisniewski, H. M. (1985b). Alzheimer's disease in Down's Syndrome: clinicopathological studies, Neurology, 35, 957-961.

Wisniewski, K. E., French, J. H., Rosen, J. F., Kozlowski, P. B. Tenner, M., & Wisniewski, H. M. (1982). Basal ganglia calcification (BCG) in Down's Syndrome (DS) - another manifestation of premature aging. Annals of the New York Academy of Science, 396, 179-189.

Wisniewski, K. E., Howe, J., Gwyn-Williams, D. & Wisniewski, H. M. (1978). Precocious aging and dementia in patients with Down's Syndrome. Biological Psychiatry, 13, 619-627.

Wisniewski, K. E., Wisniewski, H. M., & Wen, G. Y. (1985a). Occurrence of neuropathological changes and dementia of Alzheimer's disease in Down's Syndrome. Annals of Neurology, 7, 278-282.

Afterword

Down Syndrome in Psychobiological Profile

Lynn Nadel
Dept. of Psychology
University of Arizona
Tucson, Arizona

Introduction

The mental retardation observed to varying degree in virtually all individuals with Down Syndrome is perhaps the signal feature of this syndrome. Largely because of it, institutionalization has until recently been the fate of most persons with Down Syndrome. Assessments of psychobiological function in such individuals, constituting the bulk of extant research prior to this past decade, could not possibly reveal their true potential. Studies of home-reared Down Syndrome children, though in their infancy, have already shown conclusively that these children have potential in excess of that suggested by earlier work. The chapters in this volume document what is currently known of the psychobiological development of Down Syndrome individuals in a number of domains, including general central nervous system structure and function, sensory and motor capacities, cognitive development, language acquistion and function. In my comments here, I discuss some of the major points of convergence, the hints and suggestions, the doubts and uncertainties, that came out of the meeting at which these chapters were initially presented.

CNS Structure and Function

Recent work has confirmed that there is a subtle, highly selective, disorder affecting central nervous system development in Down Syndrome. A widespread loss of small neurons is evidenced in both hippocampal formation and neocortex. In the former, there is extensive malformation in the dentate gyrus, reflecting the high proportion of small, late-developing granule cells normally found in that structure. In the latter, cell loss is largely re-stricted to layer IV, which contains the cell bodies of small, <u>local circuit</u> neurons. These data are discussed in the contribution by Kemper. Galaburda and Kean (personal communication) attempted to place these raw neurological facts in a conceptual framework. They noted that 'local-circuit' neurons which project over short distances de-rive from a different part of the neural crest than do neurons which project over longer distances; that is, to a different brain system, and that this distinction be-tween local and long-distance projection systems arises very early in evolution. Down Syndrome seems to exert its influence selectively on local circuit neuron develop-ment, leaving the major input-output cells -- usually the <u>pyramidal</u> cells -- largely unscathed. In this selective action upon local-circuit neurons may lie hints to both the source of mental retardation and the mechanisms by which an extra 21st chromosome translates into Down Syn-drome.

Kemper also considers the relation between Down Syn-drome and Alzheimer's disease. They share some important features: neurofibrillary tangles and plaques are mani-fested in cortical structures, and there is, in both cases, some involvement of chromosome 21. However, they differ in other ways: the specific distribution of neuro-pathology, for example, is distinct. Further, though there is nearly 100% incidence of neuropathology in Down Syndrome by age 35 or so, only a fraction of individuals with Down Syndrome develop dementia by this age. This latter fact is most intriguing, not only for what it says about the relation between Down Syndrome and Alzheimer's disease, but also for what it says about relations be-tween the neuropathology typically associated with Alzheimer's disease and the dementia assumed to reflect that pathology. The differences in particular patterns of pathology between the two syndromes suggest the possibil-ity that there are rather specific sites which must be damaged before dementia is observed.

Whatever the conclusion concerning structural damage to

portions of the limbic system and neocortex, neurophysi-
cal studies such as those described by Courchesne indicate that problems exist at other levels of the neuraxis
as well. That problems seem more severe in the auditory
than in the visual system, as also noted by Peuschel is
his more behaviorally-oriented chapter, is of potential
importance for understanding the severity of the language
problem, and for pointing towards effective intervention
strategies. As Miller notes, there are disproportionate
difficulties with production of language, a fact that
also is consistent with the greater problems observed in
audition.

Cognitive Development

The picture presented by neurological studies is one of
subtle differences embedded in a broad context of relative normalcy. As discussed to some extent by Courchesne,
brain development is an extremely plastic process, involving an initial overproliferation of nerve cells and
synapses, followed by an activity-dependent 'pruning' of
these connections, leaving behind those that proved useful. It has been known for some time that variations in
early experiences can alter the extent of nerve cell
ramications (e.g. Rosenzweig and Bennett, 1978), suggesting that adequate stimulation is needed to promote
adequate brain development. Much the same conclusion can
be derived from recent studies of the impact of early
stimulation upon limbic system development and function
(e.g. Meaney, Aitken, van Berkel, Bhatnagar and Sapolsky,
1988; Wilson, Willner, Kurz and Nadel, 1986; Nadel and
Willner, in press). Such results suggest that the early
stimulation environment could make an important difference in the fate of Down Syndrome individuals, and every
indication from the past decades' study of individuals
that were not institutionalized indicates that this is
true (see chapter by Wisniewski, Miezejeski and Hill).
    In order to structure the early environment of Down
Syndrome individuals optimally, one needs an accurate
picture of their cognitive development, its normal and
abnormal features. Broadly speaking: few obvious differences between the Down Syndrome children and the normally

developing children appear in the earliest months of life, and all objective testing suggests that there is but a small gap between them at birth. Though there are important differences in acquisition of basic concepts about objects, Wishart's data on her youngest subjects indicates that relatively normal acquisition is within range for many of the Down Syndrome infants. The situation seems less favorable with regard to number concepts, where Gelman and Cohen demonstrate that Down Syndrome children approach the task of learning about numbers in a rote-like, non-normal fashion. As in Wishart's study, they do not appear to have access to the implicit knowledge principles that are assumed to guide effective learning in normally developing children.

Major differences emerge at around 20 months of age, generally around the age of the "vocabulary surge" in normally developing children. Down Syndrome children use the same "first words", but have great trouble going beyond simple utterances, reflecting disproportionate difficulties in grammatical aspects of language, and in production rather than comprehension. Fowler's careful study of a few children over many years provides critical information: Down Syndrome children get "stuck" on a certain plateau, often remaining there for years, when the normally developing children would hurdle it in short order. The good news is that there are signs of potential progress even in quite old adolescents. What could possibly be done to truncate these plateau periods, creating a cascade towards more rapid progress? One exciting possibility was raised by Meyers' demonstrations of improved reading and writing in older Down Syndrome individuals through the use of computer intervention programs. Her initial results indicate that major gains can be had, including important changes in motivation and, perhaps, self-esteem, through computer intervention. Much more research is needed on this, and similar approaches, but the prospects for beneficial application seem good. As we noted, difficulties with auditory information and production problems, are two prominent features of Down Syndrome. The use of computers would permit the use of video displays to overcome the first problem, and would provide alternative means of producing outputs that might help overcome the second. That is, the computer would be used alternative means of producing outputs that might help overcome the second. That is, the computer would be used in many respects as a prosthetic device, enabling the individual to express what is comprehended but cannot be produced through voice or writing. It does not seem unlikely that such techniques will come to play an extremely important role in the future handling of Down Syndrome children.

In sum, cognitive development in Down Syndrome individuals appears slower than normal, with some qualitative quirks that suggest rather selective deficits in rule-based systems, such as number and grammar. The best evidence leaves little doubt that these children can do much better than their institutionalized predecessors, and we have every reason to hope and expect that they will.

The Caregiving Environment

It is absolutely evident that rearing Down Syndrome children at home, or in similar surroundings, has contributed to the improved prognosis for future generations. All is not perfect, however, in this arrangement. As a number of the chapters document, the parents of Down Syndrome children treat these children differently, even without knowing it, even without wanting it, and even though these efforts -- which can be "meant well" -- are in fact counterproductive. Subtly expecting less, parents of Down Syndrome infants provide diminished feedback at various critical stages in early development. These data force us to be cautious in interpreting the remaining cognitive deficits discussed above. As we noted, improvements have been steady and impressive since de-institutionalization began, but real deficits persist. Are these going to be the irreducible minimum, or can further strides be made through improvements in the caregiver-infant dyad? Present understanding, as indicated by Wishart, Mervis, and Smith, von Tetzchner and Michalsen, suggests that subtle, but very important differences are at stake here, and it is hard to know what would follow from careful attention to improving the way caregivers interact with Down Syndrome children.

Conclusions

The past decade has brought great advances in our understanding of many aspects of Down Syndrome. More is known about what is going wrong in central nervous system maturation, and the consequences this has for the development of cognitive function. It is known that early intervention can have beneficial effects, but unclear what the limits are, or what kinds of intervention regimes are most likely to be successful. It is also known that older Down Syndrome individuals can make gains, and that the dementia associated with Alzheimer's disease is not the inevitable fate of all who survive past 35 years of age. There is reason, in other words, for hope; and that is the mood in which the meeting closed.

REFERENCES

Meaney, M.J, Aitken, D.H., van Berkel, C., Bhatnagar, S. and Sapolsky, R.M. Effect of neonatal handling on age-related impairments associated with the hippocampus. Science 239: 766-768, 1988.

Rosenzweig, M.R. and Bennett, E.L. Experiential influences on brain anatomy and brain chemistry in rodents. In: Studies on the development of behavior and the nervous system. Early influences, edited by G.Gottlieb, New York: Academic Press, 1978, vol. 4, 289-327.

Wilson, D.A., Willner, J., Kurz, E.M., and Nadel, L. Early handling increases hippocampal long-term potentiation in young rats. Behavioural Brain Research 21: 223-227, 1986.

Nadel, L. and Willner, J. Some implications of post-natal maturation in the hippocampal formation. In V. Chan-Palay and C. Kohler (eds.) The hippocampus: New Vistas. New York: AR Liss (in press).

BIBLIOGRAPHY

Abalan, F. (1984). Alzheimer's disease and malnutrition: an etiological hypothesis. Med. Hypotheses, 15(4), 385-393.

Abroms, K. I., & Bennett, J. W. (1983). Current findings in Down syndrome. Expectional Children, 49(5), 449-450.

Achenbach, T. M. (1970). Surprise and GSR as indicators of conservation: A new approach to developmental diagnosis demonstrated with retardates. Proceedings of the Annual Convention of the American Psychological Ass., 5(pt. 1), 281-282.

Acosta, L. K. (1982). Instructor use of total communication: effects on preschool Down's syndrome children's vocabulary acquisition and attempted verbalizations. Dissertation Abstracts International, 42(7-A), 3099.

Akita, H. (1977). Case study of the month: Down's syndrome. On adaptability of a child with Down's syndrome to group activities -- nursing assistance relating to child development. Kango. Tenbo., 2(11), 1017-1022.

Allsop, D., Kidd, M., Landon, M., & Tomlinson, A. (1986). Isolated senile plaque cores in Alzheimer's disease and Down's syndrome show differences in morphology. Journal of Neurology. Neurosurgery & Psychiatry, 49(8), 886-892.

Alpern, G. D., & Kimberlin, C. C. (1970). Short intelligence test ranging from infancy levels through childhood levels for use with the retarded. Am. J. Ment. Defic., 75(1), 65-71.

Alter, M. M. (1980). Visual exploratory behavior of Down's syndrome children. Dissertation Abstracts International, 41(4-A), 1527-1528.

Alter, M. M. (1980). Visual exploratory behavior of Down's syndrome children. Dissertation Abstracts International, 1(4-A), 1527-1528.

Alvarez-Morujo, A., & Garzon, Q. C. (1966). The terminal arteries of the brain in various cases of mental disorders. *Trab. Inst. Cajal. Invest. Biol.*, 58, 235-252.

Alvarez, N., & Rubin, L. (1986). Atlantoaxial instability in adults with Down syndrome: a clinical and radiological survey. *Applied Research in Mental Retardation*, 7(1), 67-78.

Amochaev, A. (1985). Recovery of auditory event-related potentials in normal and Down's syndrome individuals. *Dissertation Abstracts International*, 46(3-B), 995.

Anderson, C. J. (1982). Investigation of the role of manual communication in the facilitation of oral labelling skills with intellectually handicapped learners. *Dissertation Abstracts International*, 43(5-A), 1495.

Anderton, B. H., et al. (1982). Monoclonal antibodies show that neurofibrillary tangles and neurofillaments share antigenic determinants. *Nature*, 298(5869), 84-86.

Andrews, R., & Andress, J. G. (1977). A study of the spontaneous oral language of Down's syndrome children. *Exceptional Child*, 24(2), 86-94.

Antalova, J., (1978). The mental and social development of mongoloid children. *Psychologia a Patapsychologia Dietata*, 13(4), 291-299.

Antonarakis, S. E., et al. (1985). Linkage map on chromosome 21Q and the association of a DNA haplotype with a propensity to nondisjunction and trisomy 21. *Symposium of the National Down Syndrome Society: Annals of the New York Academy of Sciences*, 450, 95-107.

Anwar, F., & Hermelin, B. (1979). Kinaesthetic movement after-effects in children with Down' syndrome. *Journal of Mental Deficiency Research*, 23(4), 287-297.

Anwar, F. (1983). The role of sensory modality for the reproduction of shape by the severely retarded. *British Journal of Developmental Psychology*, 1(4), 317-327.

Argalias, A., Mavropoulou Colokytha, S., & Mavroudis, M. (1972). Unusual development in a mongoloid idiot. *Bull. Mem. Soc. Fr. Ophthalmol.*, 85, 52-56.

Armstrong, R. G. (1959). Review of the current theories and findings concerning mongolism. *Psychology Newsletter, NYU*, 10, 151-158.

Arnold, D. G. (1981). Maternal interaction with preschool handicapped children. *Dissertation Abstracts International*, 42(6-A), 2604-2605.

Aronson, M., & Fallstrom, K. (1977). Immediate and long-term effects of developmental training in children with

Down's syndrome. Developmental Medicine & Child Neurology, 19(4), 489-494.

Arshavskii, V. V., & Vaindrukh, F. H. (1969). On the electroencephalographic characteristics of Down's syndrome: A comparative study of patients with epileptiform paroxysmal manifestations and without them. Zhurnal Nevropatologii I Psikhiatrii, 69(10), 1534-1540.

Asher, S. R., Hymel, S., & Renshaw, P. D. (1984). Loneliness in children. Child Development, 55, 1456-1464.

Ashman, A. F. (1982). Coding, strategic behavior, and language performance of institutionalized mentally retarded young adults. American Journal of Mental Deficiency, 86(6), 627-636.

August, G. J., Stewart, M. A., & Tsai, L. (1981). The incidence of cognitive disabilities in the siblings of autistic children. British Journal of Psychiatry, 138, 416-422.

Aumonier, M. E., & Cunningham, C. C. (1983). Breast feeding in infants with Down's syndrome. Child Care, Health, & Development, 9(5), 247-255.

Bailey, P., et al. (1981). Social competence of Australian (Hunter Valley) Down's syndrome children using the M/P-A-C 1. British Journal of Mental Subnormality, 27(2)(53), 61-65.

Bakke, B. L. (1986). The effects of delay and difficulty on a visual recall task with adults who have Down syndrome. Dissertation Abstracts International, 47(6-B), 2651.

Balazs, R., & Brookshank, B. W. (1985). Neurochemical approaches to the pathogenesis of Down's syndrome. Journal of Mental Deficiency Research, 29(1), 1-14.

Ball, M. J., & Nuttall, K. (1981). Topography of neurofibrillary tangles and granulovacuoles in hippocampi of patients with Down's syndrome: Quantitative comparison with normal aging and Alzheimer's disease. Neuropath. Appl. Neurobiol., 7, 13-20.

Banik, N. L., Davison, A. N., Palo, J., & Savolainen, H. (1975). Biochemical studies on myelin isolated from the brains of patients with Down's syndrome. Brain, 98(2), 213-218.

Baram, T. Z., & Fishman, M. A. (1985). Top of the basilar artery stroke in an adolescent with Down's syndrome. Archives of Neurology, 42(3), 296.

Barden, H. S. (1983). Growth and development of selected hard tissues in Down syndrome: A review. Human Biology, 55, 539-576.

Barna, S., et al. (1980). The progress of developmentally delayed pre-school children in a home-training scheme. Child Care, Health & Development, 6(3), 157-164.

Barnard, K. E. (1975). Infant stimulation. In: R. Koch and F. F. DelaCruz (eds.), Down's Syndrome (Mongolism): Research, Prevention and Management, New York: Brunner/Mazel.

Barnet, A. B., Ohlrich, E. S., & Shanks, B. L. (1971). EEG-evoked responses to repetitive auditory stimulation in normal and Down's syndrome infants. Developmental Medicine & Child Neurology, 13(3), 321-329.

Baron, C. S. (1987). Autism and symbolic play. British Journal of Developmental Psychology, 5(2), 139-148.

Baron, J. (1972). Temperament profile of children with Down's syndrome. Dev. Med. Child Neurol., 14(5), 640-643.

Baron, J., Kuczynski, J., & Pydzik, T. (1966). The developmental malformations of fetuses and their relation to maternal age. (Polnisch) Ginek, Pol., 37, 1085-1094.

Baron, C. S., Leslie, A. M., & Frith, U. (1985). Does the autistic child have a theory of mind?. Cognition, 21(1), 37-46.

Baron, C. S., Leslie, A. M., & Frith, U. (1986). Mechanical, behavioral, and intentional understanding of picture stories in autistic children. British Journal of Developmental Psychology, 4(2), 113-125.

Bartels, K. J. (1987). Effects of socio-dramatic play therapy on pragmatic language skills in children with Down syndrome. Dissertation Abstracts International, 47(7-B), 2866.

Barthel, E. (1952). Diagnosis and therapeutic successes in mongolian idiocy. Psychiatry, Neurology and Medical Psychology (Leipzig), 4, 152-159.

Baur, A. M., & Shea, T. M. (1986). Alzheimer's disease and Down syndrome: a review and implications for adult services. Education & Training of the Mentally Retarded, 21(2), 144-150.

Baumanis, D. (1970). Both sides of the coin: The retarded child and his family. Canada's Mental Health, 18(3-4), 23-28.

Baumeister, A. A., & Williams, J. (1967). Relationship of physical stigmata to intellectual functioning of mongolism. American Journal of Mental Deficiency, 71, 586-592.

Bayley, N., Rhodes, L., & Gooch, B. (1966). A comparison of the development of institutionalized and home-reared mongoloids. A follow-up study. California Mental Health Research Digest, 4, 104-105.

Bazelon, M., et al. (1967). Reversal of hypotonia in infants with Down's syndrome by administration of 5-Hydroxytryptophan. Lancet, 2, 1130.

Becker, L. E., Armstrong, D. L., & Chan, F. (1986). Dendritic atrophy in children with Down's syndrome. Ann. Neurol., 20, 520-526.

Beckman, D. D., Wold, D. C., & Montague, J. C. (1984). A noninvasive acoustic method using frequency perturbations and computer-generated vocal-tract shapes. Journal of Speech & Hearing Research, 26(2), 304-314.

Beckman, P. J., & Kohl, F. L. (1984). The effects of social and isolate toys on the interactions and play of integrated and nonintegrated groups of preschoolers. Education & Training of the Mentally Retarded, 19(3) 169-174.

Beechly M., Bretherton, I., & Mervis, C. B. (1986). Mother's internal state language to toddlers. Special Issue: Language and Cognition in Early Social Interacaction. British Journal of Developmental Psychology, 4(3), 247-260.

Beidleman, B., (1945). Mongolism: a selective review. American Journal of Mental Deficiency, 50, 35-53.

Beley, A., Sevestre, P., Lecuyer, R. J., & Leroy, C. (1959). Contribution of the EEG of mongoloids. Rev. Neurol. Paris, 101, 457-459.

Beliakova, T. K. (1973). Paroxysmal syndrome and the severeness of the intellectual defect in Down's disease. Zh. Nevropatol. Psikhiatr. Im. S. S. Korsakova, 73(10), 1555-1557.

Benda, C. E. (1939). Studies in mongolism. I. Growth and physical development. Arch. Neurol. Psychiatry Chicago, 41, 83-97.

Benda, C. E. (1940). Growth disorder of the skull in mongolism. Am. J. Pathol., 16, 71-86.

Benda, C. E. (1940). The central nervous system in mongolism. Am. J. Ment. Defic., 45, 42-47.

Benda, C. E. (1949). Prenatal maternal factors in mongolism. J. Am. Med. Assoc., 139, 979-985.

Bennett, F. L. (1985). The effect of a token economy of cardiorespiratory fitness exercise behavior of individuals with Down's syndrome. Dissertation Abstracts International, 45(9-A), 2796.

Berg, J. M., & Stern, J., (1963). Observations on children with mongolism. Proceedings, 2nd International Congress Mental Retardation, Vienna, I, 367-372.

Berger, J., & Cunningham, C. C. (1986). Aspects of early social smiling by infants with Down's syndrome. Child Care, Health & Development, 12(1), 13-24.

Berger, J., & Cunningham, G. C. (1981). The development of eye contact between mothers and normal versus Down's syndrome infants. Developmental Psychology, 17(5), 678-689.

Berger, J., & Cunningham, C. C. (1983). Development of early vocal behaviors and interactions in Down's syndrome and nonhandicapped infant-mother pairs. Developmental Psychology, 19(3), 322-331.

Berkson, G. (1960). An analysis of reaction time in normal and mentally deficient young mongoloids. III: variation of stimulus and response complexity. Journal of Mental Deficiency Research, 4, 69-77.

Bernheimer, L. P., & Keogh, B. K. (1986). Developmental disabilities in preschool children. Advances in Special Education, 5, 61-93.

Berry, D. M. (1924). An investigation of fifty cases of mongolian imbecility. British Journal of Childrens Deseases, 21, 259.

Berry, P., Gunn, P., & Andrews, R. (1980). Behavior of Down syndrome infants in a strange situation. American Journal of Mental Deficiency, 85(3), 213-218.

Berry, P., Matthews, P., & Middleton, B. (1977). Pattern of interaction between and her Down's syndrome child: a single case ethological study. Exceptional Child, 24(3), 156-164.

Berry, P., Groeneweg, G., Gibson, D., & Brown, R. I. (1984). Mental development of adults with Down syndrome. American Journal of Mental Deficiency, 89(3), 252-256.

Berry, P., Gunn, P., & Andrews, R. J., (1984). The behaviour of Down's syndrome children using the lock box: a research note. Journal of Child Psychology & Psychiatry & Allied Disciplines, 25(1), 125-131.

Berry, P., & Gunn, P. (1984). Maternal influence on the task behaviors of young Down's syndrome children. Journal of Mental Deficiency Research, 28(4), 269-274.

Berry, P., Gunn, P., & Andrews, R. (1980). Behavior of Down syndrome infants in a strange situation. American Journal of Mental Deficiency, 85(3), 213-218.

Bidder, R. T., Hewitt, K. E., & Gray, O. P. (1983). Evaluation of teaching methods in a home-based training scheme for developmentally delayed preschool children. Child Care, Health & Development, 9(1), 1-12.

Bigum, H. B., Dustman, R. E., & Beck, E. C. (1970). Visual and somato-sensory evoked responses from mongoloid and normal children. Electroencephalography and Clinical Neurophysiology Journal, 28, 576-585.

Bigum, H. B. (1969). Visual and somatosensory evoked responses from mongoloid and normal children. Abstracts International, 30(4-B), 1913.

Bilovsky, D., & Share, J. (1965). The ITPA and Down's syndrome: an exploratory study. American Journal of Mental Deficiency, 70, 78-82.

Birch, H. G., & Demb, H. (1959). The formation and extinction of conditioned reflexes in 'brain-damaged' and mongoloid children. Journal of Nervous and Mental Diseases, 129, 162-170.

Blacher, J., & Meyers, C. E. (1983). A review of attachment formation and disorder of handicapped children. American Journal of Mental Deficiency, 87(4), 359-371.

Black, A. H., & Thomas, L. D. (1966). Differential effectiveness of primary, secondary, and social reinforcement in discrimination learning of mongoloids: preliminary note. Perceptual and Motor Skills, 23, 585-586.

Blacketer-Simmonds, D. A. (1953). An investigation into the supposed differences existing between mongols and other mentally defective subjects with regard to certain psychological traits. J. Ment. Sci. London, 99, 702-719.

Blake, J. N. (1969). A therapeutic construct for two seven-year-old nonverbal boys. Journal of Speech & Hearing Disorders, 34(4), 363-369.

Bleile, K. (1982). Consonant ordering in Down's syndrome

phonology. _Journal of Communication Disorders_, _15_(4) 275-285.

Bleile, D., & Schwarz, I. (1984). Three perspectives of the speech of children with Down's syndrome. _Journal of Communication Disorders_, _17_(2), 87-94.

Blessing, K. R. (1959). The middle range mongoloid in trainable classes. _American Journal of Mental Deficiency_, _63_, 812-821.

Bochner, S. (1983). The infant hospital as a setting for language acquisition in the handicapped. _Australia & New Zealand Journal of Developmental Disabilities_, _9_(2), 65-73.

Bochner, S. (1986). Development of intentionality in the vocalization of handicapped infants reared in a hospital setting. _Australia & New Zealand Journal of Developmental Disabilities_, _12_(1), 55-66.

Bokor, C. R. (1976). A comparison of musical and verbal responses of mentally retarded children. _Journal of Music Therapy_, _13_(2), 101-108.

Bonaccorsi, M. T., Gagon, J., Destooper, J., & Tousignant, F. (1968). Relationship between the genotype and phenotype for mongolism. _Revista de Psicologia General y Aplicada_, _23_(93), 467-479.

Booth, T. (1981). Educating children with Down's syndrome in an ordinary school. _Early Child Development and Care_, _10_.

Bowler, D. M., Cuffin, J., & Kierman, C. (1985). Dichotic listening of verbal and non-verbal material by Down's syndrome children and children of normal intelligence. _Cortex_, _21_(4), 637-644.

Bradley-Johnson, S., & Friedrich, D. D. (1981). Exploratory behavior in Down's syndrome and normal infants. _Applied Research in Mental Retardation_, _2_(3), 213-228.

Bradway, K. P. (1939). Hysterical mutism in mongol imbecile. _J. Abnormal Soc. Psych._, _31_, 458.

Bramza, A. F., Witt, P. A., Linford, A. G., & Jeanrenaud, C. (1969). Responses of mongoloid children to colored block presentation. _Perceptual & Motor Skills_, _29_(3), 1008.

Brandenburg, N. A. (1986). The familial aggregation of Down's syndrome, senile dementia of the Alzheimer's type, and other clinical disorders. _Dissertation Abstracts International_, _46_(11-B), 3709.

Brauner, A., & Brauner, F. (1976). Musical aids to assist therapy in mentally retarded and autistic children. Vie Medicale au Canada Francais, 5(10), 1024-1026, 1037-1039.

Bricker, W. A., & McLoughlin, C. S. (1982). Exploration of parental teaching style: technical note. Perceptual & Motor Skills, 55(3, pt. 2), 1174.

Brickey, M. P., (1978). The use of bimanual assembly methods by workers with mental retardation. Dissertation Abstracts International, 38(11-B), 5558-5559.

Bridges, A., & Smith, J. V. (1984). Synactic comprehension in Down's syndrome children. British Journal of Psychology, 75(2), 187-196.

Bridges, F. A., & Cicchetti, D. (1982). Mothers' ratings of the temperament characteristics of Down syndrome infants. Developmental Psychology, 18(2), 238-244.

Brink, M., & Grundlingh, E. M. (1976). Performance of persons with Down's syndrome on two projective techniques. Am. J. Ment. Defic., 81(3), 265-270.

Brinker, R. P., & Lewis, M. (1982). Making the world work with microcomputers: a learning prosthesis for handicapped infants. Exceptional Children, 49(2), 163-170.

Brinkworth, R., & Collins, J. E. (1969). Improving Mongol Babies and Introducing Them to School. Belfast: National Society for Mentally Handicapped Children.

Broffman, S. B. (1981). The development of positional patterns in the early multi-morphemic utterances of five Down's and two normal children: a descriptive comparison. Dissertation Abstracts International, 42(2-A) 607-608.

Brooks-Gunn, J., & Lewis, M. (1982). Development of play behavior in handicapped and normal infants. Topics in Early Childhood Special Education, 2(3), 14-27.

Brooks-Gunn, J., & Lewis, M. (1984). Maternal responsivity in interactions with handicapped infants. Child Development, 55(3), 782-793.

Brooksbank, B. W., & Balazs, R. (1984). Superoxide dismutase, glutathione peroxidase and lipoperoxidation in Down's syndrome fetal brain. Developmental Brain Research, 16(1), 37-44.

Brophy, K., & Stone-Zukowski, D. (1984). Social and play behaviour of special needs and non-special needs toddlers. Early Child Development & Care, 13(2), 137-154.

Broughton, E. D. (1976). Satisfaction of mothers of children with PKU, mongolism and autism with professional assistance. Dissertation Abstracts International, 36(8-B), 4145.

Brousseau, K., & Brainerd, M. G. (1928). Mongolism: a Study of the Psychical and Mental Characteristics of Mongoloid Imbeciles. Baltimore: Williams & Wilkins.

Brown, R. I. (1976). Psychology and Education of Slow Learners. Boston, MA: Routledge & Kegan Paul.

Brown, R. I., & Clarke, A. D. B. (1963). The effects of auditory distraction on institutionalized subnormal and severely subnormal persons. Journal of Mental Deficiency Research, 7, 1-8.

Brown, W. T., et al. (1985). Localization of chromosome 21 probes by in situ hybridization. Symposium of the National Down Syndrome Society: Molecular Structure of the Number 21 Chromosome and Down Syndrome. Annals of the New York Academy of Sciences, 450, 69-83.

Brushfield, T. (1924). Mongolism. British Journal of Children's Diseases, 21, 240.

Brzozowska, H., & Kaminska, M. (1960). Cerebral abscesses in a 4-year-old boy with mongolism and Fallot's syndrome. Pol. Tyg. Lek., 15, 1123-1124.

Buchka, M. (1971). The language of the mongoloid child. Heilpadagogik, 40(4), 308-312.

Buck, C., Valentine, G. H., & Hamilton, K. (1969). A study of microsymptoms in the parents and sibs of patients with Down's syndrome. American Journal of Mental Deficiency, 73(5), 683-692.

Buck, J. N. (1955). The sage: an unusual mongoloid. In A. Burton and R. E. Harris (eds.), Clinical Studies of Personality. New York: Harper & Rowe.

Buckhalt, J. A., Rutherford, R. B., & Goldberg, K. E. (1978). Verbal and nonverbal interaction of mothers with their Down's syndrome and nonretarded infants. Am. J. Ment. Defic., 82(4), 337-343.

Budgell, P. (1985). Integrating children with severe learning difficulties: Fantasy or reality? I. Educational & Child Psychology, 2(3), 60-68.

Buium, N., Rynders, J., & Turnure, J. (1974). Early maternal linguistic environment of normal and Down's syndrome language-learning children. American Journal of Mental Deficiency, 79, 52-58.

Bullard, W. N. (1911). Mongolian idiocy. Boston Medical Surgical Journal, 164, 56.

Buresch, M. A. (1975). Mongoloid Psychology: Questions and Principles Concerning the Down's Syndrome Child. Detroit, Michigan: Mongoloid Achievements Foundation, Troy, Michigan.

Burger, P. C., & Vogel, F. S. (1973). The development of the pathologic changes of Alzheimer's disease and senile dementia in patients with Down's syndrome. Am. J. Pathol., 73(2), 457-476.

Burr, D. B., & Rohr, A. (1978). Patterns of psycholinguistic development in the severely mentally retarded: a hypothesis. Soc. Biology, 25(1), 15-22.

Burstein, N. D. (1986). The effects of classroom organization on mainstreamed preschool children. Exceptional Children, 52(5), 425-434.

Butterworth, G., & Cicchetti, D. (1978). Visual calibration of posture in normal and motor retarded Down's syndrome infants. Perception, 7(5), 513-525.

Buttlerfield, E. C. (1961). A provocative case of over-achievement by a mongoloid. American Journal of Mental Deficiency, 66, 444-448.

Byck, M. (1968). Cognitive differences among diagnostic groups of retardates. Am. J. Ment. Defic., 73(1), 97-101.

Byrne, J. A. (1985). A descriptive study of flexibility in communicative style in a Down's syndrome child. Dissertation Abstracts International, 45(8-A), 2480.

Caccamo, J. M., & Yater, A. C. (1972). The ITPA and Negro children with Down's syndrome. Except. Child., 38(8), 642-643.

Caccamo, J. M. (1972). An investigation of psycholinguistic abilities of negro children with Down's syndrome. Dissertation Abstracts International, 33(3-A), 1041-1042.

Canal, T. M. (1979). A follow-up assessment project of a multidisciplinary intervention program for children with Down syndrome. Dissertation Abstracts International, 39(7-B), 3501.

Cantor, G. N., & Girardeau, F. L. (1959). Rhythmic discrimination ability in mongoloid and normal children. American Journal of Mental Deficiency, 63, 621-625.

Cardoso-Martins, C., Mervis, C. B., & Mervis, C. A.

(1985). Early vocabulary acquisition by children with Down syndrome. American Journal of Mental Deficiency, 90(2), 177-184.

Cardoso-Martins, C., & Mervis, C. B. (1985). Maternal speech to prelinguistic children with Down syndrome. American Journal of Mental Deficiency, 89(5), 451-458.

Carlson, B. W., & Gingland, D. R. (1961). Play Activities for the Retarded Child. New York: Abingdon Press.

Carr, J. (1970). Mental and motor development in young mongol children. Journal of Mental Deficiency Research, 14, 205-220.

Carr, J. (1971). A comparative study of the development of mongol and normal children from 0 to 4 years. Unpublished Ph.D. Thesis, University of London.

Carr, J. (1975). Young Children with Down's Syndrome: Their Development, Upbringing and Effect on Their Families. London: Butterworth and Company.

Carter, C. H. (1967). Unpredictability of mental development in Down's syndrome. Southern Medical Journal, 60, 834.

Carter, D., & Clark, L. (1973). MA intellectual assessment by operant conditioning of Down's syndrome children. Mental Retardation, 11(3), 39-41.

Casanova, M. F., Walker, L. C., Whitehouse, P. J., & Price, D. (1985). Abnormalities of the nucleus basalis in Down's syndrome. Ann. Neurol., 18, 310-313.

Castaldo, V. (1968). Electroencephalographic study of sleep patterns of mongoloids as related to degree of mental retardation. Psychophysiology, 5(2), 213.

Castaldo, V. (1969). Down's syndrome: A study of sleep patterns related to level of mental retardation. Am. J. Ment. Defic., 74(2), 187-190.

Cavalieri, S. (1957). The encephalographical picture of mongolism. Fracastoro, 50, 303-315.

Centerwall, S. W., & Centerwall, W. R. (1958). An Introduction to Your Child Who Has Mongolism. Los Angeles: College of Medical Evangelists.

Centerwall, S. W., & Centerwall, W. R. (1960). A study of children with mongolism reared in the home compared to those reared away from the home. Pediatrics, 25, 678-685.

Cernay, J., & Hudakova, G. (1976). Development of children with Down's syndrome. Cesk. Pediatr., 31(8), 453-

458.

Certo, N., Messullo, K., & Hunter, D. (1985). The effect of total task chain training on the acquisition of bus-person job skills at a full service community restaurant. Education & Training of the Mentally Retarded, 20(2), 148-156.

Chen, A. T., et al. (1969). Birth weight and mortality in Down's syndrome infants. Social Biology, 16(4), 290-291.

Chen, H., et al. (1978). A developmental assessment chart for noninstitutionalized Down syndrome children. Growth, 42(2), 157-165.

Cicchetti, D., & Sroufe, L. A. (1976). The relationship between affective and cognitive development in Down's syndrome infants. Child. Dev., 47(4), 920-929.

Cicchetti, D., & Serafica, F. C. (1981). Interplay among behavior systems: illustrations from attachment, affiliation, and wariness in young children with Down's syndrome. Developmental Psychology, 17(1),36-49.

Clark, G. N., & Seifer, R. (1983). Facilitating mother-infant communication: a treatment model for high-risk and developmentally-delayed infants. Infant Mental Health Journal, 4(2) 67-81.

Clarke, C. M., Edwards, J. H., & Smallpeice, V. (1961). Trisomy/normal mosaicism in an intelligent child with some mongoloid characters. Lancet, 1028-1030.

Clarke, C. M., Ford, C. E., Edwards, J. H., & Smallpeice, V. (1963). 21-trisomy/normal mosaicism in an intelligent child with some mongoloid characteristics. Lancet, 2, 1229.

Clausen, J. (1968). Behavioral characteristics of Down syndrome subjects. Am. J. Ment. Defic., 73(1), 118-126.

Clausen, J., Sersen, E. A., & Lidsky, A. (1977). Sleep patterns in mental retardation: Down's syndrome. Electroencephalogr. Clin. Neurophysiol., 43(2), 183-191.

Clements, P. R., Bates, M. V., & Hafer, M. (1976). Variability within Down's syndrome (trisomy-21): Empirically observed sex differences in IQs. Ment. Retard., 14(1), 30-31.

Clements, P. R., Hafer, M., & Pollock, J. L. (1978). Parental education and rate of intellectual development of Down's syndrome (Trisomy 21) individuals. Research & the Retarded, 5(1), 15-19.

388 Bibliography

Clunies-Ross, G. G. (1979). Accelerating the development of Down's syndrome infants and young children. Journal of Special Education, 13(2), 169-177.

Coggins, T. E. (1976). The classification of relational meaning expressed in the early two-word utterances of Down's syndrome children. Dissertation Abstracts International, 37(6-A), 3547-3548.

Coggins, T. E. (1979). Relational meaning encoded in the two-word utterances of stage 1 Down's syndrome children. Journal of Speech and Hearing Research, 22(1), 166-178.

Coggins, T. E., & Morrison, J. A. (1981). Spontaneous imitations of Down's syndrome children: a lexical analysis. Journal of Speech & Hearing Research, 24(2) 303-308.

Coggins, T. E., & Stoel-Gammon, C. (1982). Clarification strategies used by four Down's syndrome children for maintaining normal conversational interaction. Education & Training of the Mentally Retarded, 17(1), 65-67.

Coggins, T. E., Carpenter, R. L., & Owings, N. O. (1983). Examining early intentional communication in Down's syndrome and nonretarded children. British Journal of Disorders of Communication, 18(2), 98-106.

Coleman, T. W. (1960). A comparison of young brain-injured and mongolian mentally defective children on perception, thinking and behavior. Doctoral dissertation (unpublished), University of Michigan.

Coleman, M., et al. (1985). A double blind study of vitamin B-sub-6 in Down's syndrome infants: I. clinical and biochemical results. Journal of Mental Deficiency Research, 29(3), 233-240.

Collmann, R. D., & Stoller, A. (1969). Shift of child birth to younger mothers, and its effect on the incidence of mongolism in Victoria, Australia, 1939-1964. Journal of Mental Deficiency Research, 13(1), 13-19.

Colon, E. J. (1972). The structure of the cerebral cortex in Down's syndrome. Neuropaediatrie, 3, 362-376.

Colton, R. E. (1973). A study of pure tone thresholds and intelligence in institutionalized and non-institutionalized Down's syndrome. Dissertation Abstracts International, 34(5-A), 2420.

Conacher, D. G. (1969). Mental retardation in Angus County, Scotland. American Journal of Mental Deficiency, 73(6), 970-980.

Connolly, B., & Russell, F. (1976). Interdisciplinary early intervention program. Phys. Ther., 56(2), 155-158.

Cook, N. L. (1976). The acquisition of dimensional adjectives as a function of the underlying perceptual event. Dissertation Abstracts International, 37(5-B), 2475-2476.

Cook, A. S. & Culp, R. E. (1981). Mutual play of mothers with their Down's syndrome and normal infants. International Journal of Rehabilitation Research, 4(4), 542-544.

Cook, A. S. (1984). Developmental aspects of postural control in normal and Down's syndrome children. Dissertation Abstracts International, 44(7-A), 2082-2083.

Cooke, R. E. (1970). See in a report on premature senility found in brains of mongoloids. Pediatric News, 4, 1.

Cooke, N. L., & Heron, T. E. (1982). Integrating a Down's syndrome child in a classroom peer tutoring system: a case report. Mental Retardation, 20(1), 22-25.

Coraza, M. C. (1977). Motor development of Down's syndrome toddlers measured by the Hahnemann Pre-School Scales for Exceptional Children. Dissertation Abstracts International, 38(4-A), 2039-2040.

Coriat, L. F., & Fejirman, N. (1963). Infantile spasms in children with trisomy 21. La Semana Med. Ed. Pediat., 15, 493-500.

Coriat, L. F., de Theslenco, L., & Waksman, J. (1967). The effects of psychomotor stimulation on the IQ of young children with trisomy-21. Proceedings of the First Congress of the I.A.S.S.M.D., 377-385.

Cornwell, A. C., & Birch, H. G. (1969). Psychological and social development in home-reared children with Down's syndrome (mongolism). American Journal of Mental Deficiency, 74, 341-350.

Cornwell, A. C. (1974). Development of language, abstraction and numerical concept formation in Down's syndrome children. American Journal of Mental Deficiency, 79, 179-190.

Cottrell, D. J., & Crisp, A. H. (1984). Anorexia nervosa in Down's syndrome: a case report. British Journal of Psychiatry, 145, 195-196.

Cowie, V. (1972). Cytogenetical aspects of mental subnormality. British Journal of Mental Subnormality, 18(1), 31-35.

Cowie, V. A. (1970). A Study of the Early Development of Mongols. Oxford: Pergamon Press.

Cox, D. D., & Epstein, C. J. (1985). Comparative gene mapping of human chromosone 21 and mouse chromosome 16. Symposium of the National Down Syndrome Society: Molecular Structure of the Number 21 Chromosome and Downs Syndrome. Annals of the New York Academy of Sciences, 450, 169-177.

Coyle, J. T., Oster-Granite, M. L., & Gearhart, J. D. (1986). The neurobiologic consequences of Down syndrome. Special issue: The neurobiologic consequences of autosomal trisomy in mice and men. Brain Research Bulletin, 16(6), 773-787.

Crawlwy, S. R., & Spiker, D. (1983). Mother-child interactions involving two-year-olds with Down syndrome: a look at individual differences. Child Development, 54(5), 1312-1323.

Cronk, C. E. (1978). Growth of children with Down's syndrome: Birth to age 3 years. Pediatrics, 61(4), 564-568.

Crookshank, F. G. (1924). The Mongol in Our Midst. London: Kegan Paul.

Cullen, S. M. (1981). Social development and feeding milestones of young Down's syndrome children. American Journal of Mental Deficiency, 85(4), 410-415.

Cunningham, C. C. (1981). Hearing loss and treatment in young Down's syndrome children. Child Care, Health, and Development, 7(6), 357-374.

Cunningham, C. C. (1981). The development of eye contact between mothers and normal versus Down's syndrome infants. Developmental Psychology, 17(5), 678-689.

Cunningham, C. C., & Sloper, P. (1984). The relationship between maternal ratings of first word vocabulary and Reynell Language Scores. British Journal of Educational Psychology, 54(2), 160-167.

Cunningham, C. C., Glenn, S. M., Wilkinson, P., & Sloper, P. (1985). Mental ability, symbolic play, and receptive and expressive language of young children with Down's syndrome. Journal of Child Psychology & Psychiatry & Allied Disciplines, 26(2), 255-265.

Cutler, N. R. (1986). Cerebral metabolism as measured with positron emission tomography (PET) and (18F) 2-deoxy-D-glucose: healthy aging, Alzheimer's disease, and Down syndrome. Prog. Neuropsychopharmacol. Biol. Psychiatry, 10(3-5), 355-390.

Cutler, N. R., Heston, H. L., Davies, P., Haxby, J., & Schapiro, M. (1985). NIH conference. Alzheimer's disease and Down's syndrome: new insights. Ann. Intern. Med., 60(10), 675-689.

Dalton, A. J., & Crapper-Mclachlan, D. R. (1986). Clinical expression of Alzheimer's disease in Down's syndrome. Psychiatr. Clin. North Am., 9(4), 398-405.

Dalton, A. J., Crapper, D. R., & Schlotterer, G. R. (1974). Alzheimer's disease in Down's syndrome: Visual retention deficits. Cortex, 10(4), 366-377.

Dameron, L. E. (1963). Developmental intelligence of infants with mongolism. Child Dev., 34, 733-738.

Daniels, J. E. (1977). Family functioning of children with Down's syndrome. Dissertation Abstracts International, 37(8-A), 5360.

Davidenkova, E. F. (1966). Down's Disease: Clinical and Genetical Investigations. Leningrad: 'Medicine' Publishing House.

Davidoff, L. M. (1928). The brain in mongolian idiocy. A report of ten cases. Arch. Neurol. Psychiatry Chicago, 20, 1229-1257.

Davidson, J. N., Rumsby, G., & Niswander, L. A. (1985). Expression of genes on human chromosome 21. Symposium of the National Down Syndrome Society: Molecular Structure of the Number 21 Chromosome and Down Syndrome, Annals of the New York Academy of Sciences, 450, 43-54.

Davis, J. C., et al. (1964). Steroid excretion of dehydroepiandrosterone in young mothers of mongols. Lancet, 1, 782-785.

Davis, W. E. (1981). A vibratory system analysis of motor control in selected Down syndrome subjects. Dissertation Abstracts International, 41(9-A), 3941.

De Myer, W. (1965). Closed metopic suture with trigonocephaly in Down's syndrome. Neurology Minneapolis, 15, 756-760.

Dehaven, E. D. (1977). An experimental analysis of receptive language training. Dissertation Abstracts International, 37(10-B), 5347.

Dehaven, E. (1981). Teaching three severely retarded children to follow instructions. Education & Training of the Mentally Retarded, 16(1), 36-48.

DeLee, C., & Petre, Q. O. (1976). Eye-movement density during sleep in normal and pathological neonates and infants. Waking & Sleeping, 1, 45-48.

Demeedov, A. U. (1972). The influence of sex on the phenotypic characteristics of Down's syndrome. Defeltologia, 1, 33-37.

Desforges, M., & Lindsay, G. (1985). Integration of three to five year olds with special needs. Educational & Child Psychology, 2(3), 123-129.

Destrooper, J., Beland, C., Leblanc, L., & Zegray, W. (1970). Intellectual development of hospitalized mongoloid children. Union Med. Can., 99(2), 264-268.

Devine, E. A., et al. (1985). Molecular Quantitation of Aneuploid Conditions Using Chromosome 21 as a Model. Symposium of the National Down Syndrome Society: Molecular Structure of the Number 21 Chromosome and Down Syndrome, Annals of the New York Academy of Sciences, 450, 85-94.

Dey, J. (1971). Survey of 500 cases of Down's syndrome. Australian Journal of Mental Retardation, 1(5), 154-159.

Diamond, E. F., & Moon, M. S. (1961). Neuromuscular development in mongoloid children. American Journal of Mental Deficiency Research, 66, 218-221.

Dicks-Mireaux, M. J. (1966). Development of intelligence of children with Down's syndrome. Preliminary report. Journal of Mental Deficiency Research, 10, 89-93.

Dicks-Mireaux, M. J. (1972). Mental development of infants with Down's syndrome. American Journal of Mental Deficiency, 77(1), 26-32.

Dmitriev, V. (1972). Techniques for teaching early eye-hand coordination. Sharing Our Caring, 11(3), 11-15.

Dmitriev, V. (1974). Motor and cognitive development in early education. In: N. G. Haring (ed.), Behavior of Exceptional Children: An Introduction to Special Education. Columbus, Ohio: Charles E. Merrill.

Dmitriev, V. (1976). Modifying teacher behavior in order to decrease the self-stimulation and disruptive behavior of an eight year old Down's syndrome boy. Unpublished case study, Experimental Education Unit, Uni-

versity of Washington
Dmitriev, V. (1977). Programs for Down's syndrome child-
ren at the Experimental Education Unit. Proc. CPRI
Symp. 1975 -- Early Intervention, London, Ontario,
Canada.
Dmitriev, V. (1978). Programs and strategies for early
childhood education. In: N.G. Haring (ed.), Behavior of
Exceptional Children, 2nd Ed., Columbus, Ohio: Charles
E. Merrill.
Dmitriev, V. D. (1980). Synchronous visual reinforcement
of babbling in infants with Down's syndrome. Disserta-
tion Abstracts International, 40(12-A, pt.1), 6228.
Dmitriev, V., & Hawkins, J. (1974). Susie never used to
say a word. Teach. Except. Child., 6(2), 68-76.
Dmitriev, V., & Hayden, A. H. (1975). New perspectives on
children with Down's syndrome (Abstract). Sharing Our
Caring, 5(4), 15.
Dmitriev, V., Kuhn, P., & Hilenbrand, J. (1977). Speech
perception in infants with Down's syndrome. Model Pre-
school Center for Handicapped Children, Experimental
Education Unit, University of Washington.
Dmitriev, V., & Oelwein, P. (1977). Children with Down's
syndrome learn self-help skills in a preschool setting.
J. Prac. Approach Devel. Hand., 1(3), 7-12.
Dmitriev, V. D. (1980). Synchronous visual reinforcement
of babbling in infants with Down's syndrome. Disserta-
tion Abstracts International, 40(12-A, pt. 1), 6228.
Dodd, B. (1975). Recognition and reproduction of words by
Down's syndrome and non-Down's syndrome children. Amer-
ican Journal of Mental Deficiency, 80(3), 306-311.
Dodd, B. (1976). A comparison of the phonological systems
of mental age matched, normal, severely subnormal and
Down's syndrome children. British Journal of Disorders
of Communication, 11, 27-42.
Dodd, B. (1972). Comparison of babbling patterns in normal and Down's syndrome infants. Journal of Mental Deficiency Research, 16, 35-40.
Dogherty, P. (1978). Mental handicap. Operant conditioning: Success is sweet as John speaks up. Nurs. Mirror,
147(20), 45-48.
Domino, G. (1965). Personality traits in institutionalized mongoloids. American Journal of Mental Deficiency,
69, 568-570.

Domino, G., Goldschmid, M., & Kaplan, M. (1964). Personality traits in institutionalized mongoloid girls. Am. J. Ment. Defic., 68, 498.

Donoghue, E. C., et al. (1970). Some factors affecting age of walking in a mentally retarded population. Developmental Medicine & Child Neurology, 12(6), 781-792.

Du Verglas, G. (1985). Comparative follow-up study of Down's syndrome children who attended the model preschool program. Dissertation Abstracts International, 46(2-A), 398.

Duche, D. J., & Lecuyer, R., 1966. Psychoneurotic states in mongoloids. Annales Medico Psychologiques, 2, 107.

Duffy, L. and Wishart, J. G., 1987. A comparison of two procedures for teaching discrimination to Down's syndrome and normal children. British Journal of Educational Psychology, 57, 265-278.

Duffy, A. T., & Nietupski, J. (1985). Acquisition and maintenance of video game initiation, sustaining and termination skills. Education & Training of the Mentally Retarded, 20(2), 157-162.

Dunlop, K. H., Stoneman, Z., & Cantrell, M. L. (1980). Social interactions of exceptional and other children in a mainstreamed preschool. Exceptional Children, 47(2), 132-141.

Dunsdon, M. I., Carter, C. O., & Huntley, R. (1960). Upper end range of intelligence in mongolism. Lancet, 1, 565-568.

Dunst, C. J. (1976). Attitudes of parents with children in contrasting family education programs. Mental Retardation Bulletin, 4(3). 120-132.

Dunst, C. J. (1980). Cognitive-social aspects of communicative exchanges between mothers and their Down syndrome infants and mothers and their nonretarded infants. Dissertation Abstracts International, 41(1-B), 394.

Dunst, C. J., & Rheingrover, R. M. (1983). Structural characteristics of sensorimotor development among Down's syndrome infants. Journal of Mental Deficiency Research, 27(1), 11-22.

Dunst, C. J. (1981). Test settings and the sensorimotor performance of infants with Down's syndrome. Perceptual & Motor Skills, 53(2), 575-578.

Dunst, C. J. (1981). Social concomitants of cognitive

mastery in Down's syndrome infants. <u>Infant Mental Health Journal</u>, <u>2</u>(3), 144-154.

Durling, D., & Benda, C. E. (1952). Mental growth curves in untreated institutionalized mongoloid patients. <u>American Journal of Mental Deficiency</u>, <u>56</u>, 578.

Dustman, R. E. & Callner, D. A. (1979). Cortical evoked responses and response decrement in nonretarded and Down's syndrome individuals. <u>American Journal of Mental Deficiency</u>, <u>83</u>, 391-397.

Duthie, P. R. (1983). A biomechanical analysis of the jump of institutionalized individuals with Down's syndrome: a longitudinal and cross-sectional study. <u>Dissertation Abstracts International</u>, <u>43</u>(9-A), 2926.

Earl, C. J. C. (1934). The primitive catatonic psychoses of idiocy. <u>British Journal of Medical Psychology</u>, <u>14</u>, 3-11.

Eck, M. (1966). Psychological problems posed by trisomy-21. <u>Medicine Infantile</u>, <u>73</u>, 479-481.

Effgen, S. K. (1984). An analysis of the effects of visual and somatosensory-vestibular input on the postural reactions of infants having Down syndrome. <u>Dissertation Abstracts International</u>, <u>45</u>(5-A), 1364.

Efinski, D., et al. (1974). Klinefelter's and Down's syndrome in an adolescent with abnormal EEG. <u>Clin. Genet.</u> <u>5</u>(2), 81-85.

Eisner, D. A. (1983). Down's syndrome and aging: is senile dementia inevitable?. <u>Psychological Reports</u>, <u>52</u>(1) 119-124.

Ellingson, R. J., Menolascino, F. J., & Eisen, J. D. (1970). Clinical-EEG relationships in mongoloids confirmed by karyotype. <u>American Journal of Mental Deficiency</u>, <u>74</u>(5), 645- 650.

Elliott, D. (1985). Manual asymmetries in the performance of sequential movement by adolescents and adults with Down syndrome. <u>American Journal of Mental Deficiency</u>, <u>90</u>(1), 90-97.

Elliott, D., Weeks, D. J., & Jones, R. (1985). Lateral asymmetries in finger-tapping by adolescents and young adults with Down syndrome. <u>American Journal of Mental Deficiency</u>, <u>90</u>(4), 472-475.

Ellis, A., & Beechley, R. M. (1950). A comparison of matched groups of mongoloid and non-mongoloid feeble-minded children. <u>American Journal of Mental Deficiency</u>,

54, 464-468.

Ellis, W. G., McCulloch, J. R., & Corley, C. L. (1974). Presenile dementia in Down's syndrome. Ultrastructural identity with Alzheimer's disease. Neurology Minneaneapolis, 249(2), 101-106.

Elovaara, I. (1984). Proteins in serum and cerebrospinal fluid in demented patients with Down's syndrome. Acta Neurologica Scandinavica, 69(5), 302-305.

Engler, M. (1949). Mongolism. Bristol: John Wright & Sons.

Epstein, C. J., Cox, D. R., & Epstein, L. B. (1985). Mouse trisomy 16: an animal model of human trisomy 21 (Down syndrome). Symposium of the National Down Syndrome Society: Molecular Structure of the Number 21 Chromosome and Down Syndrome, Annals of the New York Academy of Sciences, 450, 157-168.

Ershow, A. G. (1986). Growth in black and white children with Down syndrome. American Journal of Mental Deficiency, 90(5), 507-512.

Esenther, S. E. (1984). Developmental coaching of the Down syndrome infant. American Journal of Occup. Ther., 38(7), 440-445.

Evans, D. (1976). Language development in Down's syndrome retardates: A factorial study. Contemporary Educational Psychology, 1(4), 319-328.

Evans, D. (1977). The development of language abilities in mongols: A correlational study. Journal of Mental Deficiency Research, 21(2), 103-117.

Evans, D., & Hampson, M. (1969). The language of mongols. British Journal of Disorders of Communication, 3, 171-181.

Evans, K., & Carter, C. O. (1954). Care and disposal of mongolian defectives. Lancet, 1, 960-963.

Faienza, C., & Piantoni, G. (1962). Contribution to the psychological study of the mongoloid syndrome. Lattante, 33, 795-820.

Farb, J., & Thorne, J. M. (1978). Improving the generalized mnemonic performance of a Down's syndrome child. J. Appl. Behav. Anal., 11(3), 413-419.

Fedotov, D. D., Shapiro, Y. L., & Vaindrukh, F. A. (1968). Several features of paroxysmal episodes in Down's disease. Zhurnal Nevropatologii i Psikhiatrii, 68(1), 1516-1521.

Fehr,   F.   S.   (1976).   Psychophysiological   studies   of   Down's
syndrome   children   and   the   effects   of   environmental   en-
richment.   In: R.   Karrer   (ed.),   Developmental   Psycho-
Physiology   of   Mental   Retardation,   Springfield,   Illi-
nios: C.   Thomas.
Fennell,   C.   H.   (1904).   Mongolian   imbecility.   Journal   of
Mental   Science,   50,   32.
Fewell,   R.   R.,   &   Sandall,   S.   R.   (1986).   Developmental
testing   of   handicapped   infants: a   measurement   dilemma.
Topics   in   Early   Childhood   Special   Education,   6(3),   86-
99.
Field,   T.   M.,   &   Roseman,   S.   (1982).   The   play   of   handicapped   preschool   children   with   handicapped   and   non-
handicapped   peers   in   integrated   and   nonintegated
situations.   Topics   in   Early   Childhood   Special   Education,   2(3),   28-38.
Fields,   D.   L.,   &   Gibson,   D.   (1971).   Forecasting   mental
growth   for   at-home   mongols   (Down's   syndrome).   Journal
of   Mental   Deficiency   Research,   15,   163-168.
Filler,   J.   W.   (1976).   Modifying   maternal   teaching   style:
Effects   of   task   arrangement   on   the   match-to   example
performance   of   retarded   preschool-aged   children.   American   Journal   of   Mental   Deficiency,   80(6),   602-612.
Fink,   W.   T.,   &   Brice-Gray,   K.   J.   (1979).   The   effects   of
two   teaching   strategies   on   the   acquisition   and   recall
of   an   academic   task   by   moderately   and   severely   retarded
preschool   children.   Mental   Retardation,   17(1),   8-12.
Finley,   S.   C.,   Finley,   W.   H.,   Rosecrans,   C.   J.,   &
Phillips,   C.   (1965).   Exceptional   intelligence   in   a   mongoloid   child   of   a   family   with   a   13-15/partial   21   (D/
partial   G)   translocation.   New   England   Journal   of   Medicine,   272,   1089-1092.
Fischer,   M.   A.   (1987).   Mother-child   interaction   in   preverbal   children   with   Down   syndrome.   Journal   of   Speech   &
Hearing   Disorders,   52(2),   179-190.
Fischer,   M.   A.   (1984).   An   analysis   of   preverbal   communicative   behavior   in   Down   syndrome   and   nonretarded   children.   Dissertation   Abstracts   International,   44(11-B),
3553.
Fisher,   L.   (1970).   Attention   deficit   in   brain   damaged
children.   American   Journal   of   Mental   Deficiency,   74(4),
502-508.
Fletcher,   D.   N.   (1976).   The   relationship   of   program   par-

ticipation and visitation to adaptive behavior and so-
cialization of institutionalized mentally retarded persons. Dissertation Abstracts International, 37(1-A),
219-220.

Folk, M. C., & Campbell, J. (1978). Teaching functional
reading to the TMR. Education & Training of the Mentally Retarded, 13(3), 322-326.

Ford, J. (1978). A multidisciplinary approach to early
intervention strategies for the education of the developmentally handicapped 0-3 year old: A pilot study.
Australian Journal of Mental Retardation, 5(1), 26-29.

Forman, T. M. (1967). The mongoloid child - behavioural
description. Special Education in Canada, 41, 9-11.

Foster, M. A. (1986). Families with young disabled children in family therapy. Family Therapy Collections, 18,
62-72.

Fowler, A. S. (1985). Language acquisition of Down's syndrome children: production and comprehension. Dissertation Abstracts International, 46(1-B) 324.

Fox, J., Shores, R., Lindeman, D., & Strain, P. (1986).
Maintaining social initiations of withdrawn handicapped
and nonhandicapped preschoolers through a response-
dependent fading technique. Journal of Abnormal Child
Psychology, 14(3), 387-396.

Fox, R., Karan, O. C. (1981). Regression including anorexia nervosa in a Down's syndrome adult: a seven year
follow-up. Journal of Behavior Therapy & Experimental
Psuchiatry, 12(4), 35.

Franceschi, B. F. (1963). Contribution to the study of
the psychomotor behavior of mental defectives. Evaluation by means of the Oseretzki Scale. Rass. Neuro-
psichiatr., 17, 237-251.

Francis, S. H. (1970). Behavior of low-grade institutionalized mongoloids: Changes with age. Am. J. Ment.
Defic., 75(1), 92-101.

Francis, S. H. (1971). The effects of own home and insti-
tutional-rearing on the behavioural development of normal and mongol children. J. Child Psychol. Psychiatry
Allied Discip., 12, 173-190.

Frank, H., & Fiedler, E. R. (1969). A multifactor behavioral approach to the genetic-etiological diagnosis of
mental retardation. Multivariate Behavioral Research,
4(2), 131-145.

Fraser, F. C., & Sadovnick, A. D. (1976). Correlation of IQ in subjects with Down syndrome and their parents and sibs. Journal of Mental Deficiency Research, 20(3), 179-182.

Fraser, W. I. (1978). Speech and language development of children with Down's syndrome. Dev. Med. Child. Neurol., 82(5), 429-432.

Fredericks, H. D. (1969). A comparison of the doman-delacato method and a behavior modification method upon the coordination of mongoloids. Dissertation Abstracts International, 30(4-A), 1430-1431.

Friedlander, B. Z., Sterritt, G. M., & Kirk, G. E. (1975). Exceptional Infant: III. Assessment & Intervention. New York, NY: Brunner/Mazel, XII, 242.

Frith, U., & Frith, C. D. (1974). Specific disabilities in Down's syndrome. J. Child Psychol. Psychiatry Applied Discip., 15(4), 293-301.

Frost, J. B. (1977). Provalence of mental handicap in the west of Ireland. Ir. Med. J., 70(8), 263-265.

Fukuma, E., Umezaea, Y, Kobayashi, K., & Motoike, M. (1974). Polygraphic study of the nocturnal sleep of children with Down's syndrome and endogenous mental retardation. Folia Psychihatr. Neurol. Jpn., 28(4), 333-345.

Fulton, R. T., & Lloyd, L. L. (1968). Hearing impairment in a population of children with Down's syndrome. American Journal of Mental Deficiency, 73(2), 298-302.

Gainer, R. B. (1981). The management of difficult behavior within a residential milieu. Milieu Therapy, 1(1) 17-21.

Gandhavadi, B., & Melvin J. L. (1985). Electrical blink reflex habituation in mentally retarded adults. Journal of Mental Deficiency Research, 29(1), 49-54.

Gath, A. (1972). The mental health of siblings of congenitally abnormal children. J. Child. Psychol. Psychiatry, 13(3), 211-218.

Gath, A. (1977). The impact of an abnormal child upon the parents. British Journal of Psychiatry, 130, 405-410.

Gath, A. (1986). Aging and mental handicap. Developmental Medicine & Child Neurology, 28(4), 519-522.

Gearhart, J., Singer, H. S., Moran, T. H., & Tiemeyer, M., et al. (1986). Mouse chimeras composed of trisomy 16 and normal (2N) cells: Preliminary studies. Special

issue: The neurobiologic consequences of autosomal trisomy in mice and men. Brain Research Bulletin, 16(6),
815-824.

Gibbs, E. L., Gibbs, F. A., & Hirsch, W. (1964). Rarity
of 14- and 6- per second positive spiking among mongoloids. Neurology, 14, 581-587.

Gibbs, M. V., & Thorpe, J. G. (1983). Personality stereotype of noninstitutionalized Down syndrome children.
American Journal of Mental Deficiency, 87(6), 601-605.

Gibson, D. (1966). Early developmental staging as a prophecy index in Down's syndrome. American Journal of
Mental Deficiency, 70, 825-828.

Gibson, D. (1966). Amentia level and physical concomitants of Down's syndrome: A curvilinear resolution. Am.
J. Ment. Defic., 71, 433-436.

Gibson, D. (1967). Intelligence in the mongoloid and his
parent. American Journal of Mental Deficiency, 71,
1014-1016.

Gibson, D. (1973). Karyotype variation and behavior in
Down's syndrome: methodological review. American Journal of Mental Deficiency, 78, 128-133.

Gibson, D. (1975). Chromosomal psychiatry and Down's syndrome. Canad. J. Behav. Sci/Rev. Canad. Sci. Comp.,
7(3), 167-191.

Gibson, D., & Gibbins, R. J. (1958). The relation of mongolian stigmata to intellectual status. American Journal of Mental Deficiency, 63, 345-348.

Gibson, D., & Pozsonyi, J. (1965). Morphological and behavioral consequences of chromosome subtype in mongolism. Am. J. Ment. Defic., 69, 801-804.

Gibson, D., Pozsonyi, J., & Zarfas, D. (1964). Dimensions
of mongolism: II. The interaction of clinical indices.
American Journal of Mental Deficiency, 68, 503-510.

Gibson, D., & Fields, D. L. (1984). Early infant stimulation programs for children with Down syndrome: a review
of effectiveness. Advances in Developmental and Behavioral Pediatrics, 5, 331-371.

Girardeau, F. L. (1959). The formation of discrimination
learning sets in mongoloids and normal children. Journal of Comparative and Physiological Psychology, 52,
566-570.

Giza, T., Szafran, A., Kobielowa, Z., Ostrowski, A., &
St. Epiniewski, M. (1972). Amino acids in cerebrospinal

fluid of children with Down's syndrome. Pol. Tyg. Lek., 27(4), 128-130.

Gleitman, L. R. (1981). Maturational determinants of language growth. Cognition, 10(1-3), 103-114.

Glenn, S. M., & Cunningham, C. C. (1984). Selective auditory preferences and the use of automated equipment by severely, profoundly, and multiply handicapped children. Journal of Mental Deficiency Research, 28(pt. 4), 281-296.

Glenn, S. M., & Cunningham, C. C. (1982). Recognition of the familiar words of nursery rhymes by handicapped and non-handicapped infants. Journal of Child Psychology & Psychiatry & Allied Disciplines, 23(30), 319-327.

Glenn, S. M., Cunningham, C. C. & Joyce, P. F. (1981). A study of auditory preferences in nonhandicapped infants and infants with Down's syndrome. Child Development, 52(4), 1303- 1307.

Glenn, S. M., & Cunningham, C. C. (1983). What do babies listen to most? A developmental study of auditory preferences in nonhandicapped infants and infants with Down's syndrome. Developmental Psychology, 19(3) 332-337.

Glidden, J. B., Busk, J., & Galbraith, G. C. (1975). Visual evoked responses as a function of light intensity in Down's syndrome and nonretarded subjects. Psychophysiology, 3, 263-273.

Gliddon, J. B., Galbraith, G. C., & Busk, J. (1975). Effects of preconditioning visual stimulus duration on visual-evoked responses to a subsequent test flash in Down's syndrome and nonretarded individuals. American Journal of Mental Deficiency, 80, 186-190.

Glovsky, L. (1966). Audiological assessment of a mongoloid population. Training School Bulletin, 63, 27-36.

Glovsky, L. (1972). A communication program for children with Down's syndrome. Training School Bulletin, 69, 5-9.

Godinova, A. M. (1963). Electroencephalographic changes in Down's syndrome. Zhurnal Nevropathologii i Psikhiatrii Imeni S. S. Korsakova, 63, 1058.

Golden, W., & Pashayan, H. M. (1976). The effect of parental education on the eventual mental development of noninstitutionalized children with Down syndrome. J. Pediatr., 89(4), 603-605.

Goldie, L., Curtis, J. A. H., Svendsen, U., & Robertson, N. R. C. (1968). Abnormal sleep rhythms in mongol babies. Lancet, 1, 229-230.

Goodall, E., & Corbett, J. (1982). Relationships between sensory stimulation and stereotyped behavior in severely mentally retarded and autistic children. Journal of Mental Deficiency Research, 26(3), 163-175.

Goodman, M. A. (1982). Infant affective responsiveness, affective interchange in the family, and parent perceptions of infant temperament: A family systems comparison of Down's syndrome and normal infants. Dissertation Abstracts International, 43(5-B), 1613.

Gordan, W. L., & Panagos, J. M. (1976). Developmental transformational capacity of children with Down's syndrome. Percept. Mot. Skills, 43, 967-973.

Gordon, A. M. (1944). Some aspects of sensory discrimination in mongolism. American Journal of Mental Deficiency, 49, 55.

Gordon, A. M. (1946). Some aspects of idiocy mongolism. American Journal of Mental Deficiency, 50, 402-410.

Gottsleben, R. H. (1955). The incidence of stuttering in a group of mongoloids. Training School Bulletin, 51, 209-218.

Gramza, A. F., Witt, P. A., Linford, A. G., & Jeanrenaud, C. (1969). Responses of mongoloid children to colored block presentation. Perceptual and Motor Skills, 29, 1008.

Gratz, R. T., Henderson, N. D., & Katz, S. (1972). A comparison of the functional and intellectual performance of phenylketonuric, anoxic and Down's syndrome individuals. American Journal of Mental Deficiency, 76, 710-717.

Gray, D. B. (1975). The effects of etiology, drug and visual stimuli on fixed-interval panel pushing in a population of Down's and non-Down's syndrome retarded males. Dissertation Abstracts International, 35(12-B, pt. 1), 6071-6072.

Greenberg, D. B., Wilson, W. R., Moore, J. M., & Thompson, G. (1978). Visual reinforcement audiometry (VRA) with young Down's syndrome children. Journal of Speech & Hearing Disorders, 43(4), 448-458.

Greenberg, R., & Field, T. (1982). Temperament ratings of handicapped infants during classroom, mother, and

teacher interactions. Journal of Pediatric Psychology,
7(4), 387-405.

Greenspan, S., & Delaney, K. (1983). Personal competence
of institutionalized adult males with or without Down
syndrome. American Journal of Mental Deficiency, 88(2),
218-220.

Greenwald, C. A., & Leonard, L. B. (1979). Communicative
and sensorimotor development of Down's syndrome children. American Journal of Mental Deficiency, 84(3), 296-
303.

Groner, Y., et al. (1985). Molecular structure and expression of the gene lacus on chromosome 21 encoding
the U/ZN superoxide dismutase and its relevance to Down
syndrome. Symposium of the National Down Syndrome Society, Annals of the New York Academy of Sciences, 450,
133-156.

Gropp, A. (1982). Value of an animal model for trisomy.
Virchows Arch. [Pathol. Anat.], 395(2), 117-131.

Gunn, P., Berry, P., & Andrews, R. (1977). Vocalizations
nd looking behaviour of Down's syndrome infants. British Journal of Psychology, 70(2), 259-263.

Gunn, P., Berry, P., & Andrews, R. J. (1981). The temperament of Down's syndrome infants: a research note.
Journal of Child Psych., Psychia., and Allied Disc.,
22(2), 189-194.

Gunn, P., Clark, D., & Berry, P. (1980). Maternal speech
during play with a Down's syndrome infant. Mental Retardation, 18(1), 15-18.

Gunn, P., Berry, P., & Andrews, R. J. (1983). The temperament of Down's syndrome toddlers: a research note.
Journal of Child Psychology & Psychiatry & Allied Disciplines, 24(4), 601-605.

Gunn, P., & Berry, P. (1985). The temperament of Down's
syndrome toddlers and their siblings. Journal of Child
Psychology & Psychiatry & Allied Disciplines, 26(6),
973-979.

Gunn, P., Berry, P. & Andrews, R. J. (1981). The affective response of Down's syndrome infants to a repeated
event. Child Development, 52(2), 745-751.

Gunn, P., Berry, P., & Andrews, R. J. (1982). Looking behavior of Down syndrome infants. American Journal of
Mental Deficiency, 87(3), 344-347.

Gunn, P., Berry, P. (1985). Down's syndrome temperament

and maternal response to descriptions of child behavior. Developmental Psychology, 21(5), 842-847.

Gunn, P., Clark, D., & Berry, P. (1980). Maternal speech during play with a Down's syndrome infant. Mental Retardation, 18(1), 15-18.

Gunzburg, H. C., & Sinson, J. (1973). Progress Assessment Chart of the Social Development of 'Mongol' Children. Birmingham: SEFA Publications.

Gupton, H. M. (1984). Individual differences in information processing: relationship between intellectual ability and memory for order in normal and mentally retarded individuals. Dissertation Abstracts International, 45(4-B), 1287.

Gusella, J. F., et al. (1985). Genetic Linkage Map for Chromosome 21. Symposium of the National Down Syndrome Society: Molecular Structure of the Number 21 Chromosome and Down Syndrome, Annals of the New York Academy of Sciences, 450, 25-31.

Gutmann, A. J., Rondal, J. A. (1979). Verbal operants in mothers' speech to nonretarded and Down's syndrome children matched for linguistic level. American Journal of Mental Deficiency, 83(5), 446-452.

Haberland, C. (1969). Alzheimer's disease in Down syndrome: Clinical-neuropathological observations. Acta Neurologica et Psychiatrica Belgica, 69(6), 369-380.

Haberlandt, W. F. (1966). The chromosomal pathology as a contribution to a genetically oriented psychiatry. Nervenarzt., 37(2), 45-51.

Habinakova, E., Bimkova, Z., & Cernay, J. (1976). Psychomotor development of children with Down's syndrome after administration of Encephabol and intense rehabilitation by the parents. Cesk. Pediatr., 31(4), 220-222.

Haley, S. M. (1984). Relationship between postural reactions and motor milestones in infants with Down syndrome. Dissertation Abstracts International, 44(8-A), 2415.

Halle, J. W. (1985). Enhancing social competence through language: an experimental analysis of a practical procedure for teachers. Topics in Early Childhood Special Education, 4(4), 77-92.

Hallenbeck, P. N. (1960). A survey of recent research in mongolism. American Journal of Mental Deficiency, 64,

827-834.

Halpin, S. A. (1977). A comparison of trainable mentally retarded and normal children at the preoperational reasoning level on grade-sequenced mathematics tasks. Dissertation Abstracts International, 38(2-A), 726-727.

Hanson, M. J., & Schwarz, R. H. (1978). Results of a longitudinal intervention program for Down's syndrome infants and their families. Education and Training of the Mentally Retarded, 13(4), 403-407.

Hanson, M. J., & Bellamy, G. T. (1977). Continuous measurement of progress in infant intervention programs. Education & Training of the Mentally Retarded, 12(1), 52-58.

Hanson, M. J., & Hanline, M. F. (1985). An analysis of response-contingent learning experiences for young children. Journal of the Association for Persons With Severe Handicaps, 10(1), 31- 40.

Harris, S. R. (1981). Relationship of mental and motor development in Down's syndrome infants. Physical and Occupational Therapy in Pediatrics, 1, 13-18.

Harris, J. (1983). What does mean length of utterance mean? Evidence from a comparative study of normal and Down's syndrome children. British Journal of Disorders of Communication, 18(3), 153-169.

Harris, S. R. (1980). Effects of neurodevelopmental therapy on improving motor performance in Down's syndrome infants. Dissertation Abstracts International, 41(5-A), 2059.

Harris, S. R. (1983). Comparative performance levels of female and male infants with Down syndrome. Physical & Occupational Therapy in Pediatrics, 3(2), 15-21.

Hartley, X. Y. (1982). Receptive language processing of Down's syndrome children. Journal of Mental Deficiency Research, 26(4), 263-269.

Hartley, X. Y. (1985). Receptive language processing and ear advantage of Down's syndrome children. Journal of Mental Deficiency Research, 29(2), 197-205.

Hartley, X. Y. (1986). A summary of recent research into the development of children with Down's syndrome. Journal of Mental Deficiency Research, 30(1), 1-14.

Hartley, X. Y. (1983). Receptive language processing and hemispheric dominance of Down's syndrome children. International Journal of Rehabilitation Research, 6(3),

357-358.

Haubold, H., Loew, W., & Haefele-Niemann, R. (1960). Possibilities and limitations of a postmaturation treatment of retarded and especially of mongoloid children. Landarzt, 36, 378-383.

Hawley, J. L. (1982). A descriptive study of adolescent home-reared Down's syndrome children and their families in East Tennessee. Dissertation Abstracts International, 43(2-B), 525.

Hayashi, T., Hsu, T. C., & Chao, D. (1962). A case of mosaicism in mongolism. Lancet, 1, 218-219.

Hayden, A. H. (1978). Early childhood education. In: K. E. Allen, V. Holm and R. Schiefelbusch (eds.), Early Intervention -- A Team Approach. Baltimore: University Park Press.

Hayden, A. H. (1979). Implications of infant intervention research. All. Hlth. Behav. Scie., 1(4).

Hayden, A. H., & Dmitriev, V. (1973). The multi-disciplinary preschool program for Down's syndrome children at the University of Washington model pre-school center. In: B. Z. Friedlander, G. M. Sterritt, and G. E. Kirka (eds.), Exceptional Infant, Vol. II. New York: Brunner/Mazel.

Hayden, A. H., & Dmitriev, V. (1974). New perspectives on Down's syndrome. In: Proc. 1974 Down's Syn. Cong., Milwaukee, Wisconsin.

Hayden, A. H., & Dmitriev, V. (1975). Early developmental and educational programs for the child with Down's syndrome. In: B. Z. Friedlander, G. Kirk, and G. Sterritt, (eds.), The Exceptional Infant, Vol. III. New York: Brunner/Mazel.

Hayden, A. H., & Haring, N. G. (1976). Early intervention for high risk infants and young children: programs for Down's syndrome children. In: T. D. Tjossem (ed.), Intervention Strategies for High Risk Infants and Young Children, Baltimore: University Park Press.

Hayden, A. H., & Haring, N. G. (1977). The acceleration and maintenance of developmental gains in Down's syndrome school-aged children. Proc. Intern. Assoc. Sci. Ment. Defic. Symp., 1976, Washington, D. C. Baltimore: University Park Press.

Heaton-Ward, W. A. (1960). The effects of NIAMID, a monoamine oxidase inhibitor on the IQ and behaviour of mongols. Proceedings of the London Conference on the Scientific Study of Mental Retardation.

Heaton-Ward, W. A. (1961). An interim report on a controlled trial of the effects of NIAMID on the mental age and behavior of mongols. In: J. Jancar (ed.), Stoke Park Studies: Mental Subnormality, Bristol: Johnson.

Heffernan, L., Black, F. W., & Poche, P. (1982). Temperament patterns in young neurologically impaired children. Journal of Pediatric Psychology, 7(4), 415-423.

Henderson, S. E., & Morris, J. (1981). The motor deficit in Down's syndrome children: a problem of timing?. Journal of Child Psychology & Psychiatry & Allied Disciplines, 22(3), 233-245.

Henderson, S. E., Morris, J., & Ray, S. (1981). Performance of Down syndrome and other retarded children on the Cratty Gross-motor Test. American Journal of Mental Deficiency, 85(4), 416-424.

Hermelin, B. (1969). Some behavioral studies of mongolism. Proceedings of the American Academy on Mental Retardation, San Francisco, Calif.

Hermelin, B., & O'Connor, N. (1961). Shape perception and reproduction in normal children and mongol and non-mongol imbeciles. Journal of Mental Deficiency Research, 67-71.

Herriot, P. (1972). The effect of order of labelling on the subjective organization and clustering of severely retarded adults. American Journal of Mental Deficiency, 76(6), 632-638.

Herriot, P., & Cox, A. M. (1971). Subjective organization and clustering in the free recall of intellectually-subnormal children. American Journal of Mental Deficiency, 75(6), 702-711.

Heston, L. L. (1984). Down's syndrome and Alzheimer's dementia: defining an association. Psychiatric Development, 2(4), 287-294.

Heston, L. L., & Mastri, A. R. (1977). The genetics of Alzheimer's disease: Association with hematologic malignancy and Down's syndrome. Arch. Gen. Psychiatry, 34(8), 976-981.

Heston, L. L., & White, J. (1978). Pedigrees of 30 families with Alzheimer's disease: Associations with defective organization of microfilaments and microtubules. Behavior Genetics, 8(4), 315-331.

Heumayer-Skritek, M. (1975). On the mental structure of mongolism. Paediatr. Paedol. (Suppl.), 4, 70-82.

Hewitt, K. E., Carter, G., & Jancar, J. (1985). Aging in Down's syndrome. British Journal of Psychiatry, 147, 58-62.

Hill, P. M. (1979). An analysis of the relationship between cognitive development and symbolic play in young Down's syndrome children. Dissertation Abstracts International, 40(1-A), 165-166.

Hill, P. M., & McCune-Nicolich, L. (1981). Pretend play and patterns of cognition in Down's syndrome children. Child Development, 52(2), 611-617.

Hill, S. D., & Tomlin, C. (1980). Self-recognition in retarded children. Child Development.

Himwich, H. E., & Fazekas, J. F. (1940). Cerebral metabolism in mongolism idiocy and phenylpyruvic amentia. Arch. Neurol. Psychiatry, 44, 1213.

Hirai, T. (1968). The electroencephalograph in Down's syndrome. Saishin Igaku, 24(2), 278-283.

Hirai, T., & Izawa, S. (1964). An electroencephalographic study of mongolism -- with special reference to its EEG development and intermediate fast wave. Folia Psychiatr. Neurol. Jpn., 66, 18.

Hirsch, W., Mex, A., & Vogel, F. (1969). Metabolic traits in mentally retarded children as compared with normal populations: monoaminodicarboxylic acids and their half amides and total amino acids. Journal of Mental Deficiency Research, 13(2), 130-142.

Hobson, R. P. (1984). Early childhood autism and the question of egocentrism. Journal of Autism & Developmental Disorders, 14(1) 85-104.

Hoehne, R. (1984). Fruhe krankengymnastik -- uberschatzte therapie, uberforderte therapeuten?/Early physical therapy: Overestimated therapy, overburdened therapists? Fruhforderung Interdisziplinar, 3(1), 1-6.

Hogg, J. (1981). Learning, using and generalizing manipulative skills in a preschool classroom by nonhandicapped and Down's syndrome children. Educational Psychology, 1(4), 319-340.

Hogg, J., & Moss, J. C. (1983). Prehensile development in Down's syndrome and non-handicapped preschool children. British Journal of Developmental Psychology, 1(2), 189-204.

Hogg,   J.   (1982). Motor development and performance of severely   mentally   handicapped people. Developmental Med-
icine & Child Neurology, 24(2), 188-193.
Holburn,   C.   S.,   & Dougher, M. J. (1985). The fire-alarm
game: exit   training   using negative and positive rein-
forcement   under   varied stimulus conditions. Journal of
Visual Impairment & Blindness, 79(9), 401-403.
Holdgrafer,   G.   (1980).   Facilitating syntax acquisition.
Psychological Reports, 46(2), 498.
Holdgrafer,   G.   (1981). Mode-relations in language learn-
ing   by language-deficient retarded subjects. Perceptual
& Motor Skills, 53(2), 520-522.
Holdgrafer,   G. (1982). Teaching comprehension and produc-
tion. Perceptual & Motor Skills, 55(1), 306.
Hollien,   H.,   & Hopeland, R. H. (1965). Speaking fundamen-
tal   frequency (SFF) characteristics of mongoloid girls.
Journal of Speech and Hearing Disorders, 30, 344-349.
Hook,   E.   B. (1982). Epidemiology of Down's syndrome. In:
S.   M.   Pueschel   and   J. E. Rynders (eds.), Advances in
Biomedicine   and the Behavioral Sciences. Cambridge, MA:
Ware Press.
Hooshyar,   N.   (1985). Language interactions between mothers   and   their   nonhandicapped   children,   mothers   and
their   Down   syndrome   children,   mothers and their lan-
guage-impaired   children. International Journal of Rehabilitation Research, 8(4), 475-47.
Horackova,   M.,   & Hrubcova, M. (1959). The problem of educating   mongoloid   children.   Ceskoslovenska Pediatrica,
14, 1023-1030.
Horstmeier,   D.   S. (1986). The mother-child communicative
interactions   of   educationally advantaged Down syndrome
and   normal children matched for auditory comprehension.
Dissertation   Abstracts   International, 46(12-A, pt. 1),
3701.
Howard,   W.   D.   (1985). Atlanto-axial instability in Down
syndrome: a   need   for   awareness. Mental Retardation,
23(4), 197-199.
Huang,   I. N.,   & Borter, S. J. (1987). The color isolation
effect   in   free recall by adults by with Down syndrome.
American Journal of Mental Deficiency, 92(1), 115-118.
Hubschman,   E.   W.   (1977). Language development of early-
institutionalized   Down's   syndrome subjects. Dissertation Abstracts International, 38(1-A), 137-138.

Hughes, W. (1977). Atherosclerosis, Down's syndrome, and Alzheimer's disease. (Letter) Br. Med. J., 2, 702.

Hunt, J. V. (1966). A comparison of normal infants and children with Down's syndrome (mongolism) on free play behaviour and galvanic skin response. Dissertation Abstracts International, 26(7), 4090.

Hurley, A. D., & Sovner, R. (1982). Down's syndrome: a Hunt, J. V. (1966). A comparison of normal infants and children with Down's syndrome (mongolism) on free play behaviour and galvanic skin response. Dissertation Abstracts International, 26(7), 4090.

Hurley, A. D., & Sovner, R. (1982). Down's syndrome: a psychiatric perspective. Psychiatric Aspects of Mental Retardation Newsletter, 1(9), 31-3.

Hurley, A. D., & Sovner, R. (1986). Dementia, mental retardation, and Down's syndrome. Psychiatric Aspects of Mental Retardation Reviews, 5(8) 39-44.

Jackson-Cook, C. K. (1985). The extra chromosome in trisomy-21: its parental origin and etiology. Dissertation Abstracts International, 46(3-B), 748.

Jacoby, H. B. (1971). A comparison of mongoloid and non-mongoloid trainable retarded children on tasks of intentional and incidental learning. Dissertation Abstracts International, 31(10-A), 5233.

Jago, J., Jago, A. G., & Hart, M. (1984). An evaluation of the total communication approach for teaching language skills to developmentally delayed preschool children. Education & Training of the Mentally Retarded, 19(3), 175-182.

Jakab, I. (1978). Basal ganglia calcification and psychosis in mongolism. Eur. Neurol., 17(5), 300-314.

James, R. J. (1975). Multivariate analysis of the walking behavior in institutional Down's syndrome males. Dissertation Abstracts International, 35(11-B), 5500-5501.

James, W. (1968). Mongolism, delayed fertilization and sexual behaviour. Nature, 219(5151), 279-280.

James, W. H. (1969). The effect of maternal psychological stress on the foetus. British Journal of Psychiatry, 115(524), 811-825.

Jameson-Bloom, C. (1981). Assessments, goals, and expectations of mothers of children with Down syndrome enrolled in early intervention programs. Dissertation Abstracts International, 42(2-A), 873.

Jayaraman, A., Ballweg, G. P., Donnenfeld, H., & Chusid, J. G. (1976). Hydrocephalus in Down's syndrome. Childs. Brain, 293, 202-207.

Jeffree, D., Wheldall, K., & Mittler, P. (1973). Facilitating two-word utterances in two Down's syndrome boys. American Journal of Mental Deficiency, 78, 117-122.

Jelgersma, H. C. (1958). Early senile dementia in mongoloids. Folia Psychiatr. Neerl., 61, 367-374.

Jelgersma, H. C. (1962). Dementia in mongolism. Revue Neurol., 106, 2214-2217.

Jelgersma, H. C. (1963). On the tuber flocculi in mongolian idiocy. Psychiatr. Neurol. Neurochir., 66, 131-137.

Jelgersma, H. C. (1968). Another case of early senile dementia in mongolism. Folia Psychiatr. Neerl., 61, 501-504.

Jenkins, E. C., et al. (1983). Atypical Down syndrome and partial trisomy 21. Clinical Genetics, 24, 97-102.

Jens, K. G., & Johnson, N. M. (1982). Affective development: a window to cognition in young handicapped children. Topics in Early Childhood Special Education, 2(2) 17-24.

Jervis, G. A. (1942). Recent progress in the study of mental deficiency. Mongolism: a review of the literature of the last decade. American Journal of Mental Deficiency, 47, 467.

Jervis, G. A. (1948). Early senile dementia in mongoloid idiocy. American Journal of Psychiatry, 105, 102-106.

Jervis, G. A. (1970). Report on premature senility found in brains of mongoloids'. Pediatric News, 4, 1 & 46.

Jervis, G. A. (1970). Premature senility in Down's syndrome. Annals of the New York Academy of Sciences, 171, 559-561.

Johnson, C. D., & Barnett, D. C. (1961). Relationship of physical stigmata to intellectual status in mongoloids. American Journal of Mental Deficiency, 66, 435-437.

Johnson, J. T., Jr., & Olley, J. G. (1971). Behavioral comparisons of mongoloid and nonmongoloid retarded persons: a review. Am. J. Ment. Defic., 75(5), 546-559.

Johnson, R. C., & Abelson, R. B. (1969). Intellectual, behavioral, and physical characteristics associated with trisomy, translocation, and mosaic types of Down's syndrome. Am. J. Ment. Defic., 73(6), 852-855.

Johnson, R. C., & Abelson, R. B. (1969). The behavioral

competence of mongoloid and non-mongoloid retardates. Am. J. Ment. Defic., 73(6), 856-857.

Johnson, R. C., McKean, C. M., & Shah, S. N. (1977). Fatty acid composition of lipids in cerebral myelin and synaptosomes in phenylketonuria and Down syndrome. Arch. Neurol., 34(5), 288-294.

Johnson, R. C., & Shah, S. N. (1978). Cholesterol metabolizing enzymes in human brain: Properties, subcellular distribution and relative levels in various disseased conditions. J. Neurochem., 31(4), 895-902.

Johnson, R. T., Johnson, D. W., & Rynders, J. (1981). Effect of cooperative, competetive, and individualistic experiences on self-esteem of handicapped and nonhandicapped students. Journal of Psychology, 108(1) 31-34.

Jones, B. E., Croley, H. T., & Levy, J. M. (1960). The relation between physical and mental retardation in mongolism. Research Relating to Mentally Retarded Children, U. S. Department of Education.

Jones, J., Singh, N. N., White, A. J., & Astwood, C. (1977). Treatment of a Down's syndrome child with multiple behaviour problems in a ward setting. Australian Journal of Mental Retardation, 4(8), 16-19.

Junkala, J. B. (1966). Changes in PMA relationships in noninstitutionalized mongoloids. American Journal of Mental Deficiency, 71, 460-464.

Kaariainen, R., & Dingman, H. F. (1961). The relation of the degree of mongolism to the degree of subnormality. Am. J. Ment. Defic., 66, 438-443.

Kaback, M. M. (1970). Seen in 'premature senility found in brains of mongoloids'. Pediatric News, 4, 1 & 46.

Kaplan, A. R., & Zsako, S. (1970). Biological variables associated with mothers of children affected with the G1-trisomy syndrome (Down's syndrome). American Journal of Mental Deficiency, 74(6), 745-755.

Karlinsky, H. (1986). Alzheimer's disease in Down's syndrome: A review. Journal of the American Geriatrics Society, 34(10), 728-734.

Karpova, O. B., et al. (1978). Concentration and composition of cerebral gangliosides in Down's disease. Vopr. Med. Khim., 24(4), 524-527.

Kay, D. W. (1987). Heterogeneity in Alzheimer's disease: Epidemiological and family studies. Trends in Neurosciences, 10(5), 194-195.

Kazazian, H. H., et al. (1985). Ring chromosome 21: characterization of DNA sequences at sites of breakage and reunion. Symposium of the National Down Syndrome Society: Annals of the New York Academy of Sciences, 450, 33-42.

Keegan, D. L., Pettigrew, A., & Parker, Z. (1974). Amitriptyline in the psychotic states of Down's syndrome: the comparison of two cases. Diseases of the Nervous System, 35(8), 381-383.

Keegan, D. L., Pettigrew, A., & Parker, Z. (1974). Psychosis in Down's syndrome treated with amitriptyline. (Letter) Can. Med. Ass. J., 110(10), 1128.

Keith, H. (1958). Mongolism. Postgraduate Medicine, 23, 629-635.

Kennedy, M., & Sheridan, C. (1973). Tactile-visual equivalence of shape and slant in brain-damaged and mongoloid children. Perceptual and Motor Skills, 36(2), 632.

Kennedy, A. B. (1981). Inclinations of handicapped children to help handicapped peers. Dissertation Abstracts International, 42(2-A), 657.

Keer, R., & Blais, C. (1985). Motor skill acquisition by individuals with Down syndrome. American Journal of Mental Deficiency, 90(3) 313-318.

Kinnell, H. G. (1985). Pica as a feature of autism. British Journal of Psychiatry, 147, 80-82.

Kirman, B. H. (1951). Epilepsy in mongolism. Arch. Dis. Child., 26, 501.

Klager, M. (1977). A retarded woman's graphic and verbal expression. American Journal of Art Therapy, 16(4), 145-158.

Klebba, J. T., Gershbein, L. L., & Marks, R. (1974). Correlation of bio-clinical parameters and intelligence in subjects with Down's syndrome and other retardates. Res. Commun. Chem. Pathol. Pharmacol., 8(1), 159-180.

Knights, R. M., Hyman, J. A., & Wozny, M. A. (1965). Psychomotor abilities of familial, brain-injured and mongoloid retarded children. American Journal of Mental Deficiency, 70, 454-457.

Knights, R. M., Atkinson, B. R., & Hyman, J. A. (1967). Tactual discrimination and motor skills in mongoloid and non-mongoloid retardates and normal children. American Journal of Mental Deficiency, 71, 894-900.

Knox, M. (1983). Changes in the frequency of language use

by Down's syndrome children interacting with nonretarded peers. Education & Training of the Mentally Retarded, 18(3), 185-190.

Koch, R., & De La Cruz, F. F. (1975). Down's Syndrome (Mongolism): Research, Prevention, And Management. New York, NY: Brunner/Mazel XII, 242.

Koch, R., Share, J., Webb, A., & Graliker, B. V. (1963). The predictability of Gesell development scales in mongolism. J. Pediatr., 62, 93.

Koch, R., Share, J. B., & Graliker, B. V. (1965). The effects of Cytomel on children with Down's syndrome - A double-blind longitudinal study. Pediatrics, 66, 776-778.

Kohler, C. (1975). Mongolism: An encephalopathy not like others. Ann. Med. Psychol. Paris, 2(5), 847-871.

Kohlmann, T., & Rett, A. (1975). Clinical psychological studies on adolescent and adult mongols. Paediatr. Paedol. (Suppl.), 4, 48-58.

Kohn, G., Taysi, K., Atkins, T. E., & Mellman, W. J. (1970). Mosaic mongolism. I. Clinical correlations. Journal of Pediatrics, 76, 874-879.

Kolata, G. (1985). Down syndrome-Alzheimer's linked. Science, 230(4730), 1152-1153.

Kolstoe, O. P. (1958). Language training of low-grade mongoloid children. American Journal of Mental Deficiency, 63, 17-30.

Komiya, M. (1981). An experimental study of tactual and visual discrimination in children with Down's syndrome. Japanese Journal of Special Education.

Komiya, M. (1973). Comparative studies of Down's syndrome and physiologically mentally retarded children on figure-copying ability. Japanese Journal of Special Education, 11, 31-38.

Konczak, L. J., & Johnson, C. M. (1983). Reducing inappropriate verbalizations in a sheltered workshop through differential reinforcement of other behavior. Education & Training of the Mentally Retarded, 18(2) 120-124.

Kopp, C. B., Krakwo, J. B., & Johnson, K. L. (1983). Strategy production by young Down syndrome children. American Journal of Mental Deficiency, 88(2), 164-169.

Kostrezewski, J. (1970). The dynamics of intellectual development in individuals with complete and incomplete trisomy of chromosomes group G in the karyotype. Roczniki: Filozoficzne, 18(4), 55-81.

Kostrzewski, J. (1963). Investigations on the level of mental development in Down's syndrome. Pediatria Polska, 38, 781-789.

Kostrzewski, J. (1965). The dynamics of intellectual and social development in Down's syndrome: Results of experimental investigation. Roczniki: Filozoficzne, 13(4), 5-32.

Kousseff, B. G. (1978). Trisomy 21 with average intelligence?! Birth Defects, 14(6C), 323-325.

Kovattana, P. M., & Kraemer, H. C. (1974). Response to multiple visual cues of color, size, and form by autistic children. Journal of Autism and Childhood Schiz. 80(6), 251-261.

Krakow, J. B., & Kopp, C. B. (1982). Sustained attention in young Down syndrome children. Topics in Early Childhood Special Education, 2(2), 32-42.

Krakow, J. B., & Kopp, C. B. (1983). The effects of developmental delay on sustained attention in young children. Child Development, 54(5), 1143-1155.

Kramer, B. (1953). The problems of mongolism. Mongolism, A Symposium, p. 77, New York: New York Association for the Mentally Retarded.

Kravitz, H., & Boehm, J. J. (1971). Rhythmic habit patterns in infancy: their sequence, age of onset, and frequency. Child Development, 42(2), 399-413.

Kreezer, G. (1936). Electric potentials of the brain in certain types of mental deficiency. Arch. Neurol. Psychiatry Chicago, 36, 1216-1213.

Kreezer, G. (1939). Intelligence level and occipital alpha rhythm in the mongolian type of mental deficiency. American Journal of Psychology, 52, 503-532.

Krynicki, V. (1976). The temporal and periodic organization of REM eye movements in mental retardation. Neuropsychobiology, 2(1), 9-17.

Kuenzel, M. W. (1929). A survey of mongolian traits. Training School Bulletin, 26, 49-59.

Kugel, R. B. (1970). Combatting retardation in infants with Down's syndrome. Children, 17(5), 188-192.

Kugel, R. B., & Reque, D. (1961). A comparison of mongoloid children. Journal of the American Medical Association, 175, 959-961.

Kumin, L. (1986). A survey of speech and language pathology services for Down syndrome: state of the art. Applied Research in Mental Retardation, 7(4), 491-499.

Kysela, G. M. (1973). Early childhood education for children with Down's syndrome. Mental Retardation Bulletin, 2(2), 58-63.

La Veck, B., & La Veck, G. D. (1977). Sex differences in development among young children with Down syndrome. J. Pediatr., 91(5), 767-769.

Lake, C. E., Ziegler, M. G., Coleman, M., & Kopin, I. J. (1979). Evaluation of the sympathetic nervous system in Trisomy-21 (Down's syndrome). Journal of Psychiatric Research, 15(1), 1-6.

Lang, J. L. (1974). Psychology and psychopathology of the child with Down's syndrome: structural features. Revue de Neuropsychiatrie Infantile et D'Hygiene Mentale de L'Enfance, 22, 19-39.

Langer, S. (1965). Some peculiarities in the mental development of mongoloid children. Cas. Lek. Cesk., 102, 100-105.

Lassen, N. A., Christensen, S., Hoedt-Rasmussen, K., & Stewart, B. M. (1966). Cerebral oxygen comsumption in Down's syndrome. Arch. Neurol., 15(6), 595-602.

Lasser, B. R. (1970). Teaching mothers of mongoloid children to use behavior modification procedures. Dissertation Abstracts International, 30(12-A), 5239-5240.

Launay, C., & Bayen, M. (1964). Mental development in mongoloids. Revue Du Practicien, 14, 21-31.

Lavieille, J., et al. (1967). Apropos of neuroradiology in children. Its technical and clinical peculiarities. J. Radiol. Electrol. Med. Nucl., 48(10), 577-579.

Layton, T. L., & Sharifi, H. (1979). Meaning and structure of Down's syndrome and nonretarded children's spontaneous speech. American Journal of Mental Deficiency, 83(5), 439-445.

Le Blanc, D., French, R., & Shultz, B. (1977). Static and dynamic balance skills of trainable children with Down's syndrome. Percept. Mot. Skills, 45(2), 641-642.

Leader, S., & Grozin, M. (1935). Capillary development and its relation to the intelligence of children with mongolism. Am. J. Dis. Child., 49, 1169.

LeBlanc, D., French, R., & Shultz, B. (1977). Static and dynamic balance skills of trainable children with

Down's syndrome. <u>Perceptual & Motor Skills</u>, <u>45</u>(2), 641-642.

Leddet, I., et al. (1986). Comparison of clinical diagnoses and Rimland E2 scores in severely disturbed children. <u>Journal of Autism & Developmental Disorders</u>, <u>16</u>(2), 215-225.

Lee, J. C., Ornitz, E. M., Tanguay, P. E., & Ritvo, E. R. (1969). Sleep EEG patterns in a case of Down's syndrome -- before and after 5-HTP. <u>Electroencephalogr. Clin. Neurophysiol.</u>, <u>27</u>(7), 686.

Lee, J. M. (1986). Teacher wait-time: task performance of developmentally delayed and non-delayed young children. <u>Dissertation Abstracts International</u>, <u>47</u>(4-A), 1281.

Leifer, J. S., & Lewis, M. (1983). Maternal speech to normal and handicapped children: a look at question asking behavior. <u>Infant Behavior & Development</u>, <u>6</u>(2) 175-187.

Leifer, J. S., & Lewis, M. (1984). Acquisition of conversational response skills by young Down syndrome and nonretarded young children. <u>American Journal of Mental Deficiency</u>, <u>88</u>(6) 610-618.

Lejeune, J. (1977). The mechanism of mental deficiency in chromosomal diseases. In: S. Armendartes and R. Lisker (eds.), <u>Human Genetics</u>. Amsterdam: Excerpta Medica.

Lejeune, J. (1978). Chromosomal anomalies and intelligence deficiency. (Author's translation) <u>Ann. Biol. Clin. Paris</u>, <u>36</u>(2), 121-126.

Lenneberg, E. H., Nichols, I., & Rosenberger, E. F. (1962). Primitive stages of language development in mongolism. Proceedings, <u>Ass. for Research in Nervous and Mental Dis.</u>, <u>42</u>, 119.

Leudar, I., Fraser, W. I., & Jeeves, M. A. (1981). Social familiarity and communication in Down syndrome. <u>Journal of Mental Deficiency Research</u>, <u>25</u>(2) 133-142.

Levin, J. A. (1983). The acquisition of intentional communication in young children with Down's syndrome through maternal interaction. <u>Dissertation Abstracts International</u>, <u>44</u>(5-A), 1420.

Levitt, P. (1985). Relating molecular specificity to normal and abnormal brain development. <u>Symposium of the National Down Syndrome Society: Molecular Structure of the Number 21 Chromosome and Down Syndrome. Annals of the New York Academy of Sciences</u>, <u>450</u>, 239-246.

Lewis, M., & Brooks-Gunn, J. (1984). Age and handicapped group differences in infants' visual attention.
Child Development, 55(3), 858-868.

Lewis, V., A., & Bryant, P. E. (1982). Touch and vision
in normal and Down's syndrome babies. Perception,
11(6), 691-701.

Li, A. K. (1981). Play and the mentally retarded child.
Mental Retardation, 19(3), 121-126.

Libb, J. W., Myers, G. J., Graham, E., & Bell, B. (1983).
Correlates of intelligence and adaptive behaviour in
Down's syndrome. Journal of Mental Deficiency Research,
27(3), 205-210.

Libb, J. W., et al. (1985). Hearing disorder and cognitive function of individuals with Down syndrome. American Journal of Mental Deficiency, 90(3), 353-356.

Lincoln, A. J., Courchesne, E., Kilman, B. A., &
Galambos, R. (1985). Neuropsychological correlates of
information-processing by children with Down syndrome.
American Journal of Mental Deficiency, 89(4), 403-414.

Lind, J., Vuorenkoski, V., Rosberg, G., Partanen, T. J.,
& Wasz-Hockert, O. (1970). Spectographic analysis of
vocal response to pain stimuli in infants with Down's
syndrome. Developmental Medicine and Child Neurology,
12, 478-486.

Litrownik, A. J., McInnis, E. T., Wetzel-Pritchard, A.
M., & Filipelli, D. L. (1978). Restricted stimulus control and inferred attentional deficits in autistic and
retarded children. Journal of Abnormal Psychology,
87(5), 554-562.

Loesch, M. D. (1968). Some aspects of the neurology of
Down's syndrome. Journal of Mental Deficiency Research,
12(3), 237-246.

Lombardino, L. J. (1979). Maternal speech to normal and
delayed children: a taxonomy and comparative-descrip-
tive study. Dissertation Abstracts International,
39(8-A), 4786.

Lombardino, L. J., Klein, M. P., & Saint Thomas, J.
(1982). Maternal interrogatives during discourse with
language learning normal and Down's syndrome children:
a preliminary clinical taxonomy. Education & Training
of the Mentally Retarded, 17(3) 222-226.

Longnecker, E. D., & Ferson, J. (1961). Discrimination
reversal learning in mongoloids. Am. J. Ment. Defic.,

66, 93-99.

Lonsdale, D., & Kissling, C. D. (1986). Clinical trials with thiamine tetrahydrofurfuryl disulfide (TTFD) in Down's syndrome. Journal of Orthomolecular Medicine, 1(3), 169-175.

Lorenz, S. (1985). No visible means of support: A tactical approach to the integration of children Down's syndrome into mainstream nursery provision. Educational & Child Psychology, 2(3), 116-122.

Loret, L., & Born, M. (1972). Mental deficiency, autism, and re-education. Feuillets Psychiatriques De Liege, 5(1), 45-52.

Lott, I. T. (1982). Down's syndrome, aging, and Alzheimer's disease: a clinical review. Annals of the New York Academy of Sciences, 396, 15-27.

Lott, I. T., & Lai, F. (1982). Dementia in Down's syndrome: observations from a neurology clinic. Applied Research in Mental Retardation, 3(3), 233-239.

Loveland, K. A. (1987). Behavior of young children with Down syndrome before the mirror: finding things reflected. Child Development, 58(4), 928-936.

Lowenstein, L. F. (1978). Down's syndrome: a short account of the condition known as mongolism. Lowestoft, England: Green, 8.

Ludlow, J. R., & Allen, L. M. (1979). The effect of early intervention and pre-school stimulus on the development of the Down's syndrome children. Journal of Mental Deficiency Research, 23(1), 29-44.

Lunzer, E. A., & Stratford, B. (1984). Deficits in attention in young children with specific reference to Down's syndrome and other mentally handicapped children. Early Child Development & Care, 17(2-3), 131-154.

Lure, N. B. (1971). Children with Down's syndrome and some features of their cognitive activity. Defektologiya, 3(1), 30-36.

Lydic, J. S. (1982). Motor development in children with Down syndrome. Physical & Occupational Therapy in Pediatrics, 2(4), 53-74.

Lydic, J. S., Short, M. A., & Nelson, D. L. (1983). Comparison of two scales for assessing motor development in infants with Down's syndrome. Occupational Therapy Journal of Research, 3(4), 213-221.

Lydic, J. S., Windsor, M. M., Short, M. A., & Ellis, T.

A. (1985). Effects of controlled rotary vestibular stimulation on the motor performance of infants with Down
syndrome. Special Issue: Vestibular Processing Dysfunction in Children. Physical & Occupational Therapy in
Pediatrics, 5(2-3), 93-1.

Lydic, J. S. (1985). Effects of controlled rotary vestibular stimulation on the motor performance of infants
with Down syndrome. Dissertation Abstracts International, 46(5-B) 1518.

Lyon, R. (1975). Down's syndrome: a review and critique
of literature. Research & the Retarded, 2(1), 24-45.

MacCubrey, J. (1971). Verbal operant conditioning with
young institutionalized Down's syndrome children. American Journal of Mental Deficiency, 75(6), 696-701.

MacDonald, J. E., et al. (1974). An experimental parent-
assisted treatment program for preschool language-
delayed children. Journal of Speech & Hearing Disorders, 39(4), 395-415.

Mackay, D. N. (1971). Mental subnormality in Northern
Ireland. Journal of Mental Deficiency Research, 15(1),
12-19.

Mackay, D. N., & McDonald, G. (1976). The effects of
varying digit message structures on their recall by
mongols and non-mongol subnormals. J. Ment. Defic.
Res., 29(3), 191-196.

MacKay, D. N., & Bankhead, I. (1983). Reaction times of
Down's syndrome and other mentally retarded individuals. Perceptual & Motor Skills, 56(1), 266.

MacLean, W. E., & Baumeister, A. A. (1982). Effects of
vestibular stimulation on motor development and stereotyped behavior of developmentally delayed children.
Journal of Abnormal Child Psychology, 10(2), 229-245.

MacTurk, R. H., et al. (1985). The organization of exploratory behavior in Down syndrome and nondelayed infants. Child Development, 56(3) 573-581.

MacTurk, R. H. (1985). Social mastery motivation in Down
syndrome and nondelayed infants. Topics in Early Childhood Special Education, 4(4), 93-109.

Mahoney, G., Glover, A., & Finger, I. (1981). Relationship between language and sensorimotor development of
Down syndrome and nonretarded children. American Journal of Mental Deficiency, 86(1), 21-27.

Mahoney, G. (1983). A developmental analysis of communication between mothers and infants with Down's syndrome. Topics in Early Childhood Special Education, 3(1), 63-76.

Mahoney, G., & Snow, K. (1984). The relationship of sensorimotor functioning to children's response to early language training. Mental Retardation, 21(6) 248-254.

Mann, D. M. (1983). The locus coerulus and its possible role in aging and degenerative disease of the human nervous system. Mech. Aging Dev., 23(1), 73-94.

Mann, D. M., Yates, P. O., Marcyniuk, B., & Ravindra, C. R. (1985). Pathological evidence for neurotransmitter deficits in Down's syndrome of middle age. Journal of Mental Deficiency Research, 29(2),125-135.

Mansfield, J. T. (1972). The operant conditioning of abstract motor responses to prepositional speech in mongoloids. Dissertation Abstracts International, 33(1-B), 444.

Marcell, M. M., & Armstrong, V. (1982). Auditory and visual sequential memory of Down syndrome and nonretarded children. American Journal of Mental Deficiency, 87(1), 86-95.

Marcovitch, S., Goldberg, S., Lojkasek, M., & Macgregor, D. (1987). The concept of difficult temperament in the developmentally disabled preschool child. Journal of Applied Developmental Psychology, 8(2), 151-164.

Marcovitch, S. T. (1983). Maternal stress and mother-child interactions with the developmentally delayed preschool child. Dissertation Abstracts International, 44(8-B), 2561-2562.

Marcovitch, S., Goldberg, S., MacGregor, D. L., & Lojkasek, M. (1986). Patterns of temperament variation in three groups of developmentally delayed preschool children: mother and father ratings. Journal of Developmental & Behavioral Pediatrics, 7(4), 247-252.

Marin-Padilla, M. (1976). Pyramidal cell abnormalities in the motor cortex of a child with Down's syndrome. A Golgi study. J. Comp. Neurol., 167(1), 63-81.

Markowitz, S. L. (1981). Mother-infant interactions with normal and Down syndrome infants. Dissertation Abstracts International, 41(8-A), 3530.

Marsh, R. W. (1969). Serotonin levels and intelligence in trisomy 21 type Down's syndrome. N. A. Med. J., 70, 179.

Martel, W., Uyham, R., & Stimson, C. W. (1969). Subluxation of the atlas causing spinal cord compression in a case of Down's syndrome with a manifestation of an occipital vertebra. Radiology, 93, 839-840.

Martinelli, G., et al. (1964). Electroencephalogram in adolescent mongoloid idiots (considerations on bioelectric cortical immaturity). Riv. Neurobiol, 10, 539-550.

Martins, C. C. (1985). Early vocabulary acquisition by Down syndrome children: the roles of cognitive development and maternal language input. Dissertation Abstracts International, 45(8-B), 2712.

Matey, C. M. (1982). A comparison of mother speech to 18-month and 3-year-old normal children, Down's syndrome children, and hearing-impaired children in semistructured and structured settings. Dissertation Abstracts International, 42(8-A), 3556-3557.

Mattick, P. S. (1971). Effects of three instructional conditions upon the exploratory behavior of normal and Down's syndrome infants. Dissertation Abstracts International, 32(1- A), 276.

Maurer, H. S. (1986). Context of directives given to young normally developing and Down syndrome children: mental age vs. chronological age. Dissertation Abstracts International, 46(8-B), 2838-2839.

McCall, R. B., Hagarty, P. S., & Hurlburt, N. (1972). Transitions in infant sensorimation development and the prediction of childhood IQ. Am. Psychol., 1972, 728-748.

McCarthy, M. E. (1982). Relationships among the competence of Down's syndrome infants, maternal perception of infant temperament, and maternal attitudes toward childrearing. Dissertation Abstracts International. 42(9-B), 3842-3843.

McConkey, R., & Martin, H. (1983). Mother's play with toys: a longitudinal study with Down's syndrome infants. Child Care, Health & Development, 9(4) 215-226.

McConkey, R., & Martin, H. (1984). A longitudinal study of mothers' speech to preverbal Down's syndrome infants. First Language, 5(13, pt. 1), 41-55.

McConkey, R. (1985). Changing beliefs about play and handicapped children. Special issue: children's play. Early Child Development & Care, 19(1-2), 79-94.

McCord, H. (1956). The hypno-ability of the mongoloid-type child. Journal of Clinical and Experimental Hypnosis, 4, 19-20.

McCoy, E. E., Rostafinsky, M. J., & Fishburn, C. (1968). The concentration of serotonin by platelets in Down's syndrome. Journal of Mental Deficiency Research, 12(1), 18-21.

McDade, H. L., & Adler, S. (1980). Down syndrome and short-term memory impairment: a storage or retrieval deficit?. American Journal of Mental Deficiency, 84(6), 561-567.

McDonald, G., & MacKay, D. N. (1974). The effects of proximal and distal proactive interference on recall by subnormals. Journal of Mental Deficiency Research, 18(4), 377-391.

McDonald, G., & MacKay, D. N. (1977). Pattern detection by mongol and non-mongol subnormals. Br. J. Psychol., 68(2), 223-228.

McEvoy, J., & McConkey, R. (1983). Play activities of mentally handicapped children at home and mother's perception of play. International Journal of Rehab Research, 6(2), 143-151.

McIlvane, W. J., Withstandley, J. K., & Stoddard, L. T. (1985). Positive and negative stimulus relations in severely retarded individuals' conditional discrimination. Analysis & Intervention in Developmental Disabilities, 4(3) 235-25.

McIntire, M. S., & Dutsch, S. J. (1964). Mongolism and generalized hypotonia. Am. J. Ment. Defic., 68, 699.

McIntire, M. S., Menolascino, F. J., & Wiley, J. H. (1965). Mongolism - some clinical aspects. American Journal of Mental Deficiency, 69, 794-799.

McIntosh, E. I., & Warren, S. A. (1969). Adaptive behavior in the retarded: A semi-longitudinal study. Training School Bulletin, 66(1), 12-22.

McNeill, W. D. (1955). Developmental patterns of mongoloid children: a study of certain aspects of their growth and development. Dissertation Abstracts, 15, 86-87.

McQuiston, S. (1982). The relationship between infant visual attentiveness and maternal behavior during face-to-face interaction: a longitudinal study of 3- and 6-month-old Down's syndrome and nondelayed infants. Dissertation Abstracts International, 42(8-B), 3459.

Mechem, R. S. (1970). Study of differences in measures of overprotective attitude between mothers of high and low functioning mongoloid children. Dissertation Abstracts International, 30(12-A), 5290-5291.

Meindl, J. L., Barclay, A. G., Lamp, R. E., & Yater, A. C. (1971). Mental growth in noninstitutionalized mongoloid children. Proceedings of the APA Annual Meeting, 6(2), 621-622.

Meindl, J. L., Yater, A. C., Lamp, R. E., & Barclay, A. G. (1983). Mental growth of noninstitutionalized and institutionalized children with Down's syndrome. British Journal of Mental Subnormality, 29(1), 50-56.

Melyn, M. A., & White, D. T. (1973). Mental and developmental milestones of noninstitutionalized Down's syndrome children. Pediatrics, 52, 542.

Menolascino, F. J. (1965). Psychiatric aspects of mongolism. American Journal of Mental Deficiency, 69, 653-660.

Menolascino, F. J. (1965). Psychiatric findings in a sample of institutionalized mongoloids. J. Ment. Subnorm., 13, 67-74.

Menolascino, F. J. (1974). Developmental attributes in Down's syndrome. Mental Retardation, 12(3), 13-17.

Menolascino, F. J. (1974). Changing developmental perspectives in Down's syndrome. Child Psychiatry & Human Development, 4(4), 205-215.

Merjanian, P. M. (1986). Involvement of the hippocampus and amygdala in autism. Dissertation Abstracts International, 46(10-B), 3631.

Merrill, R. E. (1970). Recreation opportunities for children with Down's syndrome. Ann. N.Y. Acad. Sci., 171, 662-665.

Mervis, C. B., & Cardoso-Martins, C. (1984). Transition from sensorimotor stage 5 to stage 6 by Down syndrome children: A response to Gibson. American Journal of Mental Deficiency, 89(1), 99-102.

Messerly, D. L. (1981). A comparison of Down's syndrome and moderately retarded children on selected gross motor skills and body somatotyping. Dissertation Abstracts International, 42(5-A), 2022.

Metcalfe, J. A., & Stratford, B. (1986). Development of perception and cognitive abilities among nonhandicapped

children and children with Down syndrome. Australia &
New Zealand Journal of Developmental Disabilities,
12(1), 65-72.
Meyer, A., & Jones, T. B. (1939). Histological changes in
the brain in mongolism. J. Ment. Sci., 85, 206.
Michaelis, C. T. (1977). The language of a Down's syn-
drome child. Dissertation Abstracts International,
37(9-A), 5747.
Michel, J. F., & Carney, R. J. (1964). Pitch character-
istics of mongoloid boys. Journal of Speech and Hearing
Disorders, 29, 121-125.
Mikkeksen, M. (1982). Parental origin of the extra chrom-
osome in Down's syndrome. Journal of Mental Deficiency
Research, 26(3), 143-151.
Millar, A. L. (1985). Effects of endurance training on
Down's syndrome adolescents and young adults. Disserta-
tion Abstracts International, 46(6-A), 1554.
Miller, D. A. (1978). Selected variables associated with
mobility training for mentally retarded adolescents.
Dissertation Abstracts International, 38(7-A), 4098-
4099.
Milunsky, A. (1970). Glucose intolerance in the parents
of children with Down's syndrome. American Journal of
Mental Deficiency, 74(4), 475-478.
Miniszek, N. A. (1982). Development of Alzheimer's dis-
ease in Down syndrome individuals. American Journal of
Mental Deficiency, 87(4), 377-385.
Mino, M. (1968). Clinical biochemistry of Down's syndrome -- energy metabolism in the brain. Saishin Igaku,
24(2), 325-328.
Miranda, S. B. (1970). Response to novel visual stimuli
by Down's syndrome and normal infants. Proceedings of
the Annual Convention of the American Psychological
Association.
Miranda, S. B., & Fantz, R. L. (1973). Visual preferences
of Down's syndrome and normal infants. Child Development, 44(3), 555-561.
Miranda, S. B. (1976). Visual attention in defective and
high-risk infants. Merrill-Palmer Quarterly, 22(3),
201-228.
Montague, J. C. (1976). Perceived age and sex characteristics of voices of institutionalized children with
Down's syndrome. Perceptual & Motor Skills, 42(1),

215-219.

Moor, L. (1967). Intellectual level in trisomy 21. Annales Meidico-Psychologiques, 2(5), 808-809.

Moore, B. C., Thuline, H. C., & Capes, L. V. (1968). Mongoloid and non-mongoloid retardates: A behavioral comparison. American Journal of Mental Deficiency, 73(3), 433-436.

Moore, B. C., Thuline, H. C., & Capes, L. (1968). Mongoloid and nonmongoloid retardates: A behavioral comparison. Am. J. Ment. Defic., 73, 433-436.

Moran, M. J., & Gilbert, H. R. (1982). Selected acoustic characteristics and listener judgement of the voice of Down syndrome adults. American Journal of Mental Deficiency, 86(5), 553-556.

Moran, M. J. (1986). Identification of Down's syndrome adults from prolonged vowel samples. Journal of Communication Disorders, 19(5), 387-394.

Morecki-O'Berg, C. (1984). Attachment behaviors and the development of the concept of permanence in young children with Down's syndrome. Dissertation Abstracts International, 45(3-A), 811-812.

Morgan, S. B. (1979). Development and distribution of intellectual and adaptive skills in Down's syndrome: implications for early intervention. Mental Retardation, 17(5), 247-249.

Moric, P. S. (1968). Mother's age and Down's syndrome. Journal of Mental Deficiency Research, 12(2), 138-143.

Morris, A. F., Vaughan, S. E., & Vaccaro, P. (1982). Measurements of neuromuscular tone and strength in Down's syndrome children. Journal of Mental Deficiency Research, 26(1), 41-46.

Morss, J. R. (1985). Early cognitive development: difference or delay? In: D. Lane and B. Stratford (eds.), Current Approaches to Down's Syndrome. London: Holt, Rinehart, and Winston.

Morss, J. R. (1983). Cognitive development in the Down's syndrome infant: slow or different?. British Journal of Educational Psychology, 53(1), 40-47.

Morss, J. R. (1984). Enhancement of object-permanence performance in the Down's syndrome infant. Child Care, Health & Development, 10(1), 39-47.

Moses, N. (1983). A model for the study of the internal regulation of spontaneous behavior in three mentally retarded children with Down's syndrome. <u>Dissertation Abstracts International</u>, <u>43</u>(11-A), 3455.

Motti, F., Cicchetti, D., & Sroufe, L. A. (1983). From infant affect expression to symbolic play: the coherence of development in Down syndrome children. <u>Child Development</u>, <u>54</u>(5), 1168-1175.

Murdoch, J. C., & Mader, N. T. (1984). Down's syndrome children and parental psychological upset. <u>J. R. Coll. Gen. Pract.</u>, <u>34</u>(259), 87-90.

Murofushi, K. (1974). Symmetrical pseudocalcium deposits in the basal ganglia and white matter of the brain with moderate leukoencephalopathy in Down's syndrome. <u>Neuropaediatrie</u>, <u>5</u>(1), 103-108.

Murofushi, K., & Arai, Y. (1968). Brain pathology in Down's syndrome. <u>Saishin Igaku</u>, <u>24</u>(2), 297-302.

Murphy, M. M. (1956). Comparison of developmental patterns of three diagnostic groups of middle grade and low grade mental defectives. <u>Am. J. Ment. Defic.</u>, <u>61</u>, 164.

Nachtsheim, H. (1963). Genetics in the service of psychiatry. Demonstrated by the example of cytogenetics of mongoloid idiocy. <u>Muench. Med. Wochenschr.</u>, <u>105</u>, 2053-2062.

Nadel, L. (1986). Down Syndrome in neurobiological perspective. In: C. J. Epstein (ed.), <u>The Neurobiology of Down Syndrome</u>. New York: Raven Press.

Nakamura, H. (1961). Nature of institutionalized adult mongoloid intelligence. <u>Am. J. Ment. Defic.</u>, <u>66</u>, 456-458.

Nakamura, H. (1965). An inquiry into systematic differences in the abilities of institutionalized adult mongoloids. <u>American Journal of Mental Deficiency</u>, <u>69</u>, 661-665.

Nakauchi, M. (1972). Analysis of personality formation of children affected with Down syndrome. <u>Psychiatr. Neurol. Jap.</u>, <u>74</u>(2), 79-97.

Nakhnikian, E. (1983). Facial expressions of emotion in Down's syndrome and normal children. <u>Dissertation Abstracts International</u>, <u>43</u>(7-B), 2348.

Nathanson, D., & Lopez, G. (1975). The maternal linguistic input of Down's syndrome and of normal Spanish-speaking Cuban-American children. <u>Revista Latin Americana De Psichologie</u>, <u>7</u>(2), 321-326.

Neumann, M. A. (1967). Langdon Down syndrome and Alzheimer's disease. J. Neuropathol. Exp. Neurol., 26(1), 149-150.

Neville, J. (1959). Paranoid schizophrenia in a mongoloid defective: some theoretical considerations derived from an unusual case. Journal of Mental Science, 105, 444-447.

Nicholls, K. (1976). Teaching visual discrimination to Down's syndrome children. Part I. Unpublished manuscript, Experimental Education Unit, University of Washington.

Nisbet, J., Zanella, K., & Miller, J. (1984). An analysis of conversations among handicapped students and a non-handicapped peer. Exceptional Children, 51(2), 156-162.

Niwa, S. I., Ohta, M., & Yamazaki, K. (1983). P300 and stimulus evaluation process in autistic subjects. Journal of Autism & Developmental Disorders, 13(1), 33-42.

Norris, D. (1971). Crying and laughing in imbeciles. Developmental Medicine and Child Neurology, 13, 756-761.

Nulman, D. M. (1978). A retrospective analysis of the relationship of age at entry into early educational interventions and subsequent intellectual achievement of Down's syndrome children. Dissertation Abstracts International, 38(12-A), 7273.

Numata, W. (1976). Training parents how to reduce tongue protrusion in a Down's syndrome child. Unpublished paper, Experimental Education Unit, University of Washington.

O'Connor, N., & Hermelin, B. (1961). Visual and stereognostic shape recognition in normal children and mongol and non-mongol imbeciles. Journal of Mental Deficiency Research, 5, 63-66.

O'Connor, L., & Schery, T. K. (1986). A comparison of microcomputer-aided and traditional language therapy for developing communication skills in non-oral toddlers. Journal of Speech & Hearing Disorders, 51(4), 356-361.

Oelwein, P. (1976). Teaching reading to Down's syndrome children. Unpublished paper, Experimental Education Unit, College of Education and Child Development and Mental Retardation Center, University of Washington.

Oelwein, P. (1977). Reading program for children with Down's syndrome. In: Devel. Prog. Down's Syndrome Child. Reston, Virginia: Council for Exceptional Children In-

stitute.
Oelwein, P. L., Fewell, R. R., & Pruess, J. B. (1985). The efficacy of intervention at outreach sites of the program for children with Down syndrome and other developmental delays. Topics in Early Childhood Special Education, 5(2), 78-87.
Ogietree, E. J. (1974). The universal child: the mongol and his education. Special Children, 1(2), 25-28.
O'Hara, P. T. (1972). Electron microscopic study of the brain in Down's syndrome. Brain, 95(4), 681-684.
O'Hare, M. G. (1966). Concept formation in children with Down's syndrome (mongolism). Dissertation Abstracts, 27(6B), 2143.
O'Kelly, C. M. (1978). Maternal linguistic environment of Down's syndrome children. Australian Journal of Mental Retardation, 5(4), 121-126.
Ong, B. H., Rosner, E., Mahanand, D., Houck, J. C., & Paine, R. S. (1967). Clinical, psychological, and radiological comparisons of trisomic and translocation Down's syndrome. Developmental Medicine and Child Neurology, 9(3), 307-312.
Ortega, D. F., Schultz, J. K., & Sanders, R. M. (1976). The use of social reinforcement to increase productivity and develop self-monitoring skills in a mentally retarded assembly-line worker. Vocational Evaluation & Work Adjustment Bulletin, 9(3), 8-1.
Oster, J. (1953). Mongolism. Copenhagen: Danish Science Press.
Owens, R. E., & MacDonald, J. D. (1982). Communicative uses of the early speech of nondelayed and Down syndrome children. American Journal of Mental Deficiency, 86(5), 503-510.
Padeh, B. (1968). Down's Syndrome. Harefuah: Journal of the Israel Medical Association, 74(1), 17-21.
Padgett, W. L., Garcia, H. D., & Pernice, M. B. (1984). A travel training program: reducing wandering in a residential center for developmentally disabled persons. Behavior Modification, 8(3), 317-330.
Palermo-Piastra, E. A. (1981). A longitudinal study of Down's syndrome, children's languages during sensorimotor stages IV through VI. Dissertation Abstracts International, 42(5-A), 2073-2074.
Palo, J., & Savolainen, H. (1973). The proteins of human

myelin in inborn errors of metabolism and in chromosomal anomalies. Acta Neuropathol. Berlin, 24(1), 56-61.

Paluck, R. J., & Esser, A. H. (1971). Controlled experimental modification of aggressive behavior in territor-
ies of severely retarded boys. American Journal of Mental Deficiency, 76(1), 23-29.

Pankratov, M. A. (1968). Sensitivity and lability of the
nervous system in patients with Down's disease. Zhurnal
Nevropatologii I Psikhiatrii, 68(10), 1513-1515.

Pantarotto, M. F. (1967). Longitudinal study of body
growth and mental development of mongoloid children
with special reference to the limits of their social
recuperability. Minerva Pediatr., 19(48), 2126-2131.

Papez, J. W., & Papez, P. (1957). Mycotic nature of brain
damage in mental deficiency. Am. J. Physiol., 70, 333-
346.

Papp, Z., Adam, B., & Szabo, Z. (1976). Prenatal growth
in Down's syndrome. Orv. Hetil., 117(5), 277-282.

Parikh, J., & Shukla, S. (1984). Mental health through
integration for children with special needs. Journal of
Psychological Research, 28(2), 77-83.

Parker, A. W., Bronks, R., & Snyder, C. W. (1986). Walking patterns in Down's syndrome. Journal of Mental Deficiency Research, 30(4), 317-330.

Parker, A. W., & James, B. (1985). Age changes in the
flexibility of Down's syndrome children. Journal of
Mental Deficiency Research, 29(3), 207-218.

Parker, G. (1984). Training for continence among children
with severe disabilities. British Journal of Mental
Subnormality, 30(1)(58), 38-43.

Parker, P. I. (1984). Auditory memory of persons with
Down's syndrome. Dissertation Abstracts International,
45(6-8), 1942.

Parmelee, A. H., Akiyama, Y., Stern, E., & Harris, M. A.
(1969). A periodic cerebral rhythm in newborn infants.
Exp. Neurol., 25(4), 575-584.

Patterson, D. (1987). The causes of Down's syndrome. Scientific American, 257, 42-48.

Patterson, D., et al. (1985). Molecular analysis of
chromosome 21 using somatic cell hybrids. Symposium of
the National Down Syndrome Society: Molecular Structure
of the Number 21 Chromosome and Down Syndrome. Annals
of the New York Academy of Sciences, 450, 109-120.

Paulson, G. W., Nance, W. E., & Son, C. D. (1968). Neurologic aspects of typical and atypical Down's syndrome.
Neurology Minneapolis, 18(3), 305-306.
Paulson, G. W., Son, C. D., & Nance, W. E. (1969). Neurologic aspects of typical and atypical Down's syndrome.
Diseases of the Nervous System, 30(9), 632-636.
Paulson, G. W. (1971). Failure of ambulation in Down's
syndrome. A clinical survey. Clin. Pediatr. Philadelphia, 10(5), 265-267.
Pecyna, P. M., & Sommers, R. K. (1985). Testing the receptive language skills of severely handicappd preschool children. Language, Speech, & Hearing Services
in the Schools, 16(1), 41.
Pesch, R. S., et al. (1978). A survey of the visual and
developmental-perceptual abilities of the Down's syndrome child. J. Am. Optom. Assoc., 49(9), 1031-1037.
Peskett, R., & Wootton, A. (1985). Turn-taking and overlap in the speech of young Down's syndrome children.
Journal of Mental Deficiency Research, 29(3), 263-273.
Peters, M. L. (1970). A comparison of the musical sensitivity of mongoloid and normal children. Journal of
Music Therapy, 7(4), 113-123.
Peterson, G. A., & Sherrod, K. B. (1981). Relationship of
maternal language to language development and language
delay of children. American Journal of Mental Deficiency, 86(4), 391-398.
Peterson, G. A. (1979). Maternal speech patterns: their
relationship to language development and language delay. Dissertation Abstracts International, 39(11-B),
5525.
Peterson, K. L. (1984). An exploration of the separation-
individuation processes in the Down syndrome child.
Dissertation Abstracts International, 45(5-A), 1530.
Peterson, N. L. (1982). Social integration of handicapped
and nonhandicapped preschoolers: a study of playmate
preferences. Topics in Early Childhood Special Education, 2(2), 56-69.
Petit, T. L., Le Boutillier, J. C., Alfano, D. P., &
Becker, L. E. (1984). Synaptic development in the human
fetus: A morphological analysis of normal and Down's
syndrome neocortex. Expr. Neurol., 83, 13-23.
Petre-Quadens, O., & Jouvet, M. (1966). Study of sleep
disorders and of oneiric activity in the mentally re-

tarded. <u>Rev. Neurol. Paris</u>, <u>115</u>(3), 530.

Philpot, M., et al. (1985). Prolactin cell autoantibodies and Alzheimer's disease. <u>Journal of Neurology, Neurosurgery & Psychiatry</u>, <u>48</u>(3), 287-288.

Pickersgill, M. J., & Pank, C. (1970). Relation of age and mongolism to lateral preferences in severely subnormal subjects. <u>Nature London</u>, <u>228</u>(278), 1342-1344.

Piessens, F. P., & Overweg, J. (1971). Alzheimer's disease in mongoloid idiocy (Down's trisomy). <u>Ned. Tijdschr. Geneeskd.</u>, <u>115</u>(48), 2018-2020.

Pipe, M. E. (1983). Dichotic-listening performance following auditory discrimination training in Down's syndrome and developmentally retarded children. <u>Cortex</u>, <u>19</u>(4), 481-491.

Pipe, M. E. (1985). Attenuation of dichotic-listening ear advantages by stimulus bias. <u>Neuropsychologia</u>, <u>23</u>(3), 437-440.

Piper, M. C., & Ramsey, M. K. (1980). Effects of early home environment on the mental development of Down's syndrome infants. <u>American Journal of Mental Deficiency</u>, <u>85</u>(1), 39-44.

Piper, M. C., & Pless, I. B. (1980). Early intervention for infants with Down's syndrome: a controlled trial. <u>Pediatrics</u>, <u>65</u>(3), 463-468.

Piper, M. C., Gosselin, C., Gendron, M., & Mazer, B. (1986). Developmental profile of Down's syndrome infants receiving early intervention. <u>Child Care, Health & Development</u>, <u>12</u>(3), 183-194.

Pisani, C. (1963). Evolutive aspects of the EEG and of the intellectual level in 35 mongoloid subjects. <u>Riv. Patol. Clin.</u>, <u>18</u>, 815-823.

Polvinale, R. A., Lutzker, J. R. (1980). Elimination of assaultive and inappropriate sexual behavior by reinforcement and social-restitution. <u>Mental Retardation</u>, <u>18</u>(1), 27-30.

Pototzky, C., & Grigg, A. E. (1942). A reversion of the prognosis in mongolism. <u>American Journal of Orthopsychiatry</u>, <u>12</u>, 503.

Potter, L. (1967). Art Activities for the Down's Syndrome Advanced Preschool. Experimental Education Unit, College of Education and Child Development and Mental Retardation Center, University of Washington.

Powers, M. (1976). Teaching addition skills to Down's

syndrome children. Unpublished paper, Experimental Education Unit, University of Washington.

Powers, M. (1976). Teaching subtraction skills to Down's syndrome children. Unpublished paper, Experimental Education Unit, University of Washington.

Prechtl, H. F., Theorell, K., & Blair, A. W. (1973). Behavioral state cycles in abnormal infants. Dev. Med. Child Neurol., 15(5), 606-615.

Price, D. L., et al. (1982). Alzheimer's disease and Down's syndrome. Annals of the New York Academy of Sciences, 396, 145-164.

Price, D. L., et al. (1985). The functional organization of the basal forebrain cholinergic system in primates and the role of this system in Alzheimer's disease. Annals of the New York Academy of Sciences, 444, 287-295.

Prior, M. R., & Chen, C. S. (1976). Short-term and serial memory in autistic, retarded, and normal children. J. Autism Child. Schizophr., 6(2), 121-131.

Pruess, J. B., Vadasy, P. F., & Fewell, R. R. (1987). Language development in children with Down syndrome: An overview of recent research. Education & Training in Mental Retardation, 22(1), 44-55.

Pueschel, S. M. (1975). Theoretical concepts of early intervention in Down's syndrome. In: R. Koch and F. F. DelaCruz (eds.), Down's Syndrome: Research, Prevention, and Management. New York: Brunner/ Mazel, Inc., 130-136.

Pueschel, S. M., Gallagher, P. L., Zartler, A. S., & Pezzullo, J. C. (1987). Cognitive and learning processes in children with Down syndrome. Research in Developmental Disabilities, 8(1), 21-37.

Pueschel, S. M., & Murphy, A. (1977). Assessment of counseling practices at the birth of a child with Down's syndrome. Am. J. Ment. Defic., 81(4), 325-330.

Purpura, D. P. (1974). Dendritic spine dysgenesis and mental retardation. Science, 186, 1126-1128.

Quaytman, W. (1953). The psychological capacities of mongoloid children in a community clinic. Q. Rev. Pediatr., 8, 255-267.

Rabensteiner, B. (1975). Social behavior, musicality and visual perception in mongoloid children. Paediatr. Paedol. (Suppl.), 4, 59-69.

Rao, B. S. (1966). Certain interesting genetical aspects of 62 mentally retarded children of different diagnostic types screened for possible biochemical anomalies. Transactions of All-India Institute of Mental Health, 6, 47-53.

Rast, M. M., & Harris, S. R. (1985). Motor control in infants with Down syndrome. Developmental Medicine & Child Neurology, 27(5), 682-685.

Read, S. G. (1982). The distribution of Down's syndrome. Journal of Mental Deficiency Research, 26(4), 215-227.

Reed, R. B., & Pueschel, S. M. (1980). Interrelationships of biological, environmental, and competency variables in young children with Down's syndrome. Applied Research in Mental Retardation, 1(3-4), 161-174.

Rees, S. (1977). The incidence of ultrastructural abnormalities in the cortex of two retarded human brains. (Down's syndrome). Acta Neuropathol. Berlin, 37(1), 65-68.

Reeves, R. H., Gearhart, J. D., & Littlefield, J. W. (1986). Genetic basis for a mouse model of Down syndrome. Special issue: The neurobiologic consequences of autosomal trisomy in mice and men. Brain Research Bulletin, 16(6), 803-814.

Rehder, H. (1976). Prenatal pathology of the Down's and Edwards' syndrome. In: A. Boue (ed.), Prenatal Diagnosis. Paris: Inserm, 117-130.

Reiber, J. L., Goetz, E. M., Baer, D. M., & Green, D. R. (1977). Increasing a Down's child's attending behavior with attention from teachers and normal preschool children. Revista Mexicana de Analisis de la Conducta, 3(1), 75-85.

Reichle, J. E. (1980). Participation in mother/child communication exchanges by sensorimotor stage six (6) Down's and normal children during three different communicatons contexts. Dissertation Abstracts International, 40(12-B, pt. 1), 5844.

Reichle J. E., Siegel, G., & Rettie, M. (1985). Matching prosodic and sound features: performance of Down's syndrome preschoolers. Journal of Communication Disorders, 18(3), 149-159.

Reid, A. H., Maloney, A. F., & Aungle, P. G. (1978). Dementia in aging mental defectives: a clinical and neuropathological study. Journal of Mental Deficiency

Research, 22(4), 223-241.

Reinecke, M. E. (1973). An analysis of the intellectual characteristics of Down's syndrome and non-Down's syndrome retarded children. Dissertation Abstracts International, 33(10-A), 5588.

Reisman, L. E. (1966). Relationship between cytogenic constitution, physical stigmata and intelligence in Down's syndrome. Proceedings of the American Association on Mental Deficiency Meeting.

Reisman, L. E., Shipe, D., & Williams, R. D. B. (1966). Mosaicism in Down's syndrome: studies in a child with an unusual chromosome constitution. American Journal of Mental Deficiency, 70, 855-859.

Resenzweig, L. E. (1953). School training of the mongoloid child. Q. Rev. Pediatr., 8, 281-289.

Rhodes, L., Gooch, B., Siegelman, E. Y., Behrns, C., & Metzger, R. (1969). A language stimulation and reading program for severely retarded mongoloid children. California Mental Health Research Monograph No. 11, State of California.

Richard, N. B. (1986). Interaction between mothers and infants with Down syndrome: infant characteristics. Topics in Early Childhood Special Education, 6(3), 54-71.

Richmond, G. (1982). Two treatment strategies for improving a profoundly retarded girl's mealtime posture. Psychological Reports, 51(3, pt. 2), 1183-1186.

Ricotti, M. P., & Zerbi, F. (1970). Cytogenetic research in a group of pupils attending a medical-psychoeducational school. Acta Neurologica, 25(6), 716-722.

Ridler, M. A., Pendrey, M. J., Faunch, J. A., & Berg, J. M. (1969). Association of D/D translocation with mongolism. Journal of Mental Deficiency Research, 13(2), 89-98.

Rietveld, C. M. (1986). The adjustment to school of eight children with Down's syndrome from an early intervention program. Australia & New Zealand Journal of Developmental Disabilities, 12(3).

Rietvald, C. M. (1983). The training of choice behaviors in Down's syndrome and nonretarded preschool children. Australia & New Zealand Journal of Developmental Disabilities, 9(3).

Riquet, C. B., & Taylor, N. D. (1981). Symbolic play in

autistic, Down's, and normal children of equivalent mental age. Journal of Autism & Developmental Disorders, 11(4), 439-448.

Rinaldi, F., et al. (1972). Spontaneous cerebral electro-activity faster than 14 c-s: electroencephalographic findings in mongoloids. Acta Neurol. Napoli, 27(3), 291-304.

Ristau, C. A. (1974). Infant vocal communication: A comparison of normal and mongoloid humans, other primates and carnivores. Dissertation Abstracts International, 35(5-B), 2411-2412.

Robenalt, K. S. (1986). Turn-taking among Down syndrome infant/mother dyads and normal infant/mother dyads. Dissertation Abstracts International, 46(11-B), 3811.

Roche, A. F. (1968). Difficulties associated with studies of growth and development in mentally retarded children. Proc. 1st Cong. Internat. Assoc. Scient. Study Ment. Defic., 845.

Rogers, G. W. (1975). Teaching parameters for the trainable mentally retarded. Dissertation Abstracts International, 35(8-A), 5179.

Roith, A. I. (1961). Psychotic depression in a mongol. J. Ment. Sub., 7, 45-47.

Rollins, H. R. (1946). Personality in mongolism with special reference to the incidence of catatonic psychosis. Am. J. Ment. Defic., 51, 219.

Romski, M. A. (1982). A comparison of the effects of speech and sign on the oral language learning of Down's syndrome children early stage I. Dissertation Abstracts International, 42(8-A), 3560.

Romski, M. A., & Ruder, K. F. (1984). Effects of speech and speech and sign instruction on oral language learning and generalization of object + object combinations by Down's syndrome children. Journal of Speech & Hearing Disorders, 49(3), 293-302.

Rondal, J. A. (1976). Maternal speech to normal and Down's syndrome children matched for mean length of utterance. Dissertation Abstracts International, 37(6-A), 3529-3530.

Rondal, J.A., Lambert, J. L., & Schier, C. (1981). Verbal and nonverbal imitation in Down's syndrome and non-Down's retarded children. Enfance, 3, 107-122.

Rondal, J. A. (1978). Patterns of correlations for various language measures in mother-child interactions for normal and Down's syndrome children. Language & Speech, 21(3), 242-252.

Rondal, J. A., Lambert, J. L., & Sohier, C. (1981). Elicited verbal and nonverbal imitation in Down's syndrome and other mentally retarded children: a replication and extension of Berry. Language & Speech, 24(3), 245-254.

Rondal, J. A. (1980). Verbal imitation by Down syndrome and nonretarded children. American Journal of Mental Deficiency, 85(3), 318-321.

Ropper, A. H., & Williams, R. S. (1980). Relationship between plagues, tangles, and dementia in Down's syndrome. Neurology, 30, 639-644.

Rosecrans, C. J. (1971). A longitudinal study of exceptional cognitive development in a partial translocation Down's syndrome child. Am. J. Ment. Defic., 76(3), 291-294.

Rosenfeld, M. J., Peterson, R. M., & Koch, R. (1969). Down's syndrome: intelligence and chromosome findings. Proceedings of the American Academy on Mental Retardation, San Francisco, CA.

Rosine, L. P., & Martin, G. L. (1983). Self-management training to decrease undesirable behavior of mentally handicapped adults. Rehabilitation Psychology, 28(4), 195-205.

Rosner, F., Steinberg, F. S., & Spriggs, H. A. (1967). Dermatoglyphic patterns in patients with selected neurological disorders. Am. J. Med. Sci., 254(5), 695-708.

Ross, L. E., Headrick, M. W., & Mackay, P. B. (1967). Classical eyelid conditioning of young mongoloid children. American Journal of Mental Deficiency, 72, 21-29.

Ross, M. H., Galaburda, A. M., & Kemper, T. L. (1984). Down's syndrome: is there a decreased population of neurons? Neurology, 34, 909-915.

Ross, R. T. (1971). A preliminary study of self-help skills and age in hospitalized Down's syndrome patients. American Journal of Mental Deficiency, 76(3), 373-377.

Ross, R. T. (1972). The mental growth of mongoloid defectives. American Journal of Mental Deficiency, 66, 736-738.

Ross, F. F. (1983). A comparison of the effects of sign language, speech, and total communication on short-term memory in Down's syndrome adolescents. <u>Dissertation Abstracts International</u>, <u>43</u>(9-A), 2964.

Rothbart, M. K., & Hanson, M. J. (1983). A caregiver report comparison of temperamental characteristics of Down syndrome and normal infants. <u>Developmental Psychology</u>, <u>19</u>(5), 766-769.

Rotundo, N., & Johnson, E. G. (1981). Verbal control of motor behavior in mentally retarded children: a re-examination of Luria's theory. <u>Journal of Mental Deficiency Research</u>, <u>25</u>(4), 281-298.

Rudrud, E. H., Ziarnik, J. P., & Colman, G. (1984). Reduction of tongue protusion of a 24-year-old woman with Down syndrome through self-monitoring. <u>American Journal of Mental Deficiency</u>, <u>88</u>(6), 647-652.

Rynders, J. E., & Horrobin, M. (1967). A mobile unit for delivering educational services to Down's syndrome (mongoloid) infants. <u>Research Report No. 30. Minn., Minneapolis Bureau of Education for the Handicapped (DHEW/OE), Wash., D.C.</u>

Rynders, J. E., Spiker, D., & Horrobin, J. M. (1976). Underestimating the educability of Down's syndrome children: Examination of methodological problems in recent literature. <u>Am. J. Ment. Defic.</u>, <u>82</u>(5), 440-448.

Rynders, J. E., Behlen, K. L., & Horrobin, J. M. (1979). Performance characteristics of preschool Down's syndrome children receiving augmented or repetitive verbal training. <u>American Journal of Mental Deficiency</u>, <u>84</u>(1), 67-73.

Rynders, J. E., & Johnson, R. T. (1980). Producing positive interaction among Down syndrome and handicapped teenagers through cooperative goal structuring. <u>American Journal of Mental Deficiency</u>, <u>85</u>(3) 268-273.

Sabsay, S. L. (1979). Communicative competence in Down's syndrome adults. <u>Dissertation Abstracts International</u>, <u>40</u>(1-A), 228.

Saito, S. (1977). Transposition of intermediate size under immediate and delayed testing conditions by normal, familially retarded, and Down's syndrome children. <u>Tohoku Psychologica Folia</u>, <u>36</u>(1-4), 32-38.

Salzberg, C. L., & Villani, T. V. (1982). Speech training by parents of Down syndrome toddlers: generalization across settings and instructional contexts. American Journal of Mental Deficiency, 87(4), 403-413.

Sand, T., Mellgren, S. I., Hestnes, A. (1983). Primitive reflexes in Down's syndrome. Journal of Mental Deficiency Research, 27(1), 39-44.

Sandler, A., & Coren, A. (1981). Integrated instruction at home and school: parent's perspective. Education & Training of the Mentally Retarded, 16(3), 183-187.

Sapon, S. M., & Reeback, R. (1966). Shaping vocal behavior in a nine-year-old mongoloid boy. University of Rochester, Verbal Behavior Laboratory Report No. 1.

Sapon, P. J. (1982). A comparison of mother-child and father-child relationships in young children with Down's syndrome. Dissertation Abstracts International, 43(1-A), 71.

Sara. V. R., et al. (1983). Somatomedins in Down's syndrome. Biological Psychiatry, 18(7), 803-811.

Sara, V. R., et al. (1984). The presence of normal receptors for somatomedin and insulin in fetuses with Down's syndrome. Biological Psychiatry, 19(4), 591-598.

Sarimski, K. (1983). Kommunikation zwischen muttern und behinderten kleinkindern./Communication between mothers and their handicapped small children. Fruhgorderung Interdisziplinar, 2(4), 167-174.

Sarimski, K. (1982). Effects of etiology and cognitive ability on observational learning of retarded children. International Journal of Rehabilitation Research, 5(1), 75-78.

Schachter, M. (1950). Psychological study of a mongolian idiot age 27 years in the light of the rorschach test. Acta Neurol. Napoli, 5, 122-127.

Schachter, M. (1961). Apropos of the psychology of parents with mongoloid children. Acta Paedopsychiatr., 38, 91-96.

Schachter, M. (1974). Long term psychologic and sociologic prognosis in mongolism. Apropos of several cases followed up for 10 years. Ann. Med. Psychol. Paris, 1(2), 195-224.

Schafer, E. W., & Peeke, H. V. (1982). Down syndrome individuals fail to habituate cortical evoked potentials. American Journal of Mental Deficiency, 87(3), 332-337.

Schauss, A. G., & Sommars, E. (1982). Children's mental retardation study is attacked: a closer look. International Journal for Biosocial Research, 3(2), 75-86.

Scheffelin, M. A. (1968). A comparison of four stimulus-response channels in paired-associate learning. American Journal of Mental Deficiency, 73(2), 303-307.

Scherer, N. J., & Owings-Nathaniel, O. (1984). Learning to be contingent: retarded children's responses to their mother's requests. Language & Speech, 27(3), 255-267.

Schlack, H. G., & Schmidt-Schuh, H. (1977). Neurophysiological and behavioral changes during mental work in children with Down's syndrome. Neuropaediatrie, 8(4), 374-386.

Schlack, H. G. (1978). Neurophysiological activation and behavior during mental achievement. Comparative studies in healthy, minimally brain damaged, and mongoloid children. Fortschr. Med., 96(18), 978-982.

Schlosser, F. D. (1972). Effect of selected combinations of stimuli on communicative responses of children with Down's syndrome. Dissertation Abstracts International, 32(8-B), 4922-4923.

Schlottmann, R. S., & Anderson, V. H. (1973). Social and play behavior of children with Down's syndrome in sexually homogeneous and heterogeneous dyads. Psychological Reports, 33, 595-600.

Schlottmann, R. S., & Anderson, V. H. (1975). Social and play behaviors of institutionalized mongoloid and non-mongoloid retarded children. Journal of Psychology, 91, 201-206.

Schmid, F., Haus, E., Moradof, S., & Dych, H. (1972). Influencing mongoloideal dyscephaly through infection implantations of fetal, heterologous brain tissue. Fortschr. Med., 90(32), 1181-1186.

Schmidt, H. S., Kaelbling, R., & Alexander, J. (1968). Sleep patterns in mental retardates: mongoloids and monozygotic twins. Psychophysiology, 5(2), 212.

Schnieder, J, W., & Brannen, E. A. (1984). A comparison of two developmental evaluation tools used to assess children with Down's syndrome. Physical & Occupational Therapy in Pediatrics, 4(4), 19-29.

Schochet, S. S., Jr., Lampert, P. W., & McCormick, W. F. (1973). Neurofibrillary tangles in patients with Down's syndrome: a light and electron microscopic study. Acta Neuropathol. Berlin, 23(4), 342-346.

Schoenfelder, T. (1965). Psychiatric aspects of mongolism. Med. Welt, 41, 2312-2314.

Scholle, N. B. (1981). A neuropsychological investigation with adult Down's syndrome subjects. Dissertation Abstracts International, 42(3-B), 1190.

Schramm, B. J. (1974). Case studies of two Down's syndrome children functioning in a Montessori environment: Research project. University of Dayton, Ohio School of Education.

Schroth, M. L. (1975). The use of IQ as a measure of problem solving ability with mongoloid and nonmongoloid retarded children. Journal of Psychology, 91(1), 9-56.

Schwarz, L. E. (1983). A comparison of procedures used to assess speech sound production in Down's syndrome children. Dissertation Abstracts International, 43(9-A), 2965.

Schweber, M. (1985). A possible unitary genetic hypothesis for Alzheimer's disease and Down syndrome. Symposium of the National Down Syndrome Society: Molecular Structure of the Number 21 Chromosome and Down Syndrome Annals of the New York Academy of Sciences, 450, 223-238.

Schwethelm, B., & Mahoney, G. (1986). Task persistance among organically impaired mentally retarded children American Journal of Mental Deficiency, 90(4), 432-439.

Scott, B. S., Petit, T. L., & Becker, L. E. (1981). Abnormal electric membrane properties of Down's syndrome DRG neurons in cell culture. Developmental Brain Research, 2(2), 257-270.

Scott, S. S., Becker, L. E., & Petit, T. L. (1983). Neurobiology of Down's syndrome. Progress in Neurobiology, 21, 199-237.

Seagoe, M. V. (1965). Verbal development in a mongoloid. Exceptional Children, 31, 269-273.

Sehgal, H. (1967). Aetiology of inability to walk in children between two and five years of age. J. Indian Med. Assoc., 48, 212-218.

Seitz, S. (1975). Language intervention - changing the language environment of the retarded child. In: R. Koch and F. F. DelaCruz (ed.), Down's Syndrome (Mongolism): Research, Prevention and Management, New York: Brunner/Mazel.

Semmel, M. I., & Dolley, D. G. (1971). Comprehension and

imitation of sentences by Down's syndrome children as a function of transformational complexity. American Journal of Mental Deficiency, 75(6), 739-745.

Semmel, M. I. (1960). Comparison of teacher ratings of brain-injured and mongoloid severely retarded (trainable) children attending community day-school classes. American Journal of Mental Deficiency, 64, 963-971.

Seppalainen, A. M., & Kivalo, E. (1967). EEG findings and epilepsy in Down's syndrome. J. Ment. Defic. Res., 11(2), 116-125.

Serafica, F. C., & Cicchetti, D. (1976). Down's syndrome children in a strange situation: Attachment and exploration behaviors. Merrill-Palmer Quarterly, 22(2), 137-150.

Sersen, E. A., Astrup, C., Floistad, I., & Wortis, J. (1970). Motor conditional reflexes and word associations in retarded children. American Journal of Mental Deficiency, 74(4), 495-501.

Seyfort, B., & Spreen, O. (1979). Two-plated tapping performance by Down's syndrome and non-Down's syndrome retardates. Journal of Child Psy., Psychia., and Allied Disc., 20(4), 351-355.

Shapiro, B. K., & Heppel, D. (1977). More on factors related to intellectual development of children with Down syndrome. (Letter) J. Pediatr., 91(2), 345-346.

Shapiro, B. L. (1975). Amplified developmental instability in Down's syndrome. Ann. Hum. Genet., 38(4), 429-437.

Shapiro, B. L. (1983). Down syndrome: a disruption of homeostasis. American Journal of Medical Genetics, 14, 241-269.

Sharav, T. (1985). High-risk population for Down's syndrome: orthodox jews in Jerusalem. American Journal of Mental Deficiency, 89(5), 559-561.

Sharav, T., & Shlomo, L. (1986). Stimulation of infants with Down syndrome: long term effects. Mental Retardation, 24(2), 81-86.

Share, J. B. (1975). Developmental progress in Down's syndrome. In: R. K. Koch and F. F. De La Cruz (eds.), Down's Syndrome (Mongolism): Research, Prevention and Management, New York: Brunner/Mazell.

Share, J. B. (1976). Review of drug treatment for Down's syndrome persons. American Journal of Mental Deficiency, 80(4), 388-393.

Share, J. B., & Veale, A. M. (1962). Developmental Landmarks for Children with Down's Syndrome (Mongolism). University of Otago Press.

Share, J. B., & Landman, G. (1972). Down's syndrome longitudinal study. Tech. Report, Serp 1972, A-7, UCLA, 91.

Share, J. B., & French, R. W. (1974). Early motor development in Down's syndrome children. Mental Retardation, 12(6), 23.

Share, J. B., & French, R. W. (1974). Guidelines of early motor development in Down's syndrome children for parents and teachers. Spec. Child., 1(2), 61-65.

Share, J., Koch, R., Webb, A., & Graliker, B. (1964). The longitudinal development of infants and young children with Down's syndrome (mongolism). American Journal of Mental Deficiency, 68, 685-692.

Share, J., Webb, A., & Koch, R. (1961). A preliminary investigation of the early developmental status of mongoloid infants. American Journal of Mental Deficiency, 66, 238-241.

Shotwell, A., & Shipe, D. (1964). Effect of out of home care on the intellectual and social development of mongoloid children. Am. J. Ment. Defic., 68, 693.

Shtilbans, I. I. (1968). The problem of polymorphism in neurogenetics. Vestn. Akad. Med. Nauk SSSR, 23(8), 59-63.

Shuttleworth, G. E. (1909). Mongolian imbecility. British Medical Journal, 2, 661-665.

Sidman, M., Kirk, B., & Willson, M. M. (1985). Six-member stimulus classes generated by conditional-discrimination procedures. Journal of the Experimental Analysis of Behavior, 43(1), 21-42.

Silverstein, A. B. (1964). An empirical test of the mongoloid stereotype. American Journal of Mental Deficiency, 68, 493-497.

Silverstein, A. B. (1966). Mental growth in mongolism. Child Development, 37, 725-729.

Silverstein, A. B., & Owens, E. P. (1968). Factor structure of the social deprivation scale for mongoloid retardates. American Journal of Mental Deficiency, 73, 315-317.

Silverstein, A. B. (1979). Imitative behavior by Down's syndrome persons. Journal of Mental Deficiency, 83(4),

409-411.

Silverstein, A. B., Herbs, D., Nasuta, R., & White, J. F. (1986). Effects of aging on the adaptive behavior of institutionalized individuals with Down's syndrome. American Journal of Mental Deficiency, 90(6), 659-662.

Silverstein, A. B., & Legutki, G. (1982). Performance of Down syndrome individuals on the Stanford-Binet Intelligence Scale. American Journal of Mental Deficiency, 86(5), 548-551.

Silverstein, A. B., Herbs, D., Nasuta, R., & White, J. F. (1986). Effects of age on the adaptive behavior of institutionalized individuals with Down syndrome. American Journal of Mental Deficiency, 90(6), 659-662.

Silverstein, A. B., et al. (1985). Adaptive behavior of institutionalized individuals with Down syndrome. American Journal of Mental Deficiency, 89(5), 555-558.

Simms, M. (1981). Outlook for the Down's syndrome child. Lancet, 2(8251), 864-865.

Simms, M., & Bridgman, G. (1984). Evaluation of progress using the context input process and product model. Child Care, Health & Development, 10(6), 359-379.

Sinef, P. M., Lejeune, J., & Jerome, H. (1979). Trisomy 21 (Down's syndrome) glutathione peroxidase, hexose monophosphate shunt and I.Q. Life Sci., 24(1), 29.

Sinex, F. M., & Myers, R. H. (1982). Alzheimer's disease, Down's syndrome, and aging: the genetic approach. Annals of the New York Academy of Sciences, 396, 3-13.

Sinson, J., & Wetherick, N. E. (1972). Cue salience and learning in severely abnormal children. Effects of varying attention value of the cues employed in a one-trial learning situation. Journal of Mental Deficiency Research, 17(3), 177-182.

Sinson, J. C., & Wetherlick, N. E. (1976). Evidence for increased mental capacity with age in Down's Syndrome. Journal of Mental Deficiency Research, 20(1), 31-34.

Sinson, J. C. (1978). Down's infants: an inter-disciplinary approach involving parents. International Journal of Rehabilitation Research, 1(1), 59-69.

Sinson, J. C., & Wetherlick, N. E. (1975). The nature of the colour retention deficit in Down's syndrome. Journal of Mental Deficiency Research, 19(2), 97-100.

Sinson, J. C., & Wetherick, N. E. (1976). Evidence for increased mental capacity with age in Down's syndrome.

J. Ment. Defic. Res., 20(1), 31-34.

Sinson, J., & Wetherick, N. E. (1973). Short-term retention of colour and shape information in mongol and other severely subnormal children. J. Ment. Defic. Res., 17(3), 177-182.

Sinson, J. C., & Wethernick, N. E. (1981). The behavior of children with Down syndrome in normal playgroups. Journal of Mental Deficiency Research, 25(2), 113-120.

Sinson, J. C., & Wethernick, N. E. (1982). Mutual gaze in preschool Down's and normal children. Journal of Mental Deficiency Research, 26(2), 123-129.

Sinson, J. C., & Wethernick, N.E. (1986). Integrating young children with Down's syndrome: gaze, play, and vocalization in the initial encounter. British Journal of Mental Subnormality, 32(2, 63), 93-101.

Skidmore, R. (1982). Home teaching for pre-school handicapped children: a cognitive approach. Child Care, Health & Development, 8(2), 105-111.

Sloper, P., Cunningham, C. C., & Arnljotsdottir, M. (1983). Parental reactions to early intervention with their Down's syndrome infants. Child Care, Health & Development, 9(6), 357-376.

Sloper, P., Glenn, S. M., & Cunningham, C. C. (1986). The effect of intensity of training on sensori-motor development in infants with Down's syndrome. Journal of Mental Deficiency Research, 30(2), 149-162.

Smith, A., & McKeown, T. (1955). Prenatal growth of mongoloid defectives. Arch. Dis. Child., 30, 257-279.

Smith, L., & Hagen, V. (1984). Relationship between home environment and sensorimotor development of Down's syndrome and nonretarded infants. American Journal of Mental Deficiency, 89(2), 124-132.

Smith, P. J. (1976). Verbal and non-verbal tasks of prediction behavior in Down's syndrome, other retarded and non-retarded populations. Dissertation Abstracts International, 36(8-A), 5204.

Smith, B. L,, & Coller, D. K. (1981). A comparative study of pre-meaningful vocalizations produced by normally developing and Down's syndrome infants. Journal of Speech & Hearing Disorders, 46(1), 46-51.

Smith, B. L. (1982). Some observation concerning pre-meaningful vocalizations of hearing-impaired infants. Journal of Speech & Hearing Disorders, 47(4), 439-441.

Smith, B. L., & Stoel, G. C. (1984). A longitudinal study of the development of stop consonant production in normal and Down's syndrome children. Journal of Speech & Hearing Disorders, 48(2), 114-118.

Smith, G. F., & Warren, S. T. (1985). The biology of Down syndrome. Symposium of the National Down Syndrome Society: Molecular Structure of the Number 21 Chromosome and Down Syndrome. Annals of the New York Academy of Sciences, 450, 1-9.

Smith, L., & Hagen, V. (1984). Relationship between the home environment and sensorimotor development of Down syndrome and retarded infants. American Journal of Mental Deficiency, 89(2), 124-130.

Smith, L., & Von Tetzchner, S. (1986). Communication, sensorimotor, and language skills of young children with Down syndrome. American Journal of Mental Deficiency, 91(1), 57-66.

Smith, M. E. (1984). An investigation into the relationship between the development of self-recognition in one to four year old children and the home environment. Dissertation Abstracts International, 44(10-A), 3020.

Snart, F., O'Grady, M., & Das, J. P. (1982). Cognitive processing by subgroups of moderately retarded children. American Journal of Mental Deficiency, 86(5), 465-472.

Solitaire, G. B., & Lamarche, J. B. (1966). Alzheimer's disease and senile dementia as seen in mongoloids: neuropathological observations. Am. J. Ment. Defic., 70(6), 840-848.

Solitare, G. B., & Lamarche, J. B. (1967). Brain weight in the adult mongol. J. Ment. Defic. Res., 11(2), 79-84.

Solitare, G. B. (1969). The spinal cord of the mongol. J. Ment. Defic. Res., 13(1), 1-7.

Somasundaram, O., Papakumari, M. (1981). A study on Down's anomaly. Child Psychiatry Quarterly, 14(3), 85-94.

Sommers, R. K., & Starkey, K. L. (1977). Dichotic verbal processing in Down's syndrome children having qualitatively different speech and language skills. Am. J. Ment. Defic., 82(1), 44-53.

Sorce, J. F., & Emde, R. N. (1982). The meaning of infant emotional expressions: regularities in caregiving responses in normal and Down's syndrome infants. Journal of Child Psychology & Psychiatry & Allied Disciplines, 86(6), 145-158.

Sovner, R., Hurley, A. D., & Labrie, R. (1985). Is mania incompatible with Down's syndrome?. British Journal of Psychiatry, 146, 319-320.

Spiker, D. K. (1980). A descriptive study of mother-child teaching interactions with high- and low-functional Down's syndrome preschoolers. Dissertation Abstracts International, 40(12-B, pt. 1), 5845.

Spiker, D. K. (1982). Parent involvement in early intervention activities with their children with Down's syndrome. Education & Training of the Mentally Retarded, (1), 24-29.

Spratlen, J., & Hamm, N. H. (1983). The use of a token economy to increase the classroom attending behavior of a Mongoloid child: a case study. Behavioral Engineering, 8(2), 59-63.

Spritzer-Griffith, S. E. (1976). Mutual visual regard of Down's syndrome and normally developing infants in interaction with a familiar and an unfamiliar adult. Dissertation Abstracts International, 36(8-B), 4181.

Squires, N., Galbraith, G., & Aine, C. (1979). Event-related potential assessment of sensory and cognitive deficits in the mentally retarded. In: D. Lehman and E. Callaway (eds.), Human Evoked Potentions. New York: Plenum Press.

Squires, N., Ollo, C., & Jordan, R. (1986). Auditory brain stem responses in the mentally retarded: audiometric correlates. Ear and Hearing, 7(2), 83-92.

Stedman, D. J., & Eichorn, D. H. (1964). A comparison of the growth and development of institutionalized and home-reared mongoloids during infancy and early childhood. American Journal of Mental Deficiency, 69, 391-401.

Stephens, M. C., & Menkes, J. H. (1969). Cerebral lipids in Down's syndrome. Dev. Med. Child Neurol., 11(3), 346-352.

Sternlight, M., & Wanderer, Z. W. (1962). Nature of institutionalized adult mongoloid intelligence. Am. J. Ment. Defic., 67, 301-302.

Stevens, H. C. (1961). The spinal fluid in mongolian idiocy. J. Am. Med. Assoc., 66, 1373-1374.

Stewart, R. M. (1927). A note on the presence of endarteritis obliterans in the brain of a mongolian imbecile. J. Neurol. Psychiatry, 7, 338, 342.

Stickland, C. A. (1954). Two mongols of unusually high mental status. Br. J. Med. Psychol., 27, 80-83.

Stimson, C. W., Kheder, N., Nicks, R. G., & Orlando, R. (1969). Nerve conduction velocity and H-reflex studies in two groups of severely retarded children. Arch. Phys. Med. Rehabil., 50(11), 626-631.

Stockert, F. B. (1964). Furthering and inhibiting influences on the development of intelligence. Nervenarzt., 35, 20-22.

Stoel-Gammon, C. (1980). Phonological analysis of four Down's syndrome children. Applied Psycholinguistics, 1(1), 31-48.

Stoller, A., & Collmann, R. D. (1969). Grandmaternal age at birth of mothers of children with Down's syndrome (mongolism). Journal of Mental Deficiency Research, 13(3), 201-205.

Stoneman, Z., Cantrell, M. L., & Hoover, D. K. (1983). The association between play materials and social behavior in a mainstreamed preschool: a naturalistic investigation. Journal of Applied Developmental Psychology, 4(2), 163-174.

Stoneman, Z., Brody, G. H., & Abbott, D. (1983). In-home observations of young Down syndrome children with their mothers and fathers. American Journal of Mental Deficiency, 87(6), 591-600.

Stonestreet, R. H. (1987). Comparisons of requesting behaviors in Down syndrome, language disordered and normal toddlers. Dissertation Abstracts International, 47(7-B), 2868.

Stratford, B. (1979). Attraction to good form in Down's syndrome. Journal of Mental Deficiency Research, 23(4), 243-251.

Stratford, B. (1979). Discrimination of size, form, and order in mongol and other mentally handicapped children. Journal of Mental Deficiency Research, 23(1), 45-53.

Stratford, B. (1980). Preferences in attention to visual cues in Down's syndrome and normal children. Journal of Mental Deficiency Research, 24(1), 57-64.

Stratford, B., & Metcalfe, J. A. (1981). Position cues in

discrimination behavior of normal Down syndrome and other mentally handicapped children. Journal of Mental Deficiency Research, 25(2), 89-103.

Stratford, B. (1980). Perception and perceptual-motor processes in children with Down's syndrome. Journal of Psychology, 104(1), 139-145.

Stratford, B., & Metcalf, J. (1982). Recognition, reproduction, and recall in children with Down's syndrome. Australia & New Zealand Journal of Developmental Disabilities, 8(3), 125-132.

Stratford, B., & Ching, E. Y. (1983). Rhythm and time in the perception of Down's syndrome children. Journal of Mental Deficiency Research, 27(1), 23-38.

Stratford, B., & Mills, K. (1984). Colour discrimination in mentally handicapped children with particular reference to Down's syndrome. Australia & New Zealand Journal of Developmental Disabilities.

Stratford, B. (1984). Down's syndrome: these our beloved children. Early Child Development & Care, 15(4), 281-289.

Stratford, B., & Steele, J. (1985). Incidence and prevalence of Down's syndrome: a discussion and report. Journal of Mental Deficiency Research, 29(1), 95-107.

Straumanis, J. J., Jr., Shagass, C., & Overton, D. A. (1970). Evoked responses in Down's syndrome of young adults. Electroencephalogr. Clin. Neurophysiol., 29(3), 24.

Straumanis, J. J., Jr., Shagass, C., & Overton, D. A. (1973). Somatosensory evoked responses in Down syndrome. Arch. Gen. Psychiatr., 29(4), 544-549.

Strazzulla, M. (1953). Speech problems of the mongoloid child. Quarterly Review of Pediatrics, 8, 268-272.

Strom, R., et al. (1984). A comparison of childrearing attitudes of parents of handicapped and non-handicapped children. Journal of Instructional Psychology, 11(2), 89-103.

Suetsugu, M., & Mehraein, P. (1980). Spine distribution along apical dendrites of the pyramidal neurons in Down's syndrome. Progress in Neurobiology, 21, 199-237.

Swaik, A. J. (1967). A study of 125 children with Langdon Down's syndrome (mongolism). II. Growth and development at preschool age. Ned. Tijdschr. Geneeskd., 111(3), 110-120.

Swanson, F. R. (1975). Preparation for employment. In: R. Koch and F. F. DelaCruz (ed.), Down's Syndrome (Mongolism): Research, Prevention and Management, New York: Brunner/Mazel.

Sylvester, P. E. (1983). The hippocampus in Down's syndrome. Journal of Mental Deficiency Research, 27(3), 227-236.

Sylvester, P.E. (1986). The anterior commissure in Down's syndrome. Journal of Mental Deficiency Research, 30(1), 19-26.

Sylvester, P. E. (1984). Nutritional aspects of Down's syndrome with special reference to the nervous system. British Journal of Psychiatry, 145, 115-120.

Szymanski, L. S., & Biederman, J. (1984). Depression and anorexia nervosa of persons with Down's syndrome. American Journal of Mental Deficiency, 89(3), 246-251.

Takashima, S., & Becker, L. E. (1985). Basal ganglia calsification in Down's syndrome. Journal of Neurology, Neurosurgery, and Psychiatry, 48, 61-64.

Takashima, S., & Becker, L. E. (1981). Abnormal neuronal development in the visual cortex of the human fetus and infant with Down's syndrome: a quantitative and qualitative Golgi study. Brain Research, 225(1), 1-21.

Talkington, L. W., & Hall, S. M. (1970). Matrix language program with mongoloids. American Journal of Mental Deficiency, 75(1), 88-91.

Talkington, L. W., Altman, R., & Grinnell, T. K. (1971). Effects of positive and negative feedback on the motor performance of mongoloids. Perceptual and Motor Skills, 33, 1075-1078.

Tamari, P. L. (1979). Language aquisition of Down's syndrome children: the development of form and meaning. Dissertation Abstracts International, 40(1-B), 1651.

Tannock, R., Kershner, J. R., & Oliver, J. (1984). Do individuals with Down's syndrome possess right hemisphere language dominance?. Cortex, 20(2), 221-231.

Tatafiore, E. (1956). Mongolism and hydrocephaly. Minerva Pediatr., 8, 503.

Tate, J. C. (1980). Comparison of attachment behaviors in Down's syndrome and normal infants. Dissertation Abstracts International, 40(9-A), 4974.

Tatekawa, H. (1969). On the traits of the children with Down's syndrome. Journal of Child Development, 5, 33-

45.
Tein, R. G. (1977). Early intervention via educational programs for parent-infant-young children with developmental delays and disabilities. Australian Journal of Mental Retardation, 4(6), 10-12.

Terplan, K. L., Sanberg, A. A., & Aceto, T. (1966). Structural anomalies in the cerebellum in association with trisomy. J. Am. Med. Assoc., 197, 557-568.

Thase, M. E. (1982). Reversible dementia in Down's syndrome. Journal of Mental Deficiency Research, 26(2), 111-113.

Thase, M. E., Liss, L., Smeltzer, D., & Maloon, J. (1982). Clinical evaluation of dementia in Down's syndrome: a preliminary report. Journal of Mental Deficiency Research, 26(4), 239-244.

Thase, M. E., Tigner, R., Smeltzer, D. J., & Liss, L., (1984). Age-related neuropsychological deficits in Down's syndrome. Biological Psychiatry, 19(4), 571-585.

Thelander, H. E., & Pryor, H. B. (1966). Abnormal patterns of growth and development in mongolism. Clinical Pediatrics, 5, 493-501.

Thompson, M. M. (1963). Psychological characteristics relevant to the education of the pre-school mongoloid child. Mental Retardation, I, 148-151.

Thompson, W. H. (1938). A mongolian with superior attainment in the language arts. Psychological Bulletin, 35, 633.

Thompson, R. A., Cicchetti, D., Lamb, M. E., & Malkin, C. (1985). Emotional responses of Down syndrome and normal infants in the strange situation: the organization of affective behavior in infants. Developmental Psychology, 21(5), 828-841.

Thorson, L. C. (1986). Mothers of disabled children: the relationship between security of mother-infant attachment and mothers' experience of social support. Dissertation Abstracts International, 47(6-B), 2636.

Thorum, A. R. (1974). A comparative study of certain audio-linguistic skills of children with two types of deficits. Dissertation Abstracts International, 34(7-B), 3555.

Topping, J. S., Thompson, H. J., & Barrios, B. A. (1976). Comparison of omission training and extinction training in mentally retarded individuals. Bulletin of the Psychonomic Society, 8(3), 211-214.

Trott, M. C. (1977). Application of Foxx and Azrin Toilet Training for the retarded in a school program. Ed. & Training of the Mentally Retarded, 12(4), 336-353.

Tsuboi, T., Inouye, E., & Kamide, H. (1968). Chromosomal mosaicism in two Japanese children with Down's syndrome. Journal of Mental Deficiency Research, 12(2), 162-172.

Tulloch, D. (1986). Object permanence and expressive language skills in visually typical, visually atypical, and Down syndrome infants. Dissertation Abstracts International, 46(9-A), 2664.

Uoashi, T. (1970). The electroencephalogram in cases with Down's syndrome. Bull. Osaka Med. Sch., 16(1), 1-22.

Valenti, C., Schutta, E. J., & Kehaty, T. (1969). Cytogenetic diagnosis of Down's syndrome in utero. Jama, 207(8), 1513-1515.

Van Gorp, E. & Baker, R. (1984). The incidence of hearing impairment in a sample of Down's syndrome school children. International Journal of Rehabilitation Research, 7(2), 198-200.

Varnhagen, C., Das, J. P., & Varnhageb, S. (1987). Auditory and visual memory span: cognitive processing by TMR individuals with Down syndrome or other etiologies. American Journal of Mental Deficiency, 91(4), 398-405.

Veall, R. M. (1974). The prevalence of epilepsy among mongols related to age. J. Ment. Defic. Res., 18(2), 99-106.

Verghese, A., & Murti, R. D. (1961). Mongolism: a review of some aspects. Transactions All India Institute Mental Health, 2, 20-36.

Verma, S. K. & Valiulla, S. (1981). Down's syndrome and other mentally retarded referrals; a study of certain variables. Child Psychiatry Quarterly, 14(3), 64-71.

Villani, T. (1980). School-based instructions and audio-recording feedback: a training package for promoting generalized use of speech teaching skills in naturalistic parent-child interactions. Dissertation Abstracts International, 41(1-B), 394.

Villiger, U., & Mathis, A. (1972). The language of mongoloids. Heilpadogogik, 41, 131-138.

Wagner, T. (1960). The mongoloid child of school age. Heilpadagogische Werkblatter, 29, 59-64.

Wakabayashi, S. (1977). The receiving process of speech sounds by a hard-of-hearing child with Down's syndrome. Japanese Journal of Psychology, 48(1), 42-48.

Wakabayaski, S. (1979). A case of infantile autism associated with Down's syndrome. Journal of Autism & Developmental Disorders, 9(1), 31-36.

Walker, N. F. (1956). A suggested association of mongolism and schizophrenia. Acta Genetica et Statistica Medica, 6, 132-142.

Walker, N. F., Carr, D. H., Sergovich, F. R., Barr, M. L., & Soltan, H. C. (1963). Trisomy-21 and 13-15/21 mongol defectives. Journal of Mental Deficiency Research, 7, 150-163.

Walker, N. G. (1956). A suggested association of mongolism and schizophrenia. Acta Genet. Basel, 6, 132-142.

Wallace, R. M., & Fehr, F. S. (1970). Heart rate, skin resistance and reaction time of mongoloid and normal children under baseline and distraction conditions. Psychophysiology, 6, 722-731.

Wallin, J. E. W. (1944). Mongolism among school children. Am. J. Orthopsychiatry, 14, 104.

Walsh, S. (1981). Keratoconus and blindness in 469 institutionalized subjects with Down syndrome and other causes of mental retardation. Journal of Mental Deficiency Research, 25(4), 243-251.

Walter, R. D., Yeager, C. L., & Rubin, H. (1955). Mongolism and convulsive seizures. Arch. Neurol. Psychiatry, 74, 559.

Waltzer, B. (1970). Comparison of institutionalized mongoloids, public school mongoloids and public school undifferentiated moderate retardates for three emotional factors. Dissertation Abstracts International, 31(3-A), 1091.

Ward, E. G. (1941). Mongolism. Proceedings of the Texas Neurological Society.

Warkany, J., Passarge, E., & Smith, L. B. (1966). Congenital malformations in autosomal trisomy syndromes. Am. J. Dis. Child., 112, 502.

Waters, J. M. (1980). The effects of parent involvement in data collection. Dissertation Abstracts International, 40(10-B), 5029.

Weather, C. (1983). Effects of nutritional supplementation on IQ and certain other variables associated with

Down syndrome. American Journal of Mental Deficiency, 88(2), 214-217.

Weinberg, B., & Zlatin, M. (1970). Speaking fundamental frequency characteristics of five- and six-year-old children with mongolism. Journal of Speech & Hearing Research, 13(2), 418-425.

Weise, P., Koch, R., Shaw, K. F., & Rosenfeld, M. J. (1974). The use of 5-HTP in the treatment of Down's syndrome. Pediatrics, 54, 165-168.

Weistuch, L., & Lewis, M. (1985). The language interaction intervention project. Special Issue: Early Intervention. Analysis & Intervention in Developmental Disabilities, 5(1-2), 97-1.

Welch, J. P. (1968). Down's syndrome and human behavior. Nature, 219(5153), 506.

Weller, E. L. (1981). A comparison of oral and signed-english communication training with Down's syndrome children in a parent-assisted language intervention program. Dissertation Abstracts International, 42(5-A), 2078.

Weller, E. L., & Mahoney, G. J. (1983). A comparison of oral and total communication modalities on the language training of young mentally handicapped children. Education & Training of the Mentally Retarded, 18(2), 103-110.

Wesenther, S. E. (1984). Developmental coaching of the Down syndrome infant. American Journal of Occupational Therapy, 38(7), 440-445.

Wesner, C. E. (1972). Induced arousal and word recognition learning by mongoloids and normals. Perceptual and Motor Skills, 35(2), 586.

Whalley, L. J. (1982). The dementia of Down's syndrome and its relevance to aetiological studies of Alzheimer's disease. Annals of the New York Academy of Sciences, 396, 39-53.

Whalley, L. J., et al. (1982). A study of familial factors in Alzheimer's disease. British Journal of Psychiatry, 140, 249-256.

White, D. (1969). IQ changes in mongoloid children during post-maturation treatment. Am. J. Ment. Defic., 73(5), 809-813.

Whitehouse, P. J. (1986). Understanding the etiology of Alzheimer's disease. Current approaches. Neurol. Clin.,

$\underline{4}$(2), 427-437.

Whiteman, B. C., Simpson, G., & Compton, W. C. (1986). Relationship of ototis media and language impairment in adolescents with Down syndrome. Mental Retardation, $\underline{24}$(6), 353-356.

Widen, J. E. (1982). The effects of intensity on the auditory brainstem response in Down's syndrome. Dissertation Abstracts International, $\underline{43}$(6-B), 1789.

Wiegel-Crump, C. A. (1981). The development of grammar in Down's syndrome children between the mental ages of 2-0 and 6-11 years. Education & Training of the Mentally Retarded, $\underline{16}$(1), 24-30.

Wilcock, J. C., & Venables, P. H. (1968). Dimensional dominance in discrimination learning: a study of severely subnormal and normal subjects. Br. J. Psychol., $\underline{59}$(3), 285-297.

Wile, I. S., & Orgel, S. T. (1928). A study of physical and mental characteristics of mongols. International Clinics, 38th Series, 1945-1947.

Wilkens, R. H., & Brody, I. A. (1971). Down's syndrome. Archives of Neurology, $\underline{25}$(1), 88.

Wimer, R. E. (1986). Two topics for further exploration. Special issue: Controversial topics on Alzheimer's disease: intersecting crossroads. Neurobiology of Aging, $\underline{7}$(6), 584.

Wing, L. (1969). The handicaps of autistic children: a comparative study. Journal of Child Psychology & Psychiatry & Allied Disciplines, $\underline{10}$(1).

Wing, L., & Wing, J. K. (1971). Multiple impairments in early childhood autism. Journal of Autism & Childhood Schizophrenia, $\underline{1}$(3), 256-266.

Wishart, J. G. (1986). The effects of step-by-step training on cognitive performance in infants with Down's syndrome. Journal of Mental Deficiency Research, $\underline{30}$(3), 233-250.

Wisniewski, H. M. (1986). Discrepancy between Alzheimer-type neuropathology and dementia in persons with Down's syndrome. Ann. N.Y. Acad. Sci., $\underline{477}$, 247-260.

Wisniewski, K., Howe, J., Williams, D. G., & Wisniewski, H. M. (1978). Precocious aging and dementia in patients with Down's syndrome. Biological Psychiatry, $\underline{13}$(5), 619-627.

Wisniewski, K. E., & Wisniewski, H. M. (1983). Age-associated changes and dementia in Down's syndrome. In: B. Reisberg (eds.), Alzheimer's Disease. New York: The Free Press.

Wisniewski, K. E., Laure-Kamionowska, M., & Wisniewski, H. M. (1984). Evidence of arrest of neurogenesis and synaptogenesis in the brains of patients with Down's syndrome. New England Journal of Medicine, 311, 1187-1188.

Wisniewski, K., Wisniewski, H. M., & Wen, G. Y. (1985). Occurrence of Alzheimer's neuropathy and dementia in Down syndrome. Annals of Neurology.

Wisniewski, K. E., Dalton, A. J., McLachen, C., Wen, G. Y., & Wisniewski, H. M. (1985). Alzheimer's disease in Down's syndrome: clinicopathologic studies. Neurology, 35(7), 957-961.

Wisniewski, K. E., Wisniewski, H. M., & Wen, G. Y. (1985). Occurence of neuropathological changes and dementia of Alzheimer's disease in Down's syndrome. Ann. Neurology, 17, 278-282.

Wisniewski, K. E., & Hill, A. L. (1985). Clinical aspects of dementia in mental retardation and developmental disabilities. In: M. Janicki and H. M. Wisiewski (eds.), Aging and Developmental Disabilities - Issues and Approaches. Baltimore: Brooks Publishing Co.

Wisniewski, K. E., Laure-Kamionowska, M., Connell, F., & Wisniewski, H. M. (1985). Quantitative determination of synaptic density and their morphology during postnatal development in visual cortex of Down syndrome brain. J. Neuropathol. Exp. Neurol., 44, 342.

Wisniewski, K. E., Laure-Kamionowska, M., and Wen, G. Y., (1985). Neuronal density and synaptogenesis in the postnatal stage of brain maturation in Down syndrome. In: C. J. Epstein (ed.), The Neurology of Down Syndrome. New York: Raven Press.

Wisniewski, K. E., & Schmidt-Sidoe, B. (1986). Myelination in Down's syndrome brains (pre-and postnatal maturation) and some clinical-pathological correlations. Ann. Neurol., 20, 429-430.

Wisniewski, K. E., & Rabe, A. (1986). Discrepancy between Alzheimer-type neuropathology and dementia in persons with Down's syndrome. Ann. N.Y. Acad. Sci., 477, 247-259.

Wisniewski, K. E., et al. (1985). Alzheimer's disease in

Down's syndrome: clinicopathologic studies. Neurology, 35(7), 957-961.

Wisniewski, K. E., & Quinn, M. R. (1984). Somatomedins and Down's syndrome. Biological Psychiatry, 19(4), 469-470.

Wolcott, G. J., & Chun, R. W. (1973). Myoclonic seizures in Down's syndrome. Dev. Med. Child Neurol., 15(6), 805-800.

Wold, D. C., & Montague, J. C. (1979). Preliminary perceived voice deviations and hearing disorders of adults with Down's syndrome. Perceptual and Motor Skills, 49(2), 564.

Wolf, J. M. (1976). The relationship of early measures of mother-child interaction and the later achievement of Down's syndrome children. Dissertation Abstracts International, 36(7-A), 4336.

Wood, J. (1909). Mongolian imbecility. Australian Medical Congress, Melbourne.

Wood, J. D. (1984). Adaptive behavior of children with infantile autism compared to children with Down's syndrome and children with schizophrenia. Dissertation Abstracts International, 45(5-A), 1350.

Woods, P. A., Corney, M. J., & Pryce, G. J. (1984). Developmental processes of preschool Down's syndrome children receiving a home-advisory service: an interim report. Child Care, Health & Development, 10(5), 287-299.

Wright, A. F. & Whalley, L. J. (1984). Genetics, aging and dementia. British Journal of Psychiatry, 145, 20-38.

Wunderlich, C. (1969). Varying social prognosis of the mentally retarded child with identical disease picture but additional different factors, demonstrated in mongolism. Med. Clin., 64(38), 2088-2096.

Wunsch, W. L. (1957). Some characteristics of mongoloids evaluated in a clinic for children with retarded mental development. American Journal of Mental Deficiency, 62, 122-130.

Yamaguchi, K. (1977). Behavior modification of retarded preschool children. RIEEC Research Bulletin, 8(14).

Yamanaka, Y. (1968). Psychological manifestations of Down's syndrome -- with special reference to psychological development. Saishin Igaku, 24(2), 283-286.

Yellin, A. M., Lodwig, A. K., & Jerison, H. J. (1980). Auditory evoked brain potentials as a function of interstimulus interval in adults with Down's syndrome. Audiology, 19(3), 255-262.

Zadikoff, C. (1977). Down's syndrome with hydrocephalus treated by compressive head binding. S. Afr. Med. J., 51(11), 353-355.

Zausmer, E. (1975). Principles and methods of early intervention. In: R. Koch and F. F. DelaCruz (eds.), Down's Syndrome: Research, Prevention, and Management. New York: Brunner/Mazel, Inc.

Zausmer, E., Pueschel, S. M., & Shea, A. (1972). A sensori-motor stimulation program for the young child with Down's syndrome. MCH Exchange, 2(1).

Zeaman, D., & House, B. J. (1962). Mongoloid MA is proportional to log CA. Child Development, 33, 481-488.

Zee-Chen, E. L., & Hardman, M. L. (1983). Postrotary nystagmus response in children with Down's syndrome. American Journal of Occupational Therapy, 37(4), 260-265.

Zekulin, Z. Y., Gibson, D., Mosley, J. L., & Brown, R. (1974). Auditory-motor chanelling in Down's syndrome subjects. American Journal of Mental Deficiency, 78, 571-577.

Zekulin-Hartley, X. Y. (1981). Hemispheric asymmetry in Down's syndrome children. Canadian Journal of Behavioural Science, 13(3), 210-217.

Zekulin-Hartley, X. Y. (1983). Selective attention to dichotic input of retarded children. Cortex, 18(2), 311-316.

Zellweger, H., Groves, B. M., & Abbo, G. (1968). Trisomy 21 with borderline mental retardation. Confin. Neurol., 30(3), 129-138.

Zimmerman, F. T., Burgemeister, B. B., & Putman, T. J. (1949). Effects of glutamic acid on intelligence of patients with mongolism. Archives of Neurology and Psychiatry, 61, 275-287.

Zimmerman, F. T., Burgemeister, B. B., & Putman, T. J. (1949). The effect of glutamic acid upon the mental and physical growth of mongols. American Journal of Psychiatry, 105, 661-668.

Zisk, P. K., & Bialer, I. (1967). Speech and language problems in mongolism: a review of the literature.

Journal of Speech and Hearing Disorders, 32(3), 228-241.

Zylstra, A. (1985). A comparison of short term memory for Down's syndrome, psycho-socially disadvantaged, and neurologically handicapped individuals on three perceptual modalities. *Dissertation Abstracts International*, 46(1-A), 126.

LISTING OF CITATIONS BY
SUBJECT AREA

EARLY INTERVENTION
IN DOWN SYNDROME

BARNA ET AL., 1980.
BIDDER ET AL., 1983.
BARNARD, 1975.
BRINKWORTH & COLLINS, 1969.
CANAL, 1979.
CONNOLLY & RUSSELL, 1976.
CORIAT ET AL., 1967.
DU VERGLAS, 1985.
ESENTHER, 1984.
FEHR, 1976.
FORD, 1978.
FRIEDLANDER ET AL., 1975.
GIBSON & FIELDS, 1984.
HAWLEY, 1982.
HANSON & SCHWARZ, 1978.
HAYDEN, 1978.
HAYDEN, 1979.
HAYDEN, & HARING, 1976.
HOEHNE, 1984.
JAMESON-BLOOM, 1981.
KUGEL, 1970.
LUDLOW & ALLEN, 1979.
MACDONALD ET AL., 1974.
MORGAN, 1979.
NULMAN, 1978.
OELWEIN ET AL., 1985
PIPER ET AL., 1986.
PIPER & PLESS, 1980.
PUESCHEL, 1975.
RYNDERS & HORROBIN, 1967.
SHARAV & SHLOMO, 1986.
SKIDMORE, 1982.

SLOPER ET AL., 1983.
SPIKER, 1982.
SINSON, 1978.
WESENTHER, 1984.
WOODS ET AL., 1984.
ZAUSMER, 1975.
ZAUSMER ET AL., 1972.

MAINSTREAM
EDUCATION PROGRAMS

BECKMAN & KOHL, 1984.
BURSTEIN, 1986.
BOOTH, 1981.
BUDGELL, 1985.
COOKE & HERON, 1982.
DESFORGES & LINDSAY, 1985.
DUNLOP ET AL., 1980.
FIELD & ROSEMAN, 1982.
LORENZ, 1985.
PARIKH & SHUKLA, 1984.
PETERSON, 1982.
PRUESS ET AL., 1987.
STONEMAN ET AL., 1983.

AUTISM AND DOWN SYNDROME

AUGUST ET AL., 1981.
BARON ET AL., 1985.
BARON ET AL., 1986.
BERNHEIMER & KEOGH, 1986.
BARON, 1987.
BRAUNER & BRAUNER, 1976.
ROUGHTON, 1976.
GOODALL & CORBETT, 1982.
HOBSON, 1984.
KINNELL, 1985.
KOVATTANA & KRAEMER, 1974.
LITROWNIK ET AL., 1978.
MERJANIAN, 1986.
NIWA ET AL., 1983.
PRIOR & CHEN, 1976.
RIGUET & TAYLOR, 1981.
WOOD, 1984.
WAKABAYASKI, 1979.
WING, 1969.
WING & WING, 1971.

ADULT INTERACTION WITH DOWN SYNDROME CHILDREN

ARNOLD, 1981.
BERRY, & GUNN, 1984.
BRICKER & MCLOUGHLIN, 1982.
BROOKS-GUNN & LEWIS, 1984.
BERGER & CUNNINGHAM, 1981.
BUCKHALT ET AL., 1978.
CARDOSO-MARTINS, 1985.
COOK, & CULP, 1981.
CRAWLEY & SPIKER, 1983.
CUNNINGHAM, 1981.
DUNST, 1980.
FILLER, 1976.
FISCHER, 1987.
GREENBERG & FIELD, 1982.
GUNN & BERRY, 1985.
GIBSON, 1967.
GUNN ET AL., 1980.
LASSER, 1970.
LOMBARDINO, 1979.
MARCOVITCH, 1983.
MARKOWITZ, 1981.
MCCARTHY, 1982.
MCCONKEY & MARTIN, 1983.
MCQUISTON, 1982.
MORECKI & O'BERG, 1984.
MECHEM, 1970.
NATHANSON & LOPEZ, 1975.
PETERSON, 1979.
RICHARD, 1986.
RONDAL, 1978.
SAPON, 1982.
SORCE & EMDE, 1982.
STONEMAN ET AL., 1983.
SARIMSKI, 1983.
SPIKER, 1980.
TATE, 1980.
THORSON, 1986.

DOWN SYNDROME AND
ALZHEIMER'S DISEASE

ANDERTON ET AL., 1982.
ABALAN, 1984.
ALLSUP ET AL., 1986.
BAUER & SHEA, 1986.
BRANDENBURG, 1986.
BALL & NUTTALL, 1981.
BURGER & VOGEL, 1973.
CASANOVA ET AL., 1985.
COOKE, 1970.
COYLE ET AL., 1986.
CUTLER, 1986.
CUTLER ET AL., 1985.
DALTON ET AL., 1974.
EISNER, 1983.
ELLIS ET AL., 1974.
ELOVAARA, 1984.
HEWITT ET AL., 1985.
HESTON, 1984.
HESTON & MASTRI, 1977.
HESTON & WHITE, 1978.
HURLEY & SOVNER, 1986.
HUGHES, 1977.
JELGERSMA, 1958.
JELGERSMA, 1962.
JELGERSMA, 1968.
JERVIS, 1948.
JERVIS, 1970.
JERVIS, 1970.
KOLATA, 1985.
KABACK, 1970.
KARLINSKY, 1986.
KAY, 1987.
LEVITT, 1985.
LOTT, 1982.
MINISZEK, 1982.
MANN, 1983.
NEUMANN, 1967.
PHILPOT ET AL., 1985.
PRICE ET AL., 1982.
PRICE ET AL., 1985.

PIESSENS & OVERWEG, 1971.
PURPURA, 1974.
ROPPER & WILLIAMS, 1980.
ROSS ET AL., 1984.
SINEX & MYERS, 1982.
SCHOCHET ET AL., 1973.
SOLITAIRE & LAMARCHE, 1966.
THASE, 1982.
THASE ET AL., 1982.
TAKASHIMA & BECKER, 1985.
WHALLEY, 1982.
WHALLEY ET AL., 1982.
WISNIEWSKI ET AL., 1985.
WRIGHT & WHALLEY, 1984.
WHITEHOUSE, 1986.
WIMER, 1986.
WISNIEWSKI, 1986.
WISNIEWSKI & HILL, 1985.
WISNIEWSKI & RABE, 1986.
WISNIEWSKI
  & WISNIEWSKI, 1983.
WISNIEWSKI ET AL., 1985.
WISNIEWSKI ET AL., 1985.
WISNIEWSKI ET AL., 1985.
WISNIEWSKI ET AL., 1985.
WISNIEWSKI ET AL., 1978.
WISNIEWSKI ET AL., 1985.

VISION AND VISUAL
PERCEPTION IN DOWN SYNDROME

ALTER, 1980.
ANWAR, 1983.
ALTER, 1980.
BAKKE, 1986.
BIGUM, 1969.
BRAMZA ET AL., 1969.
COLEMAN, 1960.
COOK, 1976.
COOK, 1976.
EFFGEN, 1984.
GUNN ET AL., 1982.
GORDAN & PANAGOS, 1976.
GRAMZA ET AL., 1969.
GRAY, 1975.
HILL & TOMLIN, 1980.
HERMELIN & O'CONNOR, 1961.
HUANG & BORTER, 1987.
KRAKOW & KOPP, 1983.
KOMIYA, 1981.
KOVATTANA & KRAEMER, 1974.
LEWIS & BROOKS-GUNN, 1984.
LEWIS & BRYANT, 1982.
LOVELAND, 1987.
METCALFE & STRATFORD, 1986.
MORSS, 1984.
MCDONALD & MACKAY, 1977.
MIRANDA, 1970.
MIRANDA, 1976.
MIRANDA & FANTZ, 1973.
NICHOLLS, 1976.
O'CONNOR & HERMELIN, 1961.
PESCH ET AL., 1978.
SINSON & WETHERICK, 1982.
STRATFORD, 1980.
STRATFORD & METCALFE, 1981.
STRATFORD, 1980.
STRATFORD & CHING, 1983.
STRATFORD & MILLS, 1984.
SINSON & WETHERLICK, 1975.
SINSON & WETHERICK, 1972.

SINSON & WETHERICK, 1973.
SPRITZER-GRIFFITH, 1976.
STRATFORD, 1979.
TULLOCH, 1986.
VARNHAGEN ET AL., 1987.
WALSH, 1981.
WILCOCK & VENABLES, 1968.

AUDITORY FUNCTION IN
DOWN SYNDROME

AMOCHAEV, 1985.
BOWLER, CUFFLIN,
  & KIERNAN, 1985.
BARNET ET AL., 1971.
BROWN & CLARKE, 1963.
COLTON, 1973.
COLTON, 1973.
CUNNINGHAM, 1981.
GLENN ET AL., 1983.
GLENN ET AL., 1981.
GLENN ET AL., 1984.
GLOVSKY, 1966.
HARTLEY 1985.
LIBB ET AL., 1985.
PARKER, 1984.
PIPE, 1983.
PIPE, 1985.
REICHLE ET AL., 1985.
SMITH, 1982.
SCHEFFELIN, 1968.
SCHLOSSER, 1972.
THORUM, 1974.
VAN GORP & BAKER, 1984.
VARNHAGEN ET AL., 1987.
WHITEMAN ET AL., 1980.
WOLD & MONTAGUE, 1979
YELLIN ET AL., 1986.
ZEKULIN-HARTLEY, 1983.

COGNITIVE DEVELOPMENT
IN DOWN SYNDROME

BERNHEIMER & KEOGH, 1986.
BERRY ET AL., 1984.
BAYLEY ET AL., 1966.
BYCK, 1968.
CARDOSO-MARTINS, 1985.
CICCHETTI & SROUFE, 1976.
CLEMENTS ET AL., 1978.
COLEMAN, 1960.
COOK, 1976.
CORNWELL, 1974.
COYLE ET AL., 1986.
DUNST, 1981.
DMITRIEV, 1974.
DMITRIEV & HAYDEN, 1975.
EVANS, 1976.
FRASER & SADOVNICK, 1976.
GIBSON, 1966.
HARRIS, 1983.
HILL & MCCUNE, 1981.
HOGG & MOSS, 1983.
HALPIN, 1977.
HARRIS, 1981.
HILL, 1979.
JACOBY, 1971.
KOMIYA, 1973.
KOSTREZEWSKI, 1970.
LIBB ET AL., 1985.
LITROWNIK ET AL., 1978.
LONGNECKER & FERSON, 1961.
LURE, 1971.
METCALFE & STRATFORD, 1986.
MORSS, 1983.
MORSS, 1985.
NADEL, 1986.
NICHOLLS, 1976.
O'HARE, 1966.
PETERSON, 1984.
PUESCHEL ET AL., 1987.
QUAYTMAN, 1953.
RABENSTEINER, 1975.

ROSECRANS, 1971.
SCHWETHELM & MAHONEY, 1986.
SIDMAN ET AL., 1985.
SIMS & BRIDGMAN, 1984.
SMITH, 1984.
SNART ET AL., 1982.
WISHART, 1986.

PLAY OF CHILDREN
WITH DOWN SYNDROME

BROOKS-GUNN & LEWIS, 1982.
BARON, 1987.
CARLSON & GINGLAND, 1961.
HILL
  & MCCUNE-NICOLICH, 1981.
HUNT, 1966.
LI, 1981.
MCCONKEY, 1985.
MCEVOY & MCCONKEY, 1983.
RIGUET & TAYLOR, 1981.
SINSON & WETHERICK, 1981.
SCHLOTTMANN
  & ANDERSON, 1973.
SCHLOTTMANN
  & ANDERSON, 1975.

DRUG THERAPY AND DOWN SYNDROME

BAZELON ET AL., 1967.
HABINAKOVA ET AL., 1976.
HEATON-WARD, 1960.
HEATON-WARD, 1961.
HIRSCH ET AL., 1969.
KEEGAN ET AL., 1974.
KOCH ET AL., 1965.
LEE ET AL., 1969.
LONSDALE & KISSLING, 1986.
SHARE, 1976.
SINEF ET AL., 1979.
WEISE ET AL., 1974.

THE DOWN SYNDROME FETUS

BROOKSBANK & BALAZS, 1984.
BARON ET AL., 1966.
BENDA, 1949.
DAVIS ET AL., 1964.
PAPP ET AL., 1976.
PETIT ET AL., 1984.
REHDER, 1976.
SARA ET AL., 1984.
SYLVESTER, 1983.
SMITH, & MCKEOWN, 1955.
TAKASHIMA & BECKER, 1981.

MEMORY IN DOWN SYNDROME

ANWAR, 1983.
BAKKE, 1986.
DODD, 1975.
DODD, 1975.
FARB & THORNE, 1978.
FARB & THRONE, 1978.
GLENN & CUNNINGHAM, 1982.
GUPTON, 1984.
MARCELL & ARMSTRONG, 1982.
MCDADE, & ADLER, 1980.
MACKAY & MCDONALD, 1976.
MCDONALD & MACKAY, 1974.
PARKER, 1984.
PRIOR & CHEN, 1976.
ROSS, 1983.
STRATFORD & METCALF, 1982.
SINSON & WETHERICK, 1973.
VARNHAGEN ET AL., 1987.
WESNER, 1972.
ZYLSTRA, 1985.

DOWN SYNDROME
AND INTELLIGENCE

ALPERN & KIMBERLIN, 1970.
BERRY ET AL., 1984.
BAUMEISTER
 & WILLIAMS, 1967.
COLEMAN ET AL., 1985.
CUNNINGHAM ET AL., 1985.
CACCAMO & YATER, 1972.
CARR, 1970.
CARTER, 1967.
CLARKE ET AL., 1961.
CLARKE ET AL., 1963.
CLEMENTS ET AL., 1976.
COLTON, 1973.
CORIAT ET AL., 1967.
DAMERON, 1963.
DEMEEDOV, 1972.
DESTROOPER ET AL., 1970.
DICKS-MIREAUX, 1966.
DUNSDON ET AL., 1960.
DURLING & BENDA, 1952.
FIELDS & GIBSON, 1971.
FINLEY ET AL., 1965.
FISHER, 1970.
FRASER & SADOVNICK, 1976.
GUPTON, 1984.
GATH, 1986.
GIBSON, 1966.
GIBSON, 1967.
GIBSON & GIBBINS, 1958.
GRATZ ET AL., 1972.
HEATON, 1960.
JOHNSON & BARNETT, 1961.
JOHNSON & ABELSON, 1969.
JUNKALA, 1966.
KLEBBA ET AL., 1974.
KOSTRZEWSKI, 1965.
KOUSSEFF, 1978.
KREEZER, 1939.
LIBB ET AL., 1983.
LEADER & GROZIN, 1935.

LEJEUNE, 1977.
LEJEUNE, 1978.
LONSDALE & KISSLING, 1986.
MEINDL ET AL., 1983.
MACCUBREY, 1970.
MCCALL ET AL., 1972.
MOOR, 1967.
NAKAMURA, 1961.
NAKAMURA, 1965.
NULMAN, 1978.
PISANI, 1963.
REINECKE, 1973.
ROSENFELD ET AL., 1969.
SCHAUSS & SOMMARS, 1982.
SILVERSTEIN
 & LEGUTKI, 1982.
SCHROTH, 1975.
SHAPIRO & HEPPEL, 1977.
SHOTWELL & SHIPE, 1964.
SINEF ET AL., 1979.
SINSON & WETHERLICK, 1976.
STERNLIGHT
 & WANDERER, 1962.
STICKLAND, 1954.
TATEKAWA, 1969.
TSUBOI ET AL., 1968.
VON STOCKERT, 1964.
WEATHERS, 1983.
WEATHERS, 1984.
WHITE, 1969.
ZEAMAN & HOUSE, 1962.
ZELLWEGER ET AL., 1968.
ZIMMERMAN ET AL., 1949.

LANGUAGE DEVELOPMENT:
INFANTS WITH DOWN SYNDROME

BERGER & CUNNINGHAM, 1983.
BOCHNER, 1983.
BOCHNER, 1986.
BUCKHALT ET AL., 1978.
CLARK & SEIFER, 1983.
CUNNINGHAM, & SLOPER. 1984.
DUNST, 1980.
DMITRIEV, 1980.
DMITRIEV, 1980.
DMITRIEV ET AL., 1977.
DODD, 1972.
DUNST, 1980.
FISCHER, 1987.
GUNN ET AL., 1980.
GUNN ET AL., 1977.
GUNN ET AL., 1980.
LENNEBERG ET AL., 1962.
MAHONEY, 1983.
MCCONKEY & MARTIN, 1984.
RISTAU, 1974.
RONDAL, 1976.
SMITH & OLLER, 1981.
TULLOCH, 1986.
WEISTUCH & LEWIS, 1985.

LANGUAGE DEVELOPMENT:
PRESCHOOL CHILDREN
WITH DOWN SYNDROME

ACOSTA, 1982.
ANDERSON, 1982.
AUMONIER
  & CUNNINGHAM, 1983.
ANDREWS & ANDRESS, 1977.
BEEGHLY ET AL., 1986.
BROFFMAN, 1981.
BYRNE-JANDACEK, 1985.
BLAKE, 1969.
BOKOR, 1976.
CARDOSO-MARTINS
  ET AL., 1985.
CARDOSO-MARTINS
  & MERVIS, 1985.
COGGINS ET AL., 1983.
COGGINS & MORRISON, 1981.
COGGINS, 1976.
COGGINS, 1976.
COGGINS, 1979.
CUNNINGHAM ET AL., 1985.
DEHAVEN, 1977.
DMITRIEV & HAWKINS, 1974.
DODD, 1975.
DODD, 1976.
DUCKER & MOONEN, 1986.
EVANS, 1976.
EVANS, 1977.
FISCHER, 1984.
FOWLER, 1985.
FRASER, 1978.
GEARHART ET AL., 1986.
GREENWALD & LEONARD, 1979.
HARRIS, 1983.
HOOSHYAR, 1985.
HORSTMEIER, 1986.
JAGO ET AL., 1984.
KNOX, 1983.
KOPP ET AL., 1983.
KOLSTOE, 1958.

PRESCHOOL (CONT.)

LEIFER & LEWIS, 1983.
LEIFER & LEWIS, 1984.
LEVIN, 1983.
LOMBARDINO ET AL., 1982.
LAYTON & SHARIFI, 1979.
LOMBARDINO, 1979.
MAHONEY & SNOW, 1984.
MAHONEY ET AL., 1981.
MATEY, 1982.
MATEY & KRETSCHMER, 1985.
MAURER, 1986.
MICHAELIS, 1977.
MONTAGUE, 1976.
O'CONNOR & SCHERY, 1986.
OWENS & MACDONALD, 1982.
PECYNA & SOMMERS, 1985.
PETERSEN & SHERROD, 1981.
REICHLE, 1980.
ROMSKI, 1982.
RONDAL ET AL., 1981.
RONDAL, 1980.
RONDAL, 1978.
SALZBERG & VILLANI, 1982.
SCHERER & OWINGS, 1984.
SMITH & STOEL-GAMMON, 1984.
SPIKER, 1980.
SEAGOE, 1965.
SEITZ, 1975.
SMITH, 1976.
SOMMERS & STARKEY, 1977.
STRAZZULLA, 1953.
TALKINGTON & HALL, 1970.
TAMARI, 1979.
THORUM, 1974.
WELLER, 1981.
WELLER & MAHONEY, 1983.
WHITEMAN ET AL., 1986.

LANGUAGE DEVELOPMENT:
SCHOOL CHILDREN
WITH DOWN SYNDROME

BLEILE & SCHWARZ, 1984.
BRIDGES & SMITH, 1984.
BARTELS, 1987.
BUCHKA, 1971.
COGGINS
 & STOEL-GAMMON, 1982.
DODD, 1976.
EVANS, 1977.
GLOVSKY, 1972.
HALLE, 1985.
HARTLEY, 1982.
HARTLEY, 1985.
HARTLEY, 1983.
HOLDGRAFER, 1980.
HOLDGRAFER, 1981.
JEFFREE ET AL., 1973.
MACCUBREY, 1971.
MACCUBREY, 1970.
MANSFIELD, 1972.
NISBET ET AL., 1984.
PALERMO-PIASTRA, 1981.
PESKETT & WOOTTON, 1985.
ROMSKI & RUDER, 1984.
RONDAL, 1980.
RHODES ET AL., 1969.
SCHWARZ, 1983.
STOEL-GAMMON, 1980.
SAPON & REEBACK, 1966.
SCHLOSSER, 1972.
SEMMEL & DOLLEY, 1971.
VILLANI, 1980.
WIEGEL-CRUMP, 1981.
WEINBERG & ZLATIN, 1970.
WING & WING, 1971.

MOTOR AND SENSORIMOTOR SKILLS IN DOWN SYNDROME

ALVAREZ & RUBIN, 1986.
AUMONIER
 & CUNNINGHAM, 1983.
ANWAR & HERMELIN, 1979.
BERKSON, 1960.
BIRCH & DEMB, 1959.
BUTTERWORTH
 & CICCHETTI, 1978.
COOK, 1984.
CARR, 1970.
CORAZA, 1977.
DAVIS, 1981.
DUNST & RHEINGROVER, 1983.
DUNST, 1981.
DUTHIE, 1983.
DMITRIEV, 1972.
DMITRIEV, 1974.
DONOGHUE ET AL., 1970.
EFFGEN, 1984.
ELLIOTT, 1985.
ELLIOTT ET AL., 1985.
FRANCESCHI-BIAGIOTTI, 1963.
FREDERICKS, 1969.
GANDHAVADI & MELVIN, 1985.
GRAY, 1975.
GREENWALD & LEONARD, 1979.
HALEY, 1984.
HARRIS, 1980.
HENDERSON & MORRIS, 1981.
HOGG, 1982.
HOWARD, 1985.
HABINAKOVA ET AL., 1976.
HARRIS, 1981.
JAMES, 1975.
KERR & BLAIS, 1985.
KNIGHTS ET AL., 1967.
KNIGHTS ET AL., 1965.
LYDIC, 1982.
LYDIC, 1985.
LYDIC ET AL., 1983.

LYDIC ET AL., 1985.
LE BLANC ET AL., 1977.
MACKAY & BANKHEAD, 1983.
MACLEAN & BAUMEISTER, 1982.
MAHONEY & SNOW, 1984.
MAHONEY ET AL., 1981.
MERVIS
 & CARDOSO-MARTINS, 1984.
MESSERLY, 1981.
MORRIS ET AL., 1982.
PARKER ET AL., 1986.
PARKER & JAMES, 1985.
PAULSON, 1971.
PICKERSGILL ET AL., 1970.
RAST & HARRIS, 1985.
RICHMOND, 1982.
ROTUNDO & JOHNSON, 1981.
SAND ET AL., 1983.
SLOPER ET AL., 1986.
SMITH & HAGEN, 1984.
SMITH
 & VON TETZCHNER, 1986.
SEHGAL, 1967.
SERSEN ET AL., 1970.
SEYFORT & SPREEN, 1979.
SHARE & FRENCH, 1974.
SMITH & HAGEN, 1984.
TALKINGTON ET AL., 1971.
ZEKULIN ET AL., 1974.

NEUROBIOCHEMISTRY
OF DOWN SYNDROME

ANDERTON ET AL., 1982.
BALAZS & BROOKSBANK, 1985.
BROOKSBANK & BALAZS, 1984.
BANIK ET AL., 1975.
COYLE ET AL., 1986.
GIZA ET AL., 1972.
HIMWICH & FAZEKAS, 1940.
HIMWICH ET AL., 1940.
JOHNSON & SHAH, 1978.
JOHNSON ET AL., 1977.
MANN ET AL., 1985.
MARSH, 1969.
MCCOY, 1968.
MINO, 1968.
NIWA ET AL., 1983.
PALO & SAVOLAINEN, 1973.
SARA ET AL., 1983.
SARA ET AL., 1984.
STEPHENS & MENKES, 1969.
THASE, 1982.
WISNIEWSKI & QUINN, 1984.
ZIMMERMAN ET AL., 1949.

EEG IN DOWN SYNDROME

ARSHAVSKII
 & VAINDRUKH, 1969.
BELEY ET AL., 1959.
CAVALIERI, 1957.
DUSTMAN & CALLNER, 1979.
EFINSKI ET AL., 1974.
GIBBS ET AL., 1964.
GLIDDEN ET AL., 1975.
GLIDDON ET AL., 1975.
GODINOVA, 1963.
HIRAI, 1968.
HIRAI & IZAWA, 1964.
KREEZER, 1939.
PISANI, 1963.
SCHAFER & PEEKE, 1982.
SQUIRES, OLLO,
 & JORDAN, 1986.
STRAUMANIS ET AL., 1970.
STRAUMANIS ET AL., 1973.
UOASHI, 1970.

NEUROPATHOLOGY IN
DOWN SYNDROME

ALVAREZ & GARZON, 1966.
ANDERTON ET AL., 1982.
BALL & NUTTALl, 1983.
BARAM & FISHMAN, 1985.
BENDA, 1940.
BROOKSBANK & BALAZS, 1984.
BRZOZOWSKI
  & KAMINSKA, 1960.
CASANOVA ET AL., 1985.
CAVALIERI, 1957.
COLON, 1972.
CORIAT & FEJIRMAN, 1963.
COYLE ET AL., 1986.
CUTLER, 1986.
DAVIDOFF, 1928.
DE MYER, 1965.
DIAMOND & MOON, 1961.
EFINSKI ET AL, 1974.
EISNER, 1983.
ELOVAARA, 1984.
EPSTEIN ET AL., 1985.
FEDOMOV ET AL., 1968.
GISA ET AL., 1972.
HEWITT ET AL., 1985.
HIMWICH & FAZEKAS, 1940.
HUGHES, 1977.
JAYARAMAN ET AL., 1976.
JELGERMAN, 1963.
JOHNSON ET AL., 1977.
JOHNSON & SHAH, 1978.
KARPOVA ET AL., 1978.
KOHLER, 1975.
LAKE ET AL., 1979.
LASSEN ET AL., 1966.
LAVIEILLE ET AL., 1967.
LEVITT, 1985.
LOESCH, 1968.
MANN ET AL., 1985.
MANN, 1983.
MERJANIAN, 1986.

MARIN-PADILLA, 1976.
MARTEL ET AL., 1969.
MCINTYRE & DEUTSCH, 1964.
MEYER & JONES, 1939.
MUROFUSHI, 1974.
MUROFUSHI & ARAI, 1968.
O'HARA, 1972.
PALO & SAVOLAINON, 1973.
PAPEZ & PAPEZ, 1957.
PARMALEE ET AL., 1969.
PAULSON ET AL., 1968.
PETIT ET AL., 1984.
PRICE ET AL., 1985.
PURPURA, 1974.
REES, 1977.
REEVES ET AL., 1986.
ROSS ET AL., 1984.
SARA ET AL., 1984.
SARA ET AL., 1983.
SCHLACK, 1978.
SCHLACK
  & SCHMIDT-SCHUH, 1977.
SCHOCHET ET AL., 1973.
SCOTT ET AL., 1981.
SHTILBANS, 1968.
SMITH & WARREN, 1985.
SOLITARE, 1969.
SOLITARE & LAMARCHE, 1967.
STEPHENS & MENKES, 1969.
STEVENS, 1961.
STEWART, 1927.
STIMSON ET AL., 1969.
SUETSUGU & MEHRAEIN, 1980.
SYLVESTER, 1983.
SYLVESTER, 1984.
SYLVESTER, 1986.
TAKASHIMA & BECKER, 1981.
TAKASHIMA & BECKER, 1985.
TANNOCK ET AL., 1984.
TATAFIORE, 1956.

NEUROPATHOLOGY (CONT.)

TERPLAN ET AL., 1966.
WISNIEWSKI
 & WISNIEWSKI, 1983.
WISNIEWSKI ET AL., 1985.
WISNIEWSKI ET AL., 1985.
WISNIEWSKI & QUINN, 1984.
ZADIKOFF, 1977.
ZEE-CHEN & HARDMAN, 1983.
ZEKULIN-HARTLEY, 1981.

PSYCHIATRIC DISORDERS
AND PERSONALITY IN
DOWN SYNDROME

BRIDGES & CICCHETTI, 1982.
BARON, 1972.
BILOVSKY & SHARE, 1965.
BLACHER & MEYERS, 1983.
BRADWAY, 1939.
BRINK & GRUNDLINGH, 1976.
BROUSSEAU & BRAINERD, 1928.
BUCK, 1955.
COTTRELL & CRISP, 1984.
DOMINO, 1965.
DOMINO, GOLDSCHMID,
 & KAPLAN, 1964.
DUCHE & LECUYER, 1966.
EARL, 1934.
FOX & KARAN, 1981.
GIBBS & THORPE, 1983.
GREENSPAN & DELANEY, 1983.
GUNN & BERRY, 1985.
GUNN ET AL., 1983.
GUNN & BERRY, 1985.
GATH, 1972.
GIBSON, 1975.
GUNN ET AL., 1981.
HEFFERNAN ET AL., 1982.
HURLEY & SOVNER, 1982.
HABERLANDT, 1966.

JAKAB, 1978.
KEEGAN ET AL., 1974.
MARCOVITCH ET AL., 1986.
MARCOVITCH ET AL., 1987.
MENOLASCINO, 1965.
NACHTSHEIM, 1963.
NAKAUCHI, 1972.
NEVILLE, 1959.
ROTHBART & HANSON, 1983.
ROITH, 1961.
ROLLINS, 1946.
SOVNER ET AL., 1985.
SZYMANSKI
 & BIEDERMAN, 1984.
SCHOLDER, 1965.
TATEKAWA, 1969.
WALKER, 1956.
WALKER, 1956.

AUTHORS

Melissa Cohen	University of Pennsylvania
Eric Courchesne	University of California, San Diego
Anne Fowler	Haskins Laboratories
Rochel Gelman	University of Pennsylvania
A. L. Hill	NYS Office of Mental Retardation and Developmental Disabilities
Thomas L. Kemper, M. D.	
Carolyn B. Mervis	University of Massachusetts, Amherst
Laura F. Meyers	University of California, Los Angeles
Bjorg Michalsen	University of Oslo
C. M. Miezejeski	NYS Office of Mental Retardation and Developmental Disabilities
Jon M. Miller	University of Wisconsin-Madison
Siegfried M. Pueschel	Brown University
Lars Smith	University of Oslo
Stephen von Tetzchner	University of Oslo
Michael E. Thase	University of Pittsburgh
Jennifer Wishart	University of Edinburgh
K. W. Wisniewski	NYS Office of Mental Retardation and Developmental Disabilities

INDEX